Methods in Neurosciences

Volume 24

Neuroimmunology

Methods in Neurosciences

Editor-in-Chief

P. Michael Conn

Methods in Neurosciences

Volume 24

Neuroimmunology

Edited by

M. Ian Phillips

Department of Physiology
College of Medicine
J. Hillis Miller Health Science Center
University of Florida
Gainesville, Florida

Dwight Evans

Department of Psychiatry
College of Medicine
J. Hillis Miller Health Science Center
University of Florida
Gainesville, Florida

ACADEMIC PRESS
San Diego New York Boston London Sydney Tokyo Toronto

Front cover photograph: The micrograph shows a ramified microglial cell in human cerebral cortex. The section was reacted with a monoclonal antibody (LN-3) directed against human major histocompatibility complex antigen class II and stained with the immunoperoxidase method. Cresyl Violet was used as a counterstain. The picture was taken by Wolfgang J. Streit (Department of Neuroscience, College of Medicine, University of Florida, Gainesville, Florida) on a Zeiss Axioplan microscope equipped with differential interference contrast optics.

This book is printed on acid-free paper. ∞

Academic Press, Inc.
A Division of Harcourt Brace & Company
525 B Street, Suite 1900, San Diego, California 92101-4495

United Kingdom Edition published by
Academic Press Limited
24-28 Oval Road, London NW1 7DX

International Standard Serial Number: 1043-9471

International Standard Book Number: 0-12-185294-6

PRINTED IN THE UNITED STATES OF AMERICA
95 96 97 98 99 00 EB 9 8 7 6 5 4 3 2 1

Table of Contents

Section II The Brain Immune System

Section III Neuroimmune System: Effects of the Brain on the Peripheral Immune System

Contributors to Volume 24

Article numbers are in parentheses following the names of contributors. Affiliations listed are current.

VIJAYABALAN BALASINGAM (14), Department of Neurobiology and Neurosurgery, Montreal Neurological Institute, McGill University, Montreal, Quebec, Canada H3A 2B4

G. A. BELOKRYLOV (12), Immunology Department, Institute for Experimental Medicine, Sankt-Petersburg 197376, Russia

WILLIAM H. BETTS (3, 10), Rheumatology Unit, The Queen Elizabeth Hospital, Woodville, South Australia 5011, Australia

J. EDWIN BLALOCK (22), Department of Physiology and Biophysics, Center for Neuroimmunology, University of Alabama at Birmingham, Birmingham, Alabama 35294

ENRI S. BORDA (7), Immunopharmacology Laboratory, Centro de Estudios Farmacologicos y Botanicos, Consejo Nacional de Investgaciones Cientificas y Tecnicas, Buenos Aires, Argentina

RICHARD H. BUCK (5), Department of Pathology and Laboratory Medicine, University of Florida, Gainesville, Florida 32610

SONIA L. CARLSON (8, 23), Department of Anatomy and Neurobiology, University of Kentucky Medical Center, Lexington, Kentucky 40536

ELLIOT P. COWAN (4), Division of Transfusion Transmitted Diseases, Office of Blood Research and Review, Center for Biologics, Evaluation, and Research, Food and Drug Administration, Rockville, Maryland 20852

JOSEP DALMAU (16), Department of Neurology, and Corzias Laboratory of Neuro-Ocology, Memorial Sloan-Kettering Cancer Center, Cornell University Medical College, New York, New York 10021

BEREE R. DARBY (21), Department of Counseling Psychology, University of Florida, Gainesville, Florida 32610

SUHAYL S. DHIB-JALBUT (4), Department of Neurology, University of Maryland at Baltimore, Baltimore, Maryland 21201

M. P. DIMARCO (6), Department of Internal Medicine, Infectious Diseases, and Immunopathology, Respiratory Allergy and Immunology Unit, IRCCS Ospendale Maggiore Policlinco, University of Milan, I-20122 Milan, Italy

Robert M. Donahoe (26), Department of Psychiatry and Behavioral Sciences, Emory University, Georgia Mental Health Institute, Atlanta, Georgia 30306

L. H. Elliott (8), Department of Microbiology and Immunology, University of Kentucky Medical Center, Lexington, Kentucky 40536

Lewis D. Fannon (18, 21), Department of Physiology, College of Medicine, University of Florida, Gainesville, Florida 32610

Dominik Felix (15), Division of Neurobiology, University of Berne, CH-3012 Bern, Switzerland

Johan Garssen (9), Laboratory of Pathology, National Institute of Public Health and Environmental Protection, University Hospital, Bilthoven 3720 BA, The Netherlands

Dale A. Halliday (10), Cardiovascular Research Institute, University of California, San Francisco, California 94143

Ronald B. Herberman (2), Department of Medicine, University of Pittsburgh School of Medicine, and the Pittsburgh Cancer Institute, Pittsburgh, Pennsylvania 15213

William F. Hickey (17), Department of Pathology, Dartmouth Hitchcock Medical School, Lebanon, New Hampshire 03756

Gloria E. Hoffman (11), Department of Neurobiology, University of Pittsburgh School of Medicine, Pittsburgh, Pennsylvania 15213

Hans Imboden (15), Division of Neurobiology, University of Berne, CH-3012 Bern, Switzerland

Howard M. Johnson (1), Department of Microbiology and Cell Science, University of Florida, Gainesville, Florida 32611

Janet Karlix (25), Department of Pharmacy Practice, College of Pharmacy, University of Florida, Gainesville, Florida 32607

Alexander Kusnecov (11), Department of Pathology, University of Pittsburgh School of Medicine, Pittsburgh, Pennsylvania 15213

Donald T. Lysle (20), Department of Psychology, University of North Carolina, Chapel Hill, North Carolina 27599

John J. Madden (26), Department of Psychiatry, Emory University, Atlanta, Georgia 30322

CURTIS C. MAIER (22), Departments of Physiology and Biophysics, Center for Neuroimmunology, University of Alabama at Birmingham, Birmingham, Alabama 35294

JOSEPH P. MCGILLIS (8, 23, 24), Department of Microbiology and Immunology, University of Kentucky Medical Center, Lexington, Kentucky 40536

JULIAN D. MCNEIL (3, 10), Department of Medicine, Royal Adelaide Hospital, Adelaide, South Australia 5000, Australia

A. MIADONNA (6), Department of Internal Medicine, Infectious Diseases, and Immunopathology, Respiratory Allergy and Immunology Unit, IRCCS Ospendale Maggiore Policlinco, University of Milan, I-20122 Milan, Italy

L. A. MORFORD (8), Department of Microbiology and Immunology, University of Kentucky Medical Center, Lexington, Kentucky 40536

CHARLES B. NEMEROFF (26), Department of Psychiatry and Behavior Sciences, Emory University, Atlanta, Georgia 30322

DOROTHY R. OLESON (26), Department of Psychiatry and Behavioral Sciences, Emory University, Atlanta, Georgia 30322

M. PALELLA (6), Department of Internal Medicine, Infectious Diseases, and Immunopathology, Respiratory Allergy and Immunology Unit, IRCCS Ospendale Maggiore Policlinco, University of Milan, I-20122 Milan, Italy

MICHAEL A. PEZZONE (11), Department of Medicine, University of Pittsburgh School of Medicine, Pittsburgh, Pennsylvania 15213

M. IAN PHILLIPS (18), Department of Physiology, College of Medicine, University of Florida, Gainesville, Florida 32610

CAROL H. PONTZER (1), Department of Microbiology, University of Maryland, College Park, Maryand 20742

ALEXANDER G. RABCHEVSKY (17), Department of Neuroscience, College of Medicine, University of Florida, Gainesville, Florida 32610

BRUCE S. RABIN (11), Department of Pathology, University of Pittsburgh School of Medicine, Pittsburgh, Pennsylvania 15213

MYRNA R. ROSENFELD (16), Department of Neurology, and Corzias Laboratory of Neuro-Ocology, Memorial Sloan-Kettering Cancer Center, Cornell University Medical College, New York, New York 10021

MARIA ELENA SALES (7), Immunopharmacology Laboratory, Centro de Estudios Farmacologicos y Botanicos, Consejo Nacional de Investigaciones Cientificas y Tecnicas, Buenos Aires, Argentina

RAFFAELE SCICCHITANO (3, 10), Department of Thoracic Medicine, Royal Adelaide Hospital, Adelaide, South Australia 5000, Australia

E. I. SOROCHINSKAYA (12), Chemistry Institute, Sankt-Petersburg State University, Sankt-Petersburg-Petrodveretz 198904, Russia

GEORGE B. STEFANO (13), Neuroscience Research Institute, State University of New York at Old Westbury, Old Westbury, New York 11568

WOLFGANG J. STREIT (17), Department of Neuroscience, College of Medicine, University of Florida, Gainesville, Florida 32610

IAN R. TEBBETT (25), Department of Pharmaceutics, University of Florida, Gainesville, Florida 32610

A. TEDESCHI (6), Department of Internal Medicine, Infectious Diseases, and Immunopathology, Respiratory Allergy and Immunology Unit, IRCCS Ospendale Maggiore Policlinco, University of Milan, I-20122 Milan, Italy

DANIEL P. THEELE (17), Department of Physiological Sciences, College of Veterinary Science, University of Florida, Gainesville, Florida 32610

SYLVIA J. USHER (3), Department of Thoracic Medicine, Royal Adelaide Hospital, Adelaide, South Australia 5000, Australia

HENK VAN LOVEREN (9), Laboratory of Pathology, National Institute of Public Health and Environmental Protection, University Hospital, Bilthoven 3720 BA, The Netherlands

ROB J. VANDEBRIEL (9), Laboratory of Pathology, National Institute of Public Health and Environmental Protection, University Hospital, Bilthoven 3720 BA, The Netherlands

DORLINDA A. VARGA-HOUSE (5), Department of Pediatrics and Pathology University of Florida, Gainesville, Florida 32610

THERESA L. WHITESIDE (2), Department of Pathology and Otolaryngology, University of Pittsburgh School of Medicine, and the Pittsburgh Cancer Institute, Pittsburgh, Pennsylvania 15213

WILLIAM E. WINTER (5), Department of Pathology and Laboratory Medicine, University of Florida, Gainesville, Florida 32610

ANDRZEJ WOZNIAK (3), Division of Clinical Sciences, The John Curtin School of Medical Research, Australian National University, Canberra, Australian Capital Territory 2601, Australia

VOON WEE YONG (14), Department of Neurology and Neurosurgery, Montreal Neurological Institute, McGill University, Montreal, Quebec, Canada H3A 2B4

BRUCE S. ZWILLING (19), Department of Microbiology, Ohio State University, Columbus, Ohio 43210

Foreword

The human, to the best of my knowledge, is the only species that (a) studies its own origins (in ontogeny and phylogeny) and (b) has the capability to markedly alter its own future development (in individual life and in species survival). At this stage in our history, it is not yet clear whether we will soon destroy our own species, or by some almost miraculous effort prolong our survival in this hostile universe.

If indeed the latter condition should obtain, then we will soon see major qualitative changes in our self-treatment of and, more urgently, our prevention of disease. Four major explosions of new information from basic research will eventually create parallel changes in clinical practice and in preventive medicine. These very rapidly expanding areas of scientific inquiry and discovery are in *nutrition*, *chronobiology*, *molecular biology–genetics*, and *neuroimmunomodulation (NIM)*. The last of these, NIM, is probably the fastest growing field in biomedical research. NIM deals with the multiple interactions among the nervous, endocrine, and immune systems. Contributions to this body of knowledge are coming from every specialty in the sciences, from the molecular to the behavioral.

Modern scientific evidence for the interactions between the nervous and immune systems dates from the late 1800s, although this concept probably was known to the ancients in Asia, Europe, Africa, and the Americas. In 1891 Savchenko, in Russia, demonstrated that a central nervous system lesion could reverse a pigeon's nonsusceptibility to anthrax. In the 1940s the Romanian researcher Baciu (still active in research in 1994!) showed that lesions in the hypothalamus could change, among other things, the rate of phagocytosis in the peripheral blood.

Within the past two decades, the mechanisms of NIM have been investigated at the cellular and subcellular levels using the modern tools of receptor and membrane physiology, biochemistry, immunology, neurophysiology, chronobiology, and genetics. Thousands of papers on this subject appear yearly in major peer-reviewed journals. Several new journals devoted exclusively to NIM research (and its subdivisions of neuroendocrine–immunology, psychoneuroimmunology, and so on) have appeared. Several other journals have sections on NIM research, and several major journals have devoted entire special editions to this subject. Within recent years, the New York Academy of Sciences has published five volumes on NIM research, with others being planned.

Ten years ago, at my suggestion, the National Institute for Neurological Disorders and Stroke, with the National Institute of Allergy and Infectious

Disorders, of the U.S. National Institutes of Health (NIH), issued a "Program Announcement" calling for grant applications in the field of NIM research. At that time we were supporting two projects in this field. In 1993, NIH was funding more than two hundred grants in NIM or NIM-related research despite the difficulties of an abysmally low budget and the frequent lack of appreciation for research that crosses the boundaries of several disparate disciplines.

For a subject that recently was considered by many scientists to be a popular expression of witchcraft, remarkable and swift progress has been made. At the annual meetings of the (North American) Society for Neuroscience, more than one hundred papers are presented each year on NIM research; only 12 years ago, there was one! At the World Congress of Immunology in Berlin, a few years ago, there were approximately one hundred and seventy papers on NIM, making it the largest single topic out of many categories, yet two congresses earlier, the topic was virtually unknown.

Not too many years ago, most immunologists believed that the immune system was entirely autonomous. One put a lymphocyte into a culture dish, added an antigen, and out came an antibody. So who needed a nervous system? However, in the assembled, living, whole organism, lymphocytes do not function independently. There are continuous interactions, at the subcellular, tissue, and organ levels, among the nervous, endocrine, and immune systems. *In vivo, veritas!*

In common usage, the term "neuroimmunology" has often been used to describe primarily clinical studies, but in its broadest sense, as used in this volume, it could refer to all areas of investigation of neuro–immune interactions. Obviously, not all techniques in this growing field could be included in one book; however, the editors of this volume have assembled a remarkably rich and diversified collection of useful source materials. The editors must be congratulated for their pioneering work. To my knowledge, this is the first book ever published on methods in neuroimmunology. For the reader who wishes to go further, the references in each chapter will lead to additional methods.

Research on NIM and its mechanisms is growing exponentially. The International Society of Neuroimmunomodulation, founded only a few years ago, now has active members in forty countries. This revolution in basic science laboratories will undoubtedly lead to a corresponding revolution in the clinic and, most importantly, in the area of preventive medicine.

NOVERA HERBERT SPECTOR

Preface

Neuroimmunology, the study of immune factors in nervous system functions, has become a very broad and constantly expanding area of neuroscience research, with an impact on psychiatry, psychology, pharmacology, immunology, anatomy, endocrinology, and physiology. The study of neuroimmunology can be approached in two ways. One is through the brain immune system, the intrinsic manner in which the brain protects itself against infection, inflammation, and threats to the balance of the brain environment. The second is through the neuroimmune system in which the peripheral immune system influences the brain and the brain influences the peripheral immune system. In this rapidly developing field, methods are needed to study the immune system in the brain and in the periphery. Many different methods have been and are being used, so the investigator is faced with the difficult choice of which techniques and procedures are appropriate and how to carry them out. In this volume we bring together diverse areas of neuroimmunology and the methodologies so that readers can select those procedures which are suitable for their own research. Some of the methods are the standard ones used in immunology which can also be applied to neuroimmunology. Other methods are specific for either the brain immune system or the effects of the brain on the peripheral immune system. Therefore, we have included contributions on both types of general methods in Section I, methods appropriate for the brain immune system in Section II, and methods for the neuroimmune system in Section III.

In the General Methods section the measurement of interferons, natural killer cells, assays for tachykinins in human neutrophils, molecular techniques for detecting gene expression in neuroimmunology, class I and class II major histocompatibility complex molecules, *in vitro* IgE-mediated histamine release from leukocytes, and immunopharmacological methods are covered. Included are methods on human and rodent lymphocytes, monocytes in neutrophils, characterization and preparation, and methods in immunotoxicology. This was not intended to be, nor could it be, an exhaustive collection of immunological methods. However, the chapters are written with both educational and practical goals. The reader should be able to use these chapters for information on often referred to immunological terms and procedures and at the same time be able to use these methods in a laboratory setting.

The brain immune system is approached through studies of stressor-activated areas in the central nervous system, neuroimmune connections in functional blocks, computer-assisted image analysis of neuroimmunology, the contribution of cytokines mediating reactive astrogliosis, immunocytochemistry of brain tissue, and characterization of neuronal antigens and antineuronal antibodies. Again, these techniques are representative only of the many techniques available.

The section on neuroimmune studies includes methods for measuring the immune response to brain manipulation and neuroimmunomodulation of macrophage function and methods for inducing the immume system by stressors in rats and by hypnosis in humans. Molecular techniques include the cloning and sequencing of immunoglobulin and T-cell receptor regions involved in neuroimmune disorders, leukocyte adhesion, and the role of neuropeptides as immunomodulators. The relevance of the immune system to drug abuse is also covered.

We hope we have put together a useful collection of methods and instructive chapters. We are at a time when the methods used in neuroimmunological research are being standardized so that results from one study to another can become more consistent and comparable. With accepted methods the startling discoveries of neuroimmunology become more comprehensible.

M. Ian Phillips
Dwight Evans

Methods in Neurosciences

Volume 1 Gene Probes
Edited by P. Michael Conn

Volume 2 Cell Culture
Edited by P. Michael Conn

Volume 3 Quantitative and Qualitative Microscopy
Edited by P. Michael Conn

Volume 4 Electrophysiology and Microinjection
Edited by P. Michael Conn

Volume 5 Neuropeptide Technology: Gene Expression and Neuropeptide Receptors
Edited by P. Michael Conn

Volume 6 Neuropeptide Technology: Synthesis, Assay, Purification, and Processing
Edited by P. Michael Conn

Volume 7 Lesions and Transplantation
Edited by P. Michael Conn

Volume 8 Neurotoxins
Edited by P. Michael Conn

Volume 9 Gene Expression in Neural Tissues
Edited by P. Michael Conn

Volume 10 Computers and Computations in the Neurosciences
Edited by P. Michael Conn

Volume 11 Receptors: Model Systems and Specific Receptors
Edited by P. Michael Conn

Volume 12 Receptors: Molecular Biology, Receptor Subclasses, Localization, and Ligand Design
Edited by P. Michael Conn

Volume 13 Neuropeptide Analogs, Conjugates, and Fragments
Edited by P. Michael Conn

Volume 14 Paradigms for the Study of Behavior
Edited by P. Michael Conn

Volume 15 Photoreceptor Cells
Edited by Paul A. Hargrave

Volume 16 Neurobiology of Cytokines (Part A)
Edited by Errol B. De Souza

Volume 17 Neurobiology of Cytokines (Part B)
Edited by Errol B. De Souza

Volume 18 Lipid Metabolism in Signaling Systems
Edited by John N. Fain

Volume 19 Ion Channels of Excitable Membranes
Edited by Toshio Narahashi

Section I

General Methods

[1] Measurement of Interferons

Carol H. Pontzer and Howard M. Johnson

The interferons (IFN) are a family of proteins that were initially identified by their ability to make cells resistant to infection by virus. Subsequently, other important IFN functions have been identified. For example, the interferons regulate cell growth and differentiation and are essential for proper functioning of the immune system. One type of interferon is necessary for establishment of pregnancy in a number of animal species, primarily ruminants.

There are three major groups of interferons called alpha (α), beta (β), and gamma (γ) based on protein structure and antigenic properties (reviewed in 1). Two additional IFN, omega (ω) and tau (τ), are related to IFNα but exhibit small distinct differences in structure and size. The IFN proteins are primarily α-helical in structure with molecular weights which vary from 16,000 to 24,000. There are more than 17 different IFNα genes, 2 to 3 IFNβ genes, and 1 IFNγ gene. IFNα and β are induced primarily by viruses and by tumor cells, while IFNγ is induced by antigens and mitogens that stimulate T cells. In response to this induction, IFNα and IFNβ are produced by a variety of cells, including fibroblasts, epithelial cells, macrophages, and B lymphocytes. Interferon γ, on the other hand, is produced by T lymphocytes and natural killer cells. IFNα, β, ω, and τ bind to the same complex receptor on cells, while IFNγ binds to a different receptor. Thus, IFNα, β, ω, and τ have been generally grouped together and called type I IFN, while IFNγ has been called a type II IFN.

All of the IFN are most commonly measured by their antiviral activity in culture. Many different antiviral assays exist, among them plaque inhibition, cytopathic effect, and virus yield (reviewed in 2). The kenetics of development of the antiviral state is rapid, occurring within minutes, in response to type I IFNs and slow, requiring hours, in response to type II IFNs (3). A variety of cells lines are commonly used for bioassay of IFNs. Among them are MDBK, WISH, and L-929 cells, all of which can be obtained from The American Type Culture Collection (Rockville, MD). While the bovine cell line MDBK can be used for assay of type I IFNs from a variety of species, WISH and L-929 cells are used for human and murine IFN assays, respectively, because of the species specificity of the IFNs. The challenge virus is usually vesicular stomatitis virus (VSV), Sindbis, or encephalomyocarditis virus. Results of antiviral assays are often expressed as units per milliliter

Methods in Neurosciences, Volume 24

as compared with international standard preparations, for example, NIH human IFNγ reference standard Gg23-901-503. The reference standards are available through the Antiviral Substances Program of the National Institutes of Health, which currently has a contract with Braton Biotech, Inc., Rockville, MD [(301) 762–5301]. Reporting units per milliliter can present some confusion between laboratories which can be resolved by reporting specific activity in units per milligram.

The production of monoclonal antibodies to the various IFNs has allowed for the development of both radioimmunoassays (RIA) and enzyme-linked immunosorbant assays (ELISA) to detect IFN. The primary advantage of the use of monoclonals is the ability to distinguish between different types of IFN. The newer methods are more rapid, producing results in 2–4 hr rather than the 16–48 hr needed for antiviral assays. Further, interference by other contaminating cytokines is eliminated. A common disadvantage of the use of antibodies to measure IFN is that both immunologically active and inactive species of the protein are detected. It has been reported that the binding affinity of certain monoclonal antibodies (MAb) for inactivated IFNα was significantly reduced relative to binding to the active IFN molecule (4). This differentiation was only apparent using soluble proteins and could be abrogated by binding of the IFN to a solid support, such as a microtiter well.

Antiviral Assay

The IFN bioassay still represents the most sensitive procedure to measure biologically active IFN. One unit of interferon activity is defined as the concentration needed to produce a 50% inhibition of either cytopathic effect (CPE) or virus plaque formation. Concentrations are determined with respect to an international reference standard (69/19, MRC Research Standard B; NIH G-023-901-527; NIH Ga23-902-530; NIH Gxa 01-901-535; NIBSC 83/514; 5). A laboratory standard IFN, the activity of which has been determined relative to the reference standard, can be prepared and used routinely. All IFN standard preparations should be stored at −70°C in small aliquots to avoid repeated freezing and thawing which can inactivate the IFN. The Indiana strain of VSV is passaged in L cells and stored frozen at −70°C in small aliquots.

1. Cells are plated in microtiter wells at approximately 6×10^4 Madin Darby bovine kidney (MDBK) cells/well in 100 μl medium [Hanks' minimum essential medium (HMEM)/10% fetal bovine serum (FBS)]. They are incubated at 37°C in 5% CO_2 for about 24 hr or until a confluent monolayer is obtained.

2. The next day samples to be assayed are diluted in medium (HMEM/2% FBS—which allows for observation of IFN effects without continued growth of the monolayer) in the first well of a row to a final volume of 150 μl. Threefold dilutions of the samples are made by transferring 50 μl serially to the end of the row. Pipette tips should be changed frequently to avoid IFN carryover. Triplicate determinations should be run for each sample.

3. Interferon standard preparations are also prepared in the range of 1–100 units/ml and 100 μl of each is added to triplicate wells.

4. Several wells on the plate serve as cell and virus controls, containing 100 μl of medium without interferon standard or sample.

5. The plate is incubated at 37°C for 1–6 hr for type I IFN or overnight for IFNγ.

6. The medium is removed, and each well (including the virus control wells, but not the cell control wells) is challenged with VSV at a dilution previously determined to produce 100% destruction of the monolayer in 24 hr in the absence of IFN (usually about 3000 plaque-forming units as assessed on L cells).

7. The plate is incubated at 37°C for an additional 16 hr or until full CPE is noted in the virus control wells.

8. The medium is removed from the wells, and the cells are stained with 100 μl of the 0.5% crystal violet in 30% methanol. After 3 min, the excess stain is removed, and the plate is rinsed thoroughly in tap water.

9. The interferon titer is calculated as the reciprocal of the dilution represented in the well in which 50% of the cell monolayer is protected. The interferon titer of the reference reagent is used to convert the sample values to absolute units.

The above procedure is used for the rapid assay of IFNα, but it is applicable also for assay of any of the other IFN types. Some modifications may be required; for example, MDBK cells are not that sensitive to human IFNβ. For the particular cell line employed, sensitivity to virus, sensitivity to IFN, time for production of monolayer, and time required for 100% CPE must be determined. Plaques can be produced by the addition of 4000 centipoise (cP) methyl cellulose 1 hr after virus challenge (0.5% final concentration; 6). The speed and the sensitivity of the assay can be adjusted as discussed in detail in Familletti *et al.* (7). Another variation on the assay is direct addition of cells to the IFN dilutions, which increases the assay speed, but reduces sensitivity. Virus challenge in the assay of type I IFNs can begin as early as 1 hr and is maximal at 6 hr after exposure to IFN, while 18–24 hr of IFN treatment is optimal for IFNγ.

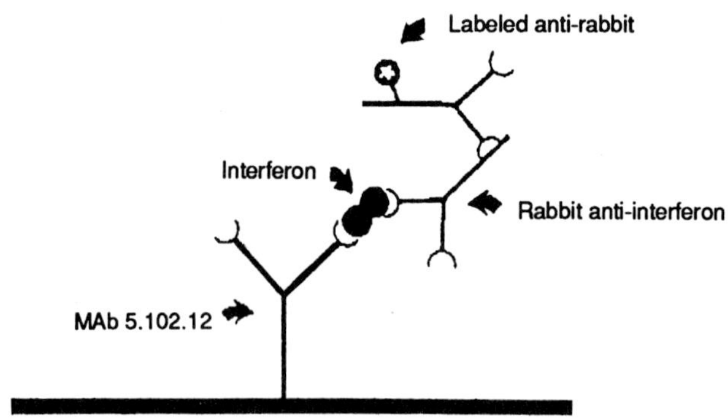

FIG. 1 A schematic of the four-tiered ELISA developed for measurement of murine IFNγ. The MAB 5.102.12, directed against the amino terminus of IFNγ, is coated on the bottom of microtiter plates. Interferon γ is added, followed by polyclonal antiserum to the carboxy terminus of the IFNγ molecule. The binding is quantified using enzyme-conjugated goat anti-rabbit IgG.

Interferon ELISA

One particularly useful type of ELISA that has been developed is based on the "antibody sandwich" principle and is summarized in Fig. 1 (8). Radioimmunoassays based on the same concept, using two antibodies that simultaneously recognize different epitopes on the IFN molecule, have also been described (9). The ELISA that is detailed here is for murine IFNγ, but can be readily modified for any assessment of any IFN subtype or species by alteration of the specific MAb or antisera used. It is sensitive to 100 pg/well (3 units IFN/100 μl) and shows no cross-reactivity with other cytokines.

Materials

96-well flat-bottom tissue culture plates (Falcon, Fisher, Pittsburgh, PA)
o-Phenylenediamine dihydrochoride (Sigma, St. Louis, MO P1526)
30% H_2O_2
2 *M* H_2SO_4
IFN standard preparation (see previous discussion)

Buffers

Binding buffer
0.1 *M* Carbonate/bicarbonate, pH 9.6
1.59 g Sodium carbonate

2.93 g Sodium bicarbonate

Q.S. to 1 liter with distilled H_2O

Wash buffer: Phosphate-buffered saline (PBS) with 0.05% (v/v) Tween 20

Blocking buffer

Adult bovine serum (100%)

Alternative buffer, 5% (w/v) instant nonfat dry milk in PBS

Substrate buffer

Solution A, 0.1 *M* citric acid (1.9 g/100 ml distilled H_2O)

Solution B, 0.1 *M* Sodium citrate (2.9 g/100 ml distilled H_2O)

Mix 9.4 ml of solution A with 10.6 ml of solution B

Antibodies

Anti-N terminal IFN MAb: Our laboratory has used hamster MAb 5.102.12 which is the product of Armenian hamster spleen cells fused with Sp2/O-Ag14 mouse myeloma cells. The donor of the spleen had been immunized with recombinant mouse IFNγ. MAb 5.102.12 binds to an epitope on the amino terminus of murine IFNγ and neutralizes the lymphokine. It is eluted from protein A–Sepharose.

Rabbit anti-C terminal murine IFNγ: This polyclonal antiserum is raised in our laboratory against a synthetic C terminal peptide of murine IFNγ and eluted from protein A–Sepharose.

Goat anti-rabbit IgG conjugated to horseradish peroxidases (Sigma).

Procedure

1. Coat wells of 96-well plate with 50 μl of anti-N terminal IFN MAb at a concentration of 60 μg/ml in binding buffer. Cover with Parafilm and incubate overnight at 37°C.
2. Wash plate by flooding with wash buffer. Flood entire plate, flick off wash, and blot excess with paper towel. Repeat four times.
3. Add 0.3 ml adult bovine serum to each well. Incubate 2 hr at room temperature. Wash four times.
4. Add 50 μl of IFN standards or samples in PBS in triplicate to wells. The standard curve for this assay ranges from 1 to 1000 units/ml of IFN activity (Fig. 2). Samples are generally diluted from between 1 : 3 and 1 : 30 to appear on the linear portion of the curve. Incubate 1 hr at room temperature. Wash four times.
5. Add 50 μl rabbit anti-IFN at a concentration of 10 mg/ml in PBS to each well. Incubate 1 hr at room temperature. Wash four times.

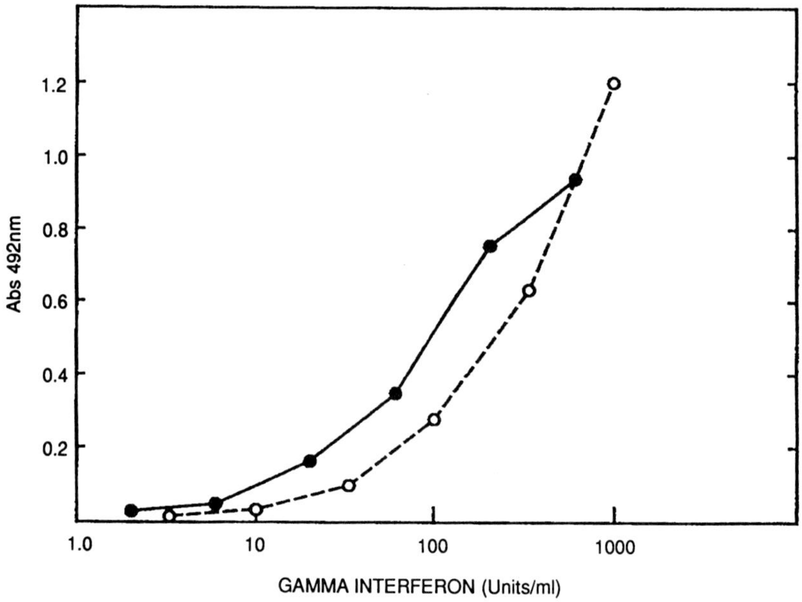

FIG. 2 Typical standard curve generated using recombinant murine IFNγ (filled circles) and natural murine IFNγ (open circles) in the ELISA. The linear portion of the curve is from approximately 30 units/ml (100 pg/well) to 1000 units/ml.

6. Add 50 μl goat anti-rabbit IgG conjugated to horseradish peroxidase (1:4000 in PBS) to each well. Incubate 1 hr at room temperature. Wash four times.

7. Prepare substrate solution by adding 8 mg *o*-phenylenediamine dihydrochloride to 20 ml of substrate buffer. Then add 8 μl 30% H_2O_2 immediately before use. Add 50 μl of substrate solution to each well. Let color develop for about 10 min or until background wells begin to change color.

8. Stop reaction with 100 μl 2 *M* H_2SO_4.

9. Read absorbance at 490 nm.

10. Absorbance values of the samples are converted to NIH antiviral reference units using the standard curve, which is created with known amounts of rMuIFNγ, the activity of which is quantified using either CPE or the plaque reduction assay.

Finally, the different types of IFNs display some different physicochemical properties, such as stability to pH. Most species of the type I IFNs are stable to pH 2. In contrast, type II is unstable below pH 5. It is also unstable at concentrations of sodium dodecyl sulfate (SDS) greater than 0.1%. The IFNs are sensitive to trypsin, chymotrypsin, and V-8 protease. They can be stored for 6 months at 4°C. Many of the IFNs are stable for 10 min at 56°C, but can be inactivated by heating at 65°C for 30–60 min. The type I IFNs are inactivated by reduction since the disulfide bond between Cys^{29} and Cys^{139} is required for biologic activity. MAb which can detect subtle structural alterations should provide the next wave of development in IFN assay.

References

1. H. M. Johnson, F. W. Bazer, B. E. Szente, and M. A. Jarpe, *Sci. Am.* **270,** 68 (1994).
2. S. Pestka (ed.), *in* "Methods in Enzymology," Vol. 78. Academic Press, New York, 1981.
3. F. Dianzani and S. Baron, *in* "Methods in Enzymology" (S. Pestka, ed.), Vol. 78, p. 409. Academic Press, New York, 1981.
4. S. Pestka, B. Kelder, J. A. Langer, and T. Staehelin. *Arch. Biochem. Biophys.* **224,** 111 (1983).
5. S. Pestka, *in* "Methods in Enzymology" (S. Pestka, ed.), Vol. 119, pp. 3–14. Academic Press, New York, 1986.
6. M. P. Langford, D. A. Weigent, G. J. Stanton, and S. Baron, *in* "Methods in Enzymology" (S. Pestka, ed.), Vol. 78, p. 339. Academic Press, New York, 1981.
7. P. C. Familletti, S. Rubinstein, and S. Pestka, *in* "Methods in Enzymology" (S. Pestka, ed.), Vol. 78, p. 387. Academic Press, New York, 1981.
8. M. A. Jarpe, M. P. Hayes, J. K. Russell, H. M. Johnson, and S. W. Russell, *J. Interferon Res.* **9,** 239 (1989).
9. B. Kelder, A. Rashidbaigi, and S. Pestka, *in* "Methods in Enzymology" (S. Pestka, ed.), Vol. 119, p. 582. Academic Press, New York, 1986.

[2] Measurements of Natural Killer Cell Numbers and Function in Humans

Theresa L. Whiteside and Ronald B. Herberman

General Characteristics of Human Natural Killer Cells

Circulating natural killer (NK) cells represent 5–15% of human peripheral blood lymphocytes (PBL) and are responsible for lysis of tumor or virus-infected cell targets without prior sensitization or major histocompatibility complex (MHC) restriction (1). Unlike T lymphocytes, which require priming or sensitization by an antigen and which recognize small (9–20 amino acid) peptides presented in the groove of the MHC class I molecules, NK cells mediate spontaneous cytotoxicity that is MHC class I unrestricted (2). The nature of a receptor responsible for recognition by the NK cell of targets susceptible to lysis remains elusive, and the mechanisms of NK cell recognition and interaction of NK cells with their targets are still poorly understood. Lysis of targets by NK cells involve several steps occurring in sequence as follows: (a) recognition of target cells; (b) binding of NK cells to target cells (conjugate formation); (c) NK cell activation, leading to rearrangements in cellular localization of cytoplasmic granules and release of pore-forming enzymes (degranulation); (d) injury and lysis of the target cell; and (e) recycling of the effector cell in preparation for another lytic event (3). The NK cell is a selective killer which does not harm normal "self" but eliminates NK-cell-susceptible targets. Only certain tumor cell lines are lysed by circulating NK cells, while many are NK cell resistant (4). The selective target cell repertoire of resting NK cells is limited to tumor cell lines, such as K562, a line established from a patient with chronic myelogenous leukemia, and only activated NK cells [e.g., lymphokine-activated killer (LAK) cells] kill fresh tumor cells (4).

Although NK cells are best known for their effector cell function, including the ability to eliminate neoplastic cells, cells infected with intracellular pathogens and certain immature or atypical normal cells, they are also active participants in a variety of normal biologic processes, ranging from hematopoiesis to reproduction, aging, neuroendocrine interactions, and immunoregulation (5). Evidence indicates that NK cells in blood or those residing in tissues can be induced to produce a spectrum of cytokines (6). It is through these cytokines that NK cells mediate and participate in physiologic responses and contribute to hematopoiesis (7). The process of NK cell activa-

Methods in Neurosciences, Volume 24

tion, followed by cytokine production, upregulation of the cytolytic function, and proliferation is initiated when the NK cell interacts through the receptors on its surface with ligands expressed on the target cell. Among various classes of surface molecules expressed on NK cells, receptors for cytokines, Fc receptors (FcR), adhesion molecules, and receptors for neuropeptides have been extensively investigated. NK cells are highly responsive to certain exogenous or endogenously produced cytokines, e.g., interleukin 2 (IL-2), because they constitutively express the intermediate-affinity IL-2 receptor (IL-2R) and rapidly upregulate the high-affinity IL-2R in the presence of IL2 (8). Natural killer cells are also inducible by interferons` and γ (9). Natural killer cells express several FcR, including FcγRIII (CD16), FcRII (CD32), and FcμR (10–12). These receptors participate in signal transduction, and signals delivered via FcR induce transcription of the genes that encode proteins relevant for NK cell functions (13). The FcR are also responsible for antibody-dependent cytotoxicity mediated by NK cells (4). Natural killer cells express a broad range of cellular adhesion molecules (CAM), including β_2 integrins involved in signal transduction and activation of NK cells (14) and β_1 integrins, specifically VLA-4 and VLA-5 (receptor for fibronectin) and VLA-6 (receptor for laminin) which participate in NK cell binding to solid substrates, extracellular matrix components, and cell targets (15). Finally, NK cells have been shown to express receptors for opioids, glucocorticoids, and other hormones or neuropeptides, which are responsible for mediating communication between the neuroendocrine system and NK cells (16, 17).

In healthy humans, the majority of circulating NK cells are in a resting state, i.e., they are not in cycle or proliferating. However, these resting NK cells are prepared to respond immediately to activating signals and are equipped to mediate the first line of defense against various pathogens (2, 18, 19). While this swift responsiveness of NK cells is a necessary attribute of the effector cell, it also requires a regulatory "check and balance" system. Natural killer cell responses have to be carefully regulated because of the potential for inappropriate activation of the lytic mechanism and for damage to normal cells or tissues. Natural killer cell activities are probably regulated in tissue by both autocrine and paracrine cytokine networks but also by the level of development, differentiation, activation, and availability of NK cells in the microenvironment. *In vivo,* NK cell development, activation, proliferation, and migration between blood and tissue may be orchestrated by the events which occur at a particular tissue site. The ability of NK cells to promptly and efficiently respond to such events qualifies them as excellent mediators of the defense and regulatory mechanisms.

Natural Killer Cells in Human Disease

The biologic role of NK cells is most likely not restricted to immunologic surveillance against infectious agents or tumor metastases. Natural killer cells appear to be an important component of pathologic processes in many human diseases, as reviewed by us recently (5). In malignancy, for example, NK cells might have a prognostic significance as, in some cases at least, low NK activity in blood has been shown to predict relapses, poor responses to therapy, and decreased survival time without metastasis (20). Decreased NK activity may also be a risk for the development of malignancy (21). Low NK activity in the blood of cancer patients seems to be significantly associated with the development of distant metastases (22). The ability of NK cells to influence (suppress or enhance) hematopoietic development translates into their crucial importance at the time of bone marrow transplantation (23). Natural killer cells, which apparently are the first cells to repopulate the marrow, might influence engraftment and control post-transplant viral infections (23, 24). In patients with leukemia treated with bone marrow or stem cell transfers, NK cells probably mediate graft-versus-leukemia effects and are important to elimination of residual tumor cells. The presence of a considerable number of activated NK cells in the normal human liver (25) and intestine (26), and newer evidence indicating that NK activity may be suppressed in these organs at the time of disease, indicate that NK cells are likely to participate in local immunologic responses. Considerable evidence exists for a relationship between low NK activity and emotional or behavioral factors, especially stress, not only in patients suffering from behavioral disorders but also in normal individuals (27, 28). Abnormalities in NK activity have also been found in patients with autoimmune disease (29).

In general, human diseases with associated NK cell abnormality can be categorized into those with low or absent NK activity (i.e., NK cell deficiency) and those in which NK activity appears to be excessive. In either category, abnormalities in NK activity can be transient or persistent. Transient decreases or increases in NK activity relative to the normal baseline level defined for each individual accompany a variety of events including exercise, stressful situations, circadian variations, mild colds, or more severe viral infections (1). Thus, transient changes from baseline in NK activity appear to be physiologically normal responses to life events. On the other hand, persistently low or high levels of NK activity are likely to be associated with disease. Frequently, but not always, the number of circulating NK cells parallels changes in NK activity (1). However, NK activity appears to be a more sensitive marker of disease progression than the absolute number of NK cells.

Although persistent abnormalities in NK activity or the number of NK cells appears to be associated with a wide spectrum of human diseases (5, 18), evidence for the causal association of abnormally low NK activity with pathogenesis is so far only available from a limited number of experimental models (30). High persistent levels of NK activity are rare, e.g., NK cell lymphoproliferations (31), and the biologic significance of chronically high NK activity is not clear. For patients with diseases associated with NK cell deficiencies, therapy with biologic response modifiers (BRM), which can restore or augment NK activity *in vivo,* offers an opportunity to demonstrate that NK cells play an important role in health. Similarly, availability of reproducible NK cell assays, allowing for serial monitoring of NK cell activity and of the number of NK cells in normal individuals and patients with various pathologic conditions, is likely to provide additional clues about the role of NK cells in human disease in the near future.

Measurements of Natural Killer Cells

In humans, the number of NK cells and NK activity are generally measured in the peripheral blood. Nevertheless, it is important to remember that NK cells are widely distributed in human tissues and that human spleen, liver, and lungs contain a considerable number of NK cells (4). Few mature NK cells are present in the lymph nodes and bone marrow, although these tissues certainly contain NK cell precursors, because considerable NK activity can be induced from lymphoid tissues and bone marrow after their incubation with IL2 (4). The ability to measure the number of NK cells or NK activity in human tissues is of course limited, and it requires dissociation of tissue biopsies with a cocktail of enzymes and separation of mononuclear cells (MNC) from tissue cells by gradient centrifugation (32). Thus, the peripheral blood has been a source of MNC, which are usually tested for NK activity in 4-hr ^{51}Cr-release assays and for the NK cell number by two-color flow cytometry, following staining of the MNC with fluorescein- or phycoerythrin-labeled monoclonal antibodies (MAb) to surface antigens on NK cells. These assays have required isolation of MNC from peripheral blood, generally on Ficoll–Hypaque gradients, and are then followed by extensive washing, counting, and dilution steps. Today, a whole-blood NK cell assay is available, which provides a more precise measure of NK activity than the conventional cytotoxicity assay performed with isolated MNC. Natural killer cell activity in blood is probably modulated by other blood cells, immunoglobulins (Ig), antigen–antibody complexes, and various soluble factors, including hormones, neuropeptides, and cytokines. Thus, separation and washing of MNC prior to NK cell assays are likely to alter both NK activity and their number, the latter due to the possibility of a loss incurred during the separation. It appears that the whole-blood assay of NK cells might better reflect their *in vivo* activity. Whole-blood flow cytometry is now routinely used to measure the number of PBL. Thus, measurements of both NK activity and the number of NK cells can be simultaneously performed on unseparated whole blood almost as soon as it is collected by venipuncture into heparinized tubes.

Assay for Natural Killer Activity in Whole Blood

The assay measures the ability of NK cells circulating in the peripheral blood to lyse an NK cell-sensitive target, K562, maintained as a cell line (33). These target cells should be in the log phase of growth at the time of the assay. They are labeled with radioactive sodium [^{51}Cr]chromate (sp act, 5 Ci/mol; NEN, Boston, MA; 100–200 μCi of ^{51}Cr/5 $\times$ 10^6 target cells) by incubating the cell pellet with ^{51}Cr for 1 hr at 37°C and using gentle mixing every 15 min. Following labeling, K562 cells are extensively washed in medium to remove any unbound radioisotope. The target cells are resuspended in fresh medium to the final concentration of 2 $\times$ 10^6/ml and refrigerated until used in the assay, but not longer than 12 hr.

Peripheral blood is collected by venipuncture into heparin (preservative-free from Gibco, Grand Island, NY; 5 to 10 U/ml blood, if possible, or into standard heparinized green-top tubes). Anticoagulated blood should be maintained at room temperature (22 to 24°C; *not* refrigerated) and tested for NK activity within a few hours of blood donation. Refrigeration of whole blood should be avoided because it has been shown to invert the CD4/CD8 T-cell ratio significantly, and it might interfere with the accuracy of NK cell determinations.

To perform the NK cell cytotoxicity assay, one begins by making a series of three 1 : 2 dilutions of the target cell suspension to obtain four target cell concentrations (2 $\times$ 10^6, 1 $\times$ 10^6, 0.5 $\times$ 10^6, and 0.025 $\times$ 10^6/ml) immediately before plating the assay. The assay is set up in 96-well, flat-bottom plastic plates (e.g., Costar 3598, Cambridge, MA) according to the plate schema shown in Fig. 1. After aliquots of 150 μl of whole blood for every patient are placed in wells of an appropriate row, 50 μl per well of target cells is added, beginning with the lowest concentration of targets and working up through the highest concentration (i.e., 2 $\times$ 10^6/well) of target cells. The assay is set up in triplicate, and the aliquots of target cells are added first to the spontaneous release (SR) wells containing target cells and medium only, then to the patient wells, and last to the maximal release wells, containing 150 μl of 5% (v/v) Triton X-100 and 50 μl of target cells. It is important to always change the automatic pipette tips and to avoid "carryover" of any blood from one well to another.

The assay plate(s) is centrifuged at 1200 rpm for 10 min at room temperature

	1	2	3	4	5	6	7	8	9	10	11	12
	MAX Release [2.0]			MAX Release [1.0]			MAX Release [0.5]			MAX Release [0.25]		
	SR [2.0]			SR [1.0]			SR [0.5]			SR [0.25]		
PT1												
PT2												
PT3												
PT4												
PT5												
PT6												

FIG. 1 A plating scheme for the NK cell assay. MAX, Maximal; SR, spontaneous release; PT, patient. The numbers in brackets refer to the number $\times$ 10^6/well of target cells. MAX release wells contain 150 μl Triton + 50 μl target suspension; SR wells contain 150 μl medium + 50 μl target suspension, and PT wells contain 150 μl whole blood + 50 μl target suspension. After incubation, 100 μl of COLD medium is added, making a total volume of 300 μl.

in a swinging-bucket-type Sorvall centrifuge equipped with adapters for plastic plates. The time and speed of centrifugation are *critical* for the formation of the interface, allowing for the optimal interaction of the target and effector cells. Following centrifugation, the plate is incubated for 4 hr at 37°C in an atmosphere of 5% CO_2 in air.

The cytotoxicity assay is stopped by the forceful addition to each well of 100 μl of *cold* RPMI 1640 medium (maintained in an ice–water bath) supplemented with 10% (v/v) fetal calf serum (FCS, Gibco, Grand Island, NY); using a multichannel Titertek dispenser. The cold medium must be added forcefully to cause mixing at the interface and to disrupt contact between effector and target cells. The plate(s) is then centrifuged at 1200 rpm for 10 min, and a 100-μl aliquot of the supernatant is *carefully* removed from each well and dispensed onto cotton filters placed in the prelabeled harvesting tubes. Great care must be taken to harvest only the supernatant and to avoid harvesting of red blood cells. The harvested supernatants are counted in a gamma counter to determine the percent specific lysis, using the formula,

$$\%\ \text{specific lysis} = \frac{(\text{ER-}b)\left[\dfrac{V_t\text{-}(V_b H)}{V_t}\right] - (\text{SR-}b)}{(\text{MR-}b) - (\text{SR-}b)},$$

where ER is the mean count per minute (cpm) of experimental release wells; SR, mean cpm of spontaneous release wells; MR, mean cpm of maximal release wells; V_t, total volume per well (300 μl in this procedure); V_b, volume of blood per well (150 μl in this procedure); H, hematocrit; and b, instrument background, which may be 0, if the gamma counter is equipped with the program which automatically subtracts background cpm in each channel.

In order to calculate the effector (E) to target (T) ratio, it is necessary to determine the white blood cell (WBC) and lymphocyte differential in every sample of peripheral blood from the patient. This requires that a small purple-top tube of blood is collected for automated cell counts. In addition, the hematocrit must be determined in each well in order to calculate the volume of supernatant (SN) in the well.

While it is acceptable to express results of cytotoxicity assays as the percentage specific lysis at different $E:T$ ratios, it may not be convenient to do so, particularly when assays performed at different $E:T$ ratios are being compared. For example, *in vitro* activated MNC which have been incubated with IL2 overnight generally have higher NK activity than resting, nonactivated NK cells, and it may be necessary to use much lower $E:T$ ratios with activated than resting NK cells to avoid measurements at the maximal level of cytotoxicity, which are uninterpretable. For this reason, an alternate way of expressing lytic activity in cytolytic units (CU) has been devised, allowing for a convenient way to quantitatively compare the relative cytotoxic activities of effector cells tested at different $E:T$ ratios in blood obtained from different individuals or the same individual repeatedly over time.

To calculate CU of NK activity for the whole-blood NK cell assay, a computer program was developed which is available on request from the Pittsburgh Cancer Institute. The program calculates CU, which are not to be equated with the lytic units (LU) obtained from the modified Van Krogh's equation, as described by Pross *et al.* (34). To calcualte CU, it is first necessary to compute the percentage of specific lysis for all the measured $E:T$ ratios. Next, the program fits a linear regression curve relating logistically transformed percentage specific lysis to the natural logarithm of the number of target cells per milliliter. If the fit is suitable, the area under the specific lysis curve between the smallest and largest cell numbers used is computed. Otherwise, the curve is reestimated, using the "pool-adjacent-violators" algorithm (35). The CU are an increasing measure of cytotoxicity, and they may range from 0 (no killing observed at any $E:T$ ratio) to a maximum of $100 \ln(RU/RL) = 208$, where the RU/RL is the ratio of the largest to smallest target cell numbers used.

The basic difference between the standard MNC NK cell assay and the whole-blood NK cell assay is that in the former, a constant number of target cells (e.g., 10^3) is used and the effector cell number is predetermined according to their expected cytolytic potency; in the latter, the $E:T$ ratios vary in all samples, and the assay seeks to establish the $E:T$ ratio that will best allow it to fit the specific lysis curve. Both the concept of the whole-blood assay (36) and the curve-fitting process are simple and easily applicable to routine clinical measurements.

As measured in the whole-blood NK cell assay, a normal range of NK activity in venous blood, established by testing 36 normal individuals in 145 independent assays, ranges from a low of 10 CU to a high of 148 CU (middle 80% range) and a mean of 70 CU. In a population of normal individuals tested sequentially at least three times, it is possible to define low and high responders. Within an individual, NK activity remains stable over time, unless an illness (e.g., infection), unusual stress, or drugs such as corticosteroids, hormones or BRM alter NK activity. Individuals with chronically low NK activity (<10 CU) should be observed and monitored serially in NK cell assays to determine how this low NK cell activity relates to their well being. Serial monitoring of NK activity can be used to measure spontaneous or treatment-induced changes in activity. Such changes can be detected only if baseline measurements (i.e., pretreatment) are available for comparisons. Similar to other cytotoxicity assays, the whole-blood NK cell assay must be performed at multiple (at least four) $E:T$ cell ratios in order to analyze the dose–response relationship accurately between the specific lysis and the number of effector cells present. While the amount of ^{51}Cr released from target cells is directly related to the proportion of target cells killed by the effectors, it is necessary to be on the linear portion of the lytic curve for this relationship to hold. When the curve flattens out at, e.g., 80% specific lysis approaching maximal lysis or when the number of effector cells in blood is too low, it is no longer possible to relate levels of cytotoxicity accurately to the number of effector cells.

Quality Control for Whole-Blood Natural Killer Cell Assay

To assure that the NK cell assay is reliable, reproducible, and free of errors, a set of control measures needs to be established and followed by every laboratory. To control for intraassay variability, a sample of peripheral blood from a normal individual is split and tested at two separate locations in the plate every time the assay is performed. If possible, it may be also advisable to similarly split patient cells for testing twice in a series of samples. When the correlation coefficients between split samples of the same individuals ($n = 10$) tested in the same assay in our laboratory were computed, a high degree of correlation ($p < 0.0001$) was obtained for intraassay CU. The other concern, especially when serial determinations of NK activity are performed, is interassay variability. To measure this parameter, samples obtained from the same individuals were retested at a minimum of 2 days and a maximum of 10 days apart in the whole-blood NK cell assays. The correlation coefficient calculated for 45 of such paired measurements was highly significant at $p < 0.001$. It is, of course, obvious that the interassay variability measured in this way may be a result not only of the assay variability but also of biologic variations in NK activity in the specimens obtained and tested several days apart. Nevertheless, a significant correlation was obtained for these measurements of CU, confirming that the whole-blood assay can be reliably performed in a clinical laboratory.

Determination of Number of Natural Killer Cells

To enumerate NK cells in whole blood, staining with MAbs, which recognize distinctive surface markers expressed on NK cells and flow cytometry, are used. Mature, circulating NK cells express the $CD3^-CD56^+CD16^+CD2^{dim}$ phenotype and are distinguishable from T cells by the lack of the T-cell receptor (TCR) expression on the cell surface or of rearranged T-cell receptor genes, which retain the germ line configuration in mature NK cells (37). Unlike B cells, NK cells do not express surface immunoglobulin (Ig); however, because NK cells are $Fc\gamma RIII^+$, they may have surface-bound Ig present (10). Surface markers expressed on NK cells or activated NK cells include IL2R (38); at least three different types of FcR (11, 12, 39); β_1 and β_2 integrins (40); various activation antigens, including HLA-DR, transferrin receptor (CD71), and CD69; and the activation-inducing molecule Leu23 (41). Many of the surface molecules expressed on NK cells are present on other hematopoietic cells, and, therefore, what distinguishes NK cells from other MNC in blood is a unique combination of several markers, such as CD56, CD16, and CD2, as well as the absence of certain other markers such as CD3, CD14, and surface Ig. Not all NK cells express the consensus phenotype described above, and subsets of NK cells which are $CD56^+CD16^-$ or $CD56^-CD16^+$ have been recognized and may represent functionally distinct subpopulations of NK cells (10, 42). Furthermore, activated NK cells may be present in blood of certain individuals, and since such activated NK cells express several distinctive "activation markers," they can be quantified by flow cytometry as, e.g., $CD3^-$ $CD56^+HLA\text{-}DR^+$; $CD3^-CD56^+CD25^+$; or $CD56^+CD16^+CD69^+$ populations. Since this requires three-color flow cytometry, a precise quantification of activated NK cells is more difficult and less commonly performed than two-color analysis of $CD56^+HLA\text{-}DR^+$ or $CD56^+CD25^+$ subsets. The latter may, of course, not all be NK cells.

The percentage of circulating $CD3^-CD56^+$ NK cells determined by two-color flow cytometry of healthy individuals is $12 \pm 6\%$ (mean $\pm$ SD; $n =$

107), with a middle 80% range of 6 to 21%. The mean absolute number ± SD of these effector cells in the peripheral circulation is 279 ± 245/mm^3, with a middle 80% range of 96–425 cells/mm^3. To calculate the absolute number of NK cells in whole blood, the absolute number of lymphocytes is first computed from the total WBC and the differential count is obtained from a small purple-top tube collected simultaneously with the heparinized blood for NK cell cytotoxicity assay. The absolute number of lymphocytes multiplied by the percentage of NK cells determined in the lymphogate by flow cytometry gives the absolute count of NK cells.

The quantification of total NK cells or NK cell subsets by flow cytometry must always be performed with appropriate controls and under strict quality control rules that apply to flow cytometry as performed in a clinical laboratory (43). Negative controls should include staining with isotype-matched irrelevant antibodies and a phosphate-buffered saline (PBS) control tube for autofluorescence. A positive control is necessary when patient samples are evaluated and generally includes blood or MNC of a repeatedly tested normal individual, whose total number of NK cells in peripheral blood is known.

It is important to realize that enumeration of NK cells by flow cytometry cannot substitute for the assessment of NK activity. The correlation between the number of circulating NK cells and NK activity for normal individuals is significant but not particularly strong (1). This probably means that NK cells vary in their state of activation or that not all NK cells in blood mediate effector cell function. Indeed, human NK cells are functionally heterogeneous, and subsets of NK cells with distinct functions have been recognized in peripheral blood (44). Therefore assessments of both the number of total NK cells and their activity are necessary to adequately evaluate natural immunity or to monitor changes during disease, therapy, or other interventions.

Recommendations for Performing Natural Killer Cells Assays

There has been a great deal of interest among neurobiologists, psychologists, and psychiatrists in NK cells and assays for measurements of NK activity. A growing body of evidence indicating that emotional distress can reduce NK activity (45, 46) has undoubtedly contributed to this interest. Additionally, it has been observed that NK cells express both receptors for certain neuroendocrine hormones and neuropeptides as well as neural adhesion molecules (NCAM), such as CD56 (47). This antigen shares epitopes with macromolecules present in the brain and neuroendocrine tissues. The possibility of direct interactions between the neuroendocrine system and NK cells has been considered (16, 46). The activities of NK cells are highly regulated, and factors produced by the neuroendocrine system have been reported to modulate cytotoxic activity (48, 49). This might be mediated through specific receptors for neuroendocrine hormones on NK cells, and it is possible that signals delivered via these receptors positively or negatively regulate NK activity. While reasons for measuring NK cell activity and numbers in cohorts of individuals undergoing emotional or physical stress are sound, it is apparent that reliable assays performed under carefully controlled conditions are necessary to establish and study effects of the neuroendocrine system on NK cells. The choice of an NK cell assay for these studies is particularly important. Thus, as pointed out in the preceding section, measuring of the numbers of NK cells is not sufficient, because it does not always correlate with NK activity. As discussed above, NK activity is a more sensitive indicator of changes in the NK cell functional status than is expression of the activation markers on NK cells. Therefore, both NK activity and number should be measured and not the number alone, even though flow cytometry is widely used and MAbs to various surface antigen on NK cells are widely available.

The whole-blood NK cell cytotoxicity assay is recommended to neurobiologists for several reasons. First, the whole-blood NK cell assay allows for the effector cells to remain in the milieu as close to that existing *in vivo* as possible during the 4-hr procedure. Thus, soluble factors, Ig, cytokines, or peptides present in blood are present in the well during the incubation of effector cells with their targets. Using this assay, it is possible to avoid separation of NK cells from erythrocytes and granulocytes which have been shown to have effects on NK activity (50). The assay is performed in autologous plasma, which probably contains all of the relevant factors listed above. This opportunity to be able to measure "native" NK activity should be attractive to neurobiologists. Second, for those who are interested in correlating NK activity with the number of total NK cells, NK cell subsets, or activated NK cells as determined by flow cytometry, the ability to perform both assays on whole blood, using the same specimens, should allow for more meaningful and stronger correlations to be made. Third, the opportunity of using whole blood allows for a much shorter time to elapse between the blood donation and assay than with the standard cytotoxicity assay performed on separated MNC. This aspect of *in vitro* testing is particularly critical when NK activity is measured after an *in vivo* intervention and when the intent is to observe changes in NK activity from the baseline level. It has been demonstrated that changes in NK activity occur very rapidly following, e.g., a stressful event (51). Therefore, it appears to be advisable to shorten the time between an intervention and assay, particularly when studies of kinetics of change in NK activity are performed. Last, the whole-blood NK cell assay offers savings of time and cost without compromising quality.

In our view, the whole-blood NK cell assay should replace the standard ^{51}Cr-release assay performed with isolated MNC as a more informative, less expensive, and faster laboratory procedure.

Having described advantages of the whole-blood NK cell assay, it is necessary to give a word of caution to those neurobiologists who are willing to use it. The assay is not as easy to perform reliably as it seems. The best approach is to have it performed in a laboratory experienced with cytotoxicity tests and with quality controls that were described above and that are obligatory. Performed by experienced and knowledgeable personnel, the assay has excellent intra- and interassay reproducibility and is applicable to serial monitoring of NK activity. The results of this assay, whether expressed as percentage specific lysis or as CU are not comparable to those obtained in the standard 4-hr ^{51}Cr-release assays performed with the gradient-separated MNC. The whole-blood NK cell assay is performed under different experimental conditions than the MNC assay, and the lytic events that occur under these conditions are obviously not comparable to those in the MNC assay. As always, each laboratory will be obliged to establish a normal range of NK activity and define coefficients of variation for intra- and interassay variability before the assay can be used experimentally. Finally, the approach to calculating the CU developed by Dr. John Bryant at our Institute is different and simpler than the LU program based on the calculations of Pross (34). At our institution, the whole-blood NK cell assay is now being used for serial studies of NK activity in patients with various diseases, including viral infections or cancer and in normal volunteers participating in various intervention studies.

Acknowledgments

The authors are grateful to Dr. Sheldon Cohen of the Department of Psychology, Carnegie–Mellon University, for making available the correlation data for inter- and intraassay reproducibility of the whole-blood NK cells assays. These assays were performed at the Immunologic Monitoring and Diagnostic Laboratory, and the staff of the laboratory is acknowledged for expert technical performance. We thank Dr. John Bryant, of the Department of Mathematics and Pittsburgh Cancer Institute, for his interest and help in establishing the whole-blood NK cell assay, in performing statistical analyses, and in developing a computer program for calculating CU.

This manuscript was supported in part by the Pathology Education and Research Foundation.

References

1. T. L. Whiteside and R. B. Herberman, *Clin. Immunol. Immunopathol.* **53,** 1 (1989).

2. G. Trinchieri, *Adv. Immunol.* **47,** 187 (1989).
3. B. Bonavida and S. C. Wright, *J. Clin. Immunol.* **6,** 1 (1986).
4. T. L. Whiteside and R. B. Herberman, *Immunol. Allergy Clin. North Am.* **10,** 663 (1990).
5. T. L. Whiteside and R. B. Herberman, *Clin. Diagn. Lab. Immunol.* **1,** 1 (1994).
6. B. Perussia, *Curr. Opinion Immunol.* **3,** 49 (1991).
7. M. C. Cuturi, I. Anegon, F. Sherman, R. Loudon, S. C. Clark, B. Perussia, and G. Trinchieri, *J. Exp. Med.* **169,** 569 (1989).
8. M. A. Caligiuri, A. Zmuidzinas, T. J. Manley, H. Levine, K. A. Smith, and J. Ritz, *J. Exp. Med.* **171,** 1509 (1990).
9. R. B. Herberman, J. R. Ortaldo, and G. D. Bonnard, *Nature (London)* **277,** 221 (1979).
10. A. Nagler, L. L. Lanier, S. Cwirla, and J. H. Phillips, *J. Immunol.* **143,** 3183 (1989).
11. D. Metes, A. Sulica, W. Chambers, T. Whiteside, P. Morel, and R. B. Herberman, submitted for publication.
12. L. Pricop, H. Rabinowich, A. Sulica, R. B. Haberman, and T. L. Whiteside, *FASEB J.* **6,** 1622 (1992).
13. P. Anderson, M. Caligiuri, C. O'Brien, T. Manley, and J. Ritz, *Proc. Natl. Acad. Sci. U.S.A.* **87,** 2274 (1990).
14. M. J. Robertson, M. A. Caliguiri, T. J. Manley, H. Levine, and J. Ritz, *J. Immunol.* **145,** 3194 (1990).
15. A. Gismondi, S. Morrone, M. J. Humphries, M. Piccoli, L. Frati, and A. Santoni, *J. Immunol.* **146,** 384 (1991).
16. Y. Shavit, J. W. Lewis, W. Terman, R. P. Gale, and J. C. Liebskind, *Science* **223,** 188 (1984).
17. L. Matera, G. Muccioli, A. Cesano, G. Bellussi, and E. Genazzani, *Brain Behav. Immun.* **2,** 1 (1988).
18. M. J. Robertson and J. Ritz, *Blood* **76,** 2421 (1990).
19. R. M. Welsh, *Nat. Immun. Cell Growth Regul.* **5,** 160 (1986).
20. S. V. Schantz, B. W. Brown, E. Lira, D. L. Taylor, and N. Beddingfield, *Cancer Immunol. Immunother.* **141** (1987).
21. D. T. Purtilo, R. S. Strobach, M. Okano, and J. R. Davis, *Lab. Invest.* **67,** 5 (1992).
22. E. H. Steinhauer, A. T. Doyle, J. Reed, and A. S. Kadish, *J. Immunol.* **129,** 2255 (1982).
23. W. J. Murphy, C. W. Reynolds, P. Tiberghien, and D. L. Longo, *J. Natl. Cancer Inst.* **85,** 1475 (1993).
24. C. Xun, S. A. Brown, C. D. Jennings, P. J. Henslée-Downey, and J. S. Thompson, *Transplantation* **56,** 409 (1993).
25. K. Hata, X. R. Zhang, S. Iwatsuki, D. H. Van Thiel, R. B. Herberman, and T. L. Whiteside, *Clin. Immunol. Immunopathol.* **56,** 401 (1990).
26. F. Shanahan, M. Brogan, and S. Targan, *Gastroenterology* **92,** 1951 (1987).
27. A. O'Leary, *Psychol. Bull.* **108,** 363 (1990).
28. S. M. Levy, R. B. Herberman, A. Simons, T. L. Whiteside, J. Lee, R. McDonald, and M. Beadle, *Nat. Immun. Cell Growth Regul.* **8,** 173 (1989).

29. C. J. Froelich, S. Guiffaut, M. Sosenko, and K. Muth, *Clin. Immunol. Immunopathol.* **50,** 132 (1989).
30. E. Gorelik and R. B. Herberman, *in* "Cancer Immunology: Innovative Approaches to Therapy," (R. B. Herberman, ed.), p. 151. Martius Nijhoft Press, New York, 1986.
31. N. Imamura, Y. Kusunoki, K. Kawa-Ha, K. Yumura, J. Hara, K. Oda, K. Abe, H. Dohy, T. Inada, H. Kajihara, and A. Kuramoto, *Br. J. Hematol.* **75,** 49 (1990).
32. T. L. Whiteside, "Tumor-Infiltrating Lymphocytes in Human Malignancies." R. G. Landes Co., Austin, 1993.
33. T. L. Whiteside, J. Bryant, R. Day, and R. B. Herberman, *J. Clin. Lab. Anal.* *2,* 102 (1990).
34. H. F. Pross, M. G. Baines, P. Rubin, P. Shragge, and M. S. Patterson, *J. Clin. Immunol.* **1,** 51 (1981).
35. B. Barlow and B. Brenner, "Statistical Inference Under Order Restrictions." Wiley, New York, 1972.
36. M. A. Fletcher, G. C. Baron, M. R. Ashman, M. A. Fischl, and N. G. Klimas, *Diagn. Clin. Immunol.* **5,** 69 (1987).
37. L. L. Lanier, S. Cwirla, and N. Federspiel, *J. Exp. Med.* **163,** 209 (1986).
38. A. Nagler, L. L. Lanier, and J. H. Phillips, *J. Exp. Med.* **171,** 1527 (1990).
39. L. Pricop, H. Rabinowich, P. A. Morel, A. Sulica, T. L. Whiteside, and R. B. Herberman, *J. Immunol.* **151,** 3018 (1993).
40. T. L. Whiteside and R. B. Herberman, *Invasion Metastasis* **12,** 128 (1992).
41. H. Rabinowich, R. B. Herberman, and T. L. Whiteside, *Cell. Immunol.* **152,** 481 (1993).
42. L. L. Lanier, A. M. Le, C. I. Civin, M. R. Loken, and J. H. Phillips, *J. Immunol.* **136,** 4480 (1986).
43. A. L. Landay and K. A. Muirhead, *Clin. Immunol. Immunopathol.* **52,** 48 (1989).
44. N. L. Vujanovic, H. Rabinowich, Y. J. Lee, L. Jost, R. B. Herberman, and T. L. Whiteside, *Cell. Immunol.* **151,** 133 (1993).
45. S. M. Levy, R. B. Herberman, J. Lee, T. L. Whiteside, M. Beadle, L. Heiden, and A. Simons, *Nat. Immun. Cell Growth Regul.* **10,** 289 (1991).
46. R. Dantzer and K. W. Kelley, *Life Sci.* **44,** 1995 (1989).
47. L. L. Lanier, C. Chang, M. Azuma, J. J. Ruitenberg, J. J. Hemperly, and J. H. Phillips, *J. Immunol.* **146,** 4421 (1991).
48. M. P. Yeager, C. T. Yu, A. S. Campbell, M. Moschella, and P. M. Guyre, *Clin. Immunol. Immunopathol.* **62,** 336 (1992).
49. S. M. Levy, J. Fernstrom, R. B. Herberman, T. L. Whiteside, J. Lee, M. Ward, and M. Massoudi, *Life Sci.* **48,** 107 (1991).
50. H. Shau, R. K. Gupta, and S. H. Golub, *Cell. Immunol.* **147,** 1 (1993).
51. W. J. Sieber, J. Rodin, L. Larson, S. Ortega, N. Cummings, S. Levy, T. L. Whiteside, and R. B. Herberman, *Brain Behav. Immun.* **6,** 141 (1992).

[3] Functional Assays to Determine Effects of Mammalian Tachykinins on Human Neutrophils

Raffaele Scicchitano, Andrzej Wozniak, Julian McNeil, Sylvia J. Usher, and William H. Betts

Introduction

Neutrophilic granulocytes play an important role in immunity and inflammation and contribute to tissue destruction in chronic inflammatory diseases such as rheumatoid arthritis and asthma. We have shown that tachykinins including substance P (SP) prime human neutrophils for enhanced superoxide anion (O_2^-) production in response to *N*-formylmethionylleucylphenylalanine (fMLP), platelet activating factor (PAF), and 12-phorbol 12-myristate acetate (PMA) (1, 2). In addition SP stimulates neutrophil antibody-dependent cell-mediated cytotoxicity (ADCC) (1). Other workers have shown that SP is chemotactic for human neutrophils (3) and monocytes (4, 5) and facilitates neutrophil chemotaxis in response to other stimuli (6) as well as promoting granule exocytosis and neutrophil aggregation (7–9).

In this chapter we describe a number of functional assays and methodologies which we have used to investigate the effects of tachykinins on human neutrophils. We also describe an enzyme-linked immunosorbent assay (ELISA) which we have developed to measure SP extracted from tissues and fluids.

Materials and Methods

Peptides

Tachykinins and their fragments may be purchased from AUSPEP, Melbourne, Australia. All peptides are shown to be endotoxin free by the *Limulus* amebocyte lysate assay (E-Toxate, Sigma Chemicals, St. Louis, MO). Stock solutions of 1 m*M* are prepared in 1 m*M* acetic acid. Aliquots (10–100 μl) are stored under nitrogen at -70°C, to prevent oxidation, and they are thawed only once before use. Any unused material is discarded. Subsequent dilutions are prepared using cold buffer and kept on ice until used.

Methods in Neurosciences, Volume 24

Isolation of Human Neutrophils

Two different methods may be used to isolate human neutrophils. The Lymphoprep gradient is simple and consistently yields high purity of cells with low basal activity. Neutrophils prepared by this method are used in the O_2^- and ADCC assays as well as for the measurements of intracellular free calcium concentration ($[Ca^{2+}]_i$). However, for the studies of leukotriene B_4 (LTB_4) production, neutrophils isolated by Percoll gradient yield more consistent results.

We use EDTA as blood anticoagulant, as heparin has been found to have an inhibitory effect on some neutrophil functions [A. Wozniak and R. Scicchitano, unpublished observation, 1989 (10)]. Use extreme care when resuspending and mixing cells throughout the isolation procedures to avoid neutrophil activation. After centrifugation the cell pellets are always resuspended first in a small volume of buffer (1 ml) by gentle pipetting and subsequently diluted to the required volume. We have noted that vigorous or extensive washing and mixing activates the cells, and this could compromise their response to neuropeptides. We recommend the use of soft rubber-top vortex mixers (Maxi Mix II, Thermolyne, Sybron Corporation, IA) and low-adherence polyvinyl tubes (Disposable Products, Adelaide, Australia) for neutrophil isolation and experiments. Always use neutrophils within 30 min of preparation.

Lymphoprep Gradient

Neutrophils are isolated from peripheral blood anticoagulated with 0.09% EDTA. The leukocyte-rich fraction (buffy coat) may be obtained by sedimenting erythrocytes with 1% dextran T-500 (2 ml dextran/10 ml blood) (Pharmacia, Uppsala, Sweden) for 40 min at room temperature. The buffy coat cells are washed twice by centrifugation at 400*g* for 10 min at room temperature which also removes most of the platelets. Neutrophils are isolated by density-gradient centrifugation using Lymphoprep (NYCOMED AS, Oslo, Norway). Buffy coat cells (10^8) in 10 ml RPMI (RPMI 1640) supplemented with 20 m*M* HEPES, 1 m*M* sodium pyruvate, 2 mg/ml sodium carbonate, 2 m*M* L-glutamine, 60 μg/ml penicillin, and 8 μg/ml gentamicin in a 50-ml conical tube are carefully underlaid with 10 ml of Lymphoprep using a 10-ml syringe with an 18-gauge needle, and the gradient is centrifuged at 400*g* for 20 min at 22°C. Neutrophils mixed with erythrocytes form pellets at the bottom of the tube. Residual erythrocytes are removed by hypotonic lysis: 5 ml of ice-cold 0.2% NaCl is mixed with each pellet by vortexing for 25 sec, and then 5 ml of 1.6% NaCl is added. The cells are washed twice in 20 ml of RPMI and resuspended to the required concentration. Neutrophils isolated by this method are always >96% pure, as determined by Grunwald–Giemsa staining, and >98% viable by trypan blue exclusion.

Percoll Gradient

Neutrophils are isolated from peripheral blood using Percoll (Pharmacia, Uppsala, Sweden) as described previously by McColl *et al.* (11) and EDTA as an anticoagulant. The leukocyte-rich fraction is obtained by sedimenting erythrocytes with 1% dextran T-500 for 40 min at 37°C, washed, and resuspended in modified Dulbecco's phosphate-buffered saline (DPBS; 138 m*M* NaCl, 2.7 m*M* KCl, 16.2 m*M* Na_2HPO_4, 1.4 m*M* KH_2PO_4, 0.5 m*M* $MgSO_4$, 0.6 m*M* $CaCl_2$, and 7.5 m*M* glucose, pH 7.3). A total of 10 ml of buffy coat cells (10^8) suspended in DPBS are then carefully layered on the top of Percoll gradients consisting of two layers of Percoll with different densities. The gradients are prepared by placing 10 ml of 1.092 g/ml Percoll in a 50-ml conical tube and then, using 10-ml syringes with attached 21-gauge needles, overlaying it gently with 10 ml of 1.070 g/ml Percoll. The gradients are centrifuged at 450*g* for 20 min at 22°C. Neutrophils are collected from the interface between the two Percoll layers, washed twice in DPBS (Ca^{2+}, Mg^{2+}-free), and resuspended in DPBS to a concentration of $1–2 \times 10^6$/ml. Occasionally, when small numbers of red blood cells copurify with the neutrophils, they are removed as described in the Lymphoprep method above. The purity and viability of neutrophils obtained using this method are the same as those for neutrophils obtained by Lymphoprep gradient.

Percoll Solutions

Percoll 150 is prepared by mixing nine parts of Percoll stock solution with one part (v/v) of 10× DPBS and adjusting the pH to 7.0 with NaOH. Percoll concentrations of 1.070 and 1.092 g/ml are prepared by mixing 5.85 ml of Percoll 150 with 4.15 ml of DPBS, and 7.65 ml of Percoll 150 with 2.35 ml of DPBS, respectively.

Superoxide Anion Production

Neutrophil O_2^- production is measured as superoxide dismutase (SOD)-inhibitable reduction of ferricytochrome *c* (Cyt *c*, type IV, horse heart, Sigma Chemicals). This is determined by the addition of 10 μl of 2 mg/ml SOD (Boehringer-Mannheim, Germany) to duplicate samples in all preliminary experiments. Measurements are made in real time, to enable determination of rates of O_2^- production, and by end point, to enable calculation of total O_2^- production by any given stimulus/manipulation as described below. All end point experiments are performed in triplicate in low-absorbance tubes (MiniSorp, Nunc, Denmark). The final concentration of cells in all experiments is adjusted to 10^6/ml.

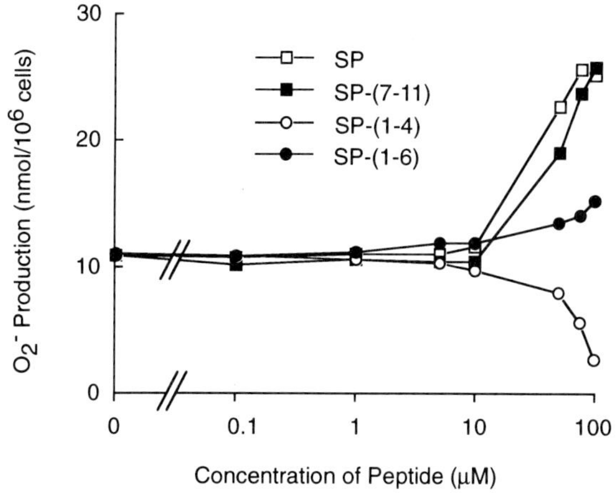

FIG. 1 Effect of substance P fragments on neutrophil fMLP-stimulated O_2^- production. Neutrophils were preincubated with (○) SP(1–4), (●) SP(1–6), (■) SP(7–11), or (□) SP for 30 min at 37°C before fMLP stimulation. Values represent means of three experiments. Reproduced with permission from A. Wozniak, W. H. Betts, G. McLennan, and R. Scicchitano, *Immunology* **78,** 629 (1993).

In the dose–response experiments, 10^6 neutrophils are incubated in triplicate with 100 μM Cyt *c* in DPBS (± SOD) containing varying concentrations of peptides (0.01 to 100 μM) in a final volume of 1.0 ml. Since the peptides are dissolved in acetic acid, our medium control includes the highest possible concentration (0.1 mM) of acetic acid. This does not affect basal or stimulated O_2^- production. Cells are incubated for 30 min at 37°C and then 0.1 μM of fMLP (Sigma Chemicals), 10 ng/ml of PMA (Sigma Chemicals), or medium is added and the mixture incubated for a further 6 min. The reaction is stopped by addition of SOD (10 μl of 2 mg/ml) and by placing the tubes on ice. The cells are pelleted by centrifugation at 1500 rpm for 5 min at 4°C and O_2^- production is quantified in cell supernatants by changes in absorption at 550 nm using an extinction coefficient of 21.1 mM^{-1} cm^{-1} (12). The priming effect of SP and its fragments on neutrophil O_2^- production assessed using this assay is illustrated in Fig. 1.

In the time-course experiments, and in experiments where the effect of SP on the dose–response to fMLP and PMA is studied, neutrophils (5×10^6 cell/ml) are incubated with medium or the stated concentration(s) of peptides for various times at 37°C. After incubation, 200 μl of cells (10^6) is transferred to a tube containing 800 μl of a prewarmed mixture of 100 μM Cyt *c* and different concentration(s) of stimulus or medium as a control. The mixture is incubated for a further 10 min at 37°C. The reaction is stopped by addition of SOD and by immersion of the tubes in ice. The O_2^- production is quantified in cell supernatants as described above.

The kinetics of O_2^- production are measured by following OD changes continuously in a thermostatted (37°C) spectrophotometer. Neutrophils (5 × 10^6 cells) are preincubated with the stated concentration of neuropeptide, or medium as a control, for 10 min at 37°C, then 200 μl of cells (10^6) is transferred to cuvettes in the spectrophotometer containing 800 μl of a prewarmed mixture containing 100 μ*M* Cyt *c* and a stimulus (e.g., fMLP or PMA), and changes in OD at 550 nm are monitored. The OD measurement is converted to nanomoles of O_2^- as explained above. The kinetics of SP-primed versus unprimed PMA-stimulated neutrophils are shown in Fig. 2.

Antibody-Dependent Cell-Mediated Cytotoxicity (ADCC)

The assay described here is based on the method of Vadas *et al.* (13). Experiments have been performed in triplicate in RPMI 1640 medium containing 0.1% (w/v) bovine serum albumin (BSA).

Preparation of P815 Target Cells

P815 (DBA/2 mastocytoma) target cells are passaged the day before by transferring 1 ml of a dense cell suspension to a 25-cm^2 tissue culture flask containing 10 ml of fresh culture medium [5% fetal calf serum (FCS)/RPMI]. The cells (usually 5–8 × 10^6) are then pelleted by centrifugation at 1500 rpm for 5 min, and the cell pellet is suspended in 100 μl of culture medium to which 200 μCi of ^{51}Cr (10–35 mCi/ml, sodium [^{51}Cr] chromate in 0.9% NaCl solution, Amersham, Australia) is added. After 1 hr incubation at 37°C in a water bath with occasional mixing, the cells are washed once in PBS and centrifuged at 1500 rpm for 5 min, and the cell pellet is suspended in 400 μl of PBS. The ^{51}Cr-labeled cells are then opsonized with trinitrophenol (TNP) by mixing with 100 μl of 10 mg/ml TNP and incubating for 20 min at room temperature. As addition of TNP changes the pH of the buffer to acidic, the pH is adjusted back to neutral with 0.1 *M* NaOH, in the presence of one drop of 0.5% phenol red. After the incubation, the cells are washed in 10 ml of 5% FCS/RPMI and resuspended in 1 ml of culture medium. They are then carefully underlaid with 1 ml of FCS and centrifuged at 1000 rpm for 10 min. After centrifugation, the supernatant and FCS are carefully removed; the cells suspended in 0.1% (w/v) BSA/RPMI to a concentration of 10^5 cells/ml and used immediately.

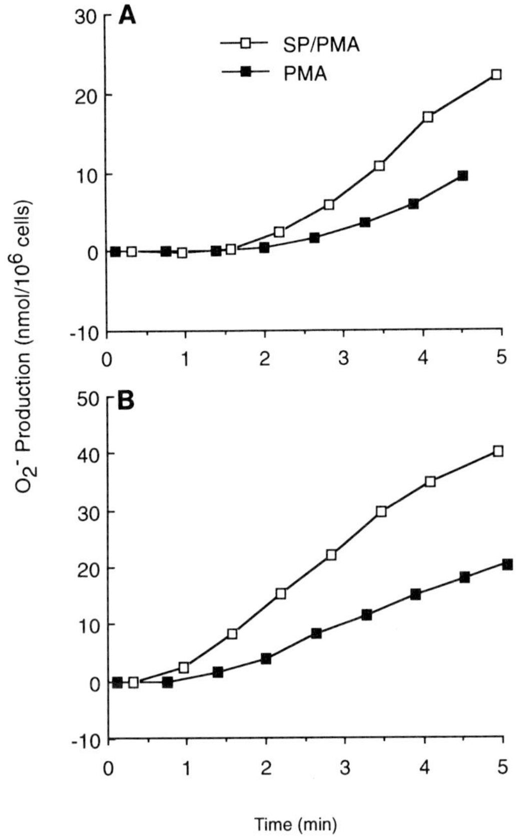

FIG. 2 Effect of SP on PMA-stimulated O_2^- production. Neutrophils (5×10^6) were preincubated with medium or 50 μM SP for 15 min at 37°C and then 10^6 cells were transferred to prewarmed cuvettes containing (A) 10 ng/ml PMA or (B) 50 ng/ml PMA in which the O_2^- production was measured continuously. The results are from a representative experiment.

Procedure for ADCC Assay

A total of 40 μl (4×10^3) of ^{51}Cr-labeled TNP-coupled P815 target cells is mixed with 80 μl (1.2×10^5) neutrophils as effector cells; 24 μl of rabbit IgG anti-DNP antibody (Miles-Yeda, Rehovot, Israel) that is cross-reacting with TNP, and 16 μl of the appropriate peptide (stimulus) in V-bottomed, 96-well microtiter plates. The final assay volume is 160 μl. After incubation of the reaction mixture for 2.5 hr at 37°C, 80 μl of the supernatant is carefully removed without disturbing the plate, and the radioactivity counted using a gamma counter (LKB, 1282 Commugamma, Turku, Finland). Percentage cytotoxicity is calculated as

$$\% \text{ cytotoxicity} = \frac{\text{experimental cpm} - \text{spontaneous release cpm}}{\text{total cpm} - \text{spontaneous release cpm}},$$

where cpm is counts per minute, spontaneous release is the ^{51}Cr released from P815 cells in the presence of medium alone, and the total count is the ^{51}Cr released from the P815 cells lysed by the addition of 4% (v/v) Triton X-100.

We have found that both the baseline and the stimulated ADCC depend on the concentration of the anti-TNP antibody. Concentrations of up to 3 μg/ml of anti-TNP are optimal and result in small baseline responses and good stimulated responses for neutrophils isolated from normal subjects. However, when neutrophils isolated from asthmatic subjects are used, lower concentrations (1–0.1 μ/ml) yield better results due to enhanced baseline activity of these cells as shown in Fig. 3.

Measurements of Intracellular Free Calcium Concentration ($[Ca^{2+}]_i$)

Changes in intracellular free calcium ($[Ca^{2+}]_i$) are measured using Fura-2-loaded neutrophils. After separation, 10^7 neutrophils are incubated with 2 μM Fura-2AM (Calbiochem, LaJolla, CA) for 30 min at 37°C in Hanks' buffer. During this time the Fura-2AM enters the cells where it is hydrolyzed to the acid form Fura-2 and trapped inside the cells. The cells are washed twice with Hanks' buffer to remove any unesterified Fura-2AM. The cells (10^6/ml) are then placed in a spectrophotofluorimeter (Perkin-Elmer LS-50). The various test components are added and changes in fluorescence (excitation, 340 nm; emission, 510 nm; slit widths, 10 nm) monitored continuously. Levels of intracellular calcium are then calculated using the equation developed by Tsein and colleagues (14, 15).

$$[Ca^{2+}]_i = K_d(F - F_{min})/(F_{max} - F),$$

where F is the fluorescence of the cell sample; F_{max}, the maximum fluorescence signal (obtained at the end of each measurement by releasing all intracellular calcium by treatment of the cell suspension with excess Triton (0.1%); and F_{min}, the minimum fluorescence value (the value obtained when there is no calcium bound to Fura-2), obtained by the addition of excess

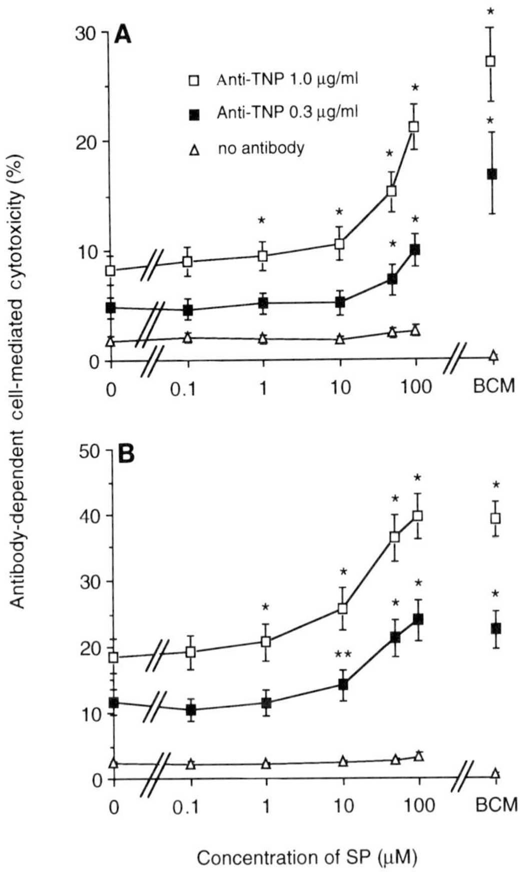

FIG. 3 Effect of SP on neutrophil ADCC in (A) normal and (B) asthmatic subjects. Neutrophils and target cells were incubated together with various concentrations of SP (or medium control) for 2.5 hr at 37°C and the indicated concentrations of antibody. Bladder carcinoma cell line U5637 conditioned medium (BCM) was used as a positive control.* $p < 0.0001$ and ** $p < 0.002$ indicate values which differ significantly from the medium control.

EGTA (2 mM buffered with 25 mM Tris) to the above. K_d is the dissociation constant for Fura-2 (220 nM). A typical fluorescence trace from fMLP-stimulated neutrophils is shown in Fig. 4.

We have found that although there are small variations in responses, both SP and its fragment SP (7–11) consistently increase $[Ca^{2+}]_i$ in neutrophils (Fig. 5).

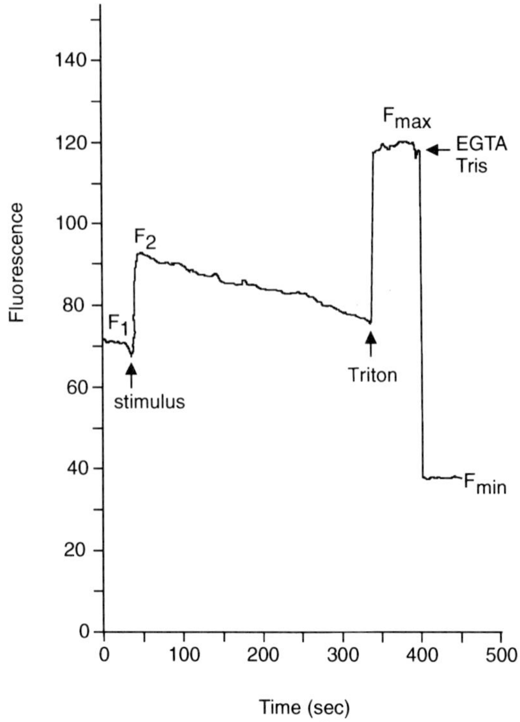

FIG. 4 Fluorescence trace from Fura-2-loaded fMLP-stimulated human neutrophils measured in presence of 2 m*M* EGTA. F_{max} and F_{min} were determined in each experiment. F_1 is used to determine the basal level of calcium concentration in the cells, and F_2 the concentration to which it increases after stimulation. The results are a representative experiment.

Leukotriene B_4 (LTB_4) and 5-Hydroxy-eicosatetrenoic Acid (5-HETE) Production

LTB_4 and 5-HETE production is measured by high-performance liquid chromatography (HPLC) as described previously by McColl *et al.* (11). We performed all experiments in quadruplicate using neutrophils isolated on Percoll gradient.

The assay is performed in 13-ml glass tubes that have been chromic acid washed before each experiment. Neutrophils (0.9 ml) suspended in DPBS (1–2 × 10^6 cells/ml) are transferred into the tubes and prewarmed to 37°C for 5 min, in a water bath. SP (100 μl) is added to the prewarmed cells to a final concentration of 0.1 or 50 μM and incubated for 15 min at 37°C. Two minutes before the end of the incubation time, 5 μl of 2 m*M* arachidonic

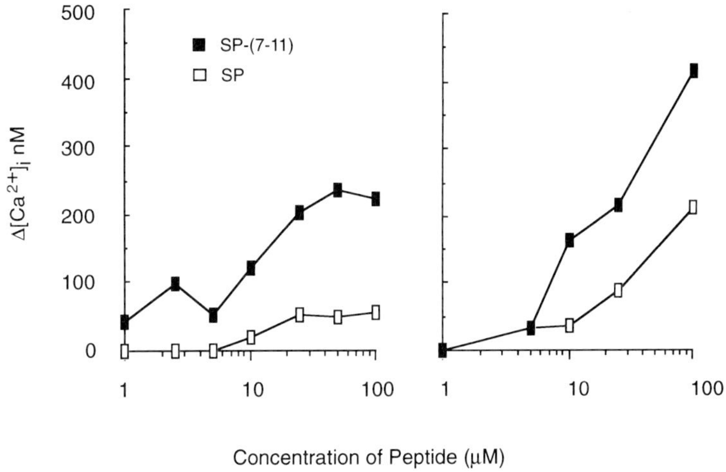

FIG. 5 Effect of (□) SP and (■) SP(7–11) on $\Delta[Ca^{2+}]_i$. For the study of changes in $\Delta[Ca^{2+}]_i$, Fura-2-loaded neutrophils were stimulated with various concentrations of SP or SP(7–11). The results are two representative experiments.

acid (AA, Sigma Chemicals) (10 μM final) is added to the samples and 5 μl of methanol (AA diluent) to the controls. After 15 min of incubation with SP, the cells are then stimulated with 5 μM A23187 (Sigma Chemicals) or 0.1 μM fMLP for an additional 5 min at 37°C. The reaction is terminated by the addition of 100 μl of 100 mM citric acid which lowers the pH of the aqueous phase to pH 3, necessary for the subsequent extraction of LTB_4 and 5-HETE into an organic phase. This is very important and the pH of several samples should be checked to ensure that there is pH $\leq$ 3. At this point in the assay, 30 ng of prostaglandin B_2 and 124.5 ng of 15-HETE (both from Sigma Chemicals) are added to each tube as the internal standards for LTB_4 and 5-HETE, respectively, and the samples are mixed. LTB_4 and 5-HETE (and the internal standards) are extracted with 5 ml of chloroform/methanol (7 : 3). The tubes are vortexed vigorously for 1 min and then centrifuged for 10 min at 2000 rpm to separate the aqueous and the organic phases. The lower chloroform layer (containing leukotrienes and HETEs) is transferred to 5-ml borosilicate glass tubes and the chloroform evaporated under vacuum, at room temperature, using a centrifugal evaporator (Savant, Hicksville, NY). The samples are reconstituted in 100 μl of the LTB_4 mobile phase, transferred to Waters low volume inserts (Waters Millipore, Milford, MA) and analyzed by HPLC.

The effect of SP on LTB4 and 5-HETE production is summarized in Table I.

TABLE I Effect of SP on LTB_4 and 5-HETE Production by Neutrophils Stimulated with fMLP and A23187[a]

Concentration of SP (μM)	Stimulus	AA	5-HETE (ng/10^6 cells)	LTB_4 (ng/10^6 cells)
0	A23187	−	29.8 ± 4.2	7.3 ± 1.0
0		+	104.7 ± 13.2	12.3 ± 1.4
0.1	A23187	−	30.6 ± 8.7	6.0 ± 1.2
0.1		+	110.1 ± 11.6	12.1 ± 2.0
50	A23187	−	43.2 ± 12.1	8.7 ± 2.0
50		+	117.8 ± 10.7	14.5 ± 2.7
0	fMLP	−	ND	ND
0		+	23.4 ± 6.2	3.5 ± 0.8
0.1	fMLP	−	ND	ND
0.1		+	26.7 ± 6.8	4.3 ± 1.1
50	fMLP	−	ND	ND
50		+	43.1 ± 7.4[b]	7.0 ± 1.4[b]

[a] Neutrophils (10^6) were incubated with 0.1 or 50 μM SP for 15 min at 37°C and then stimulated with 0.1 μM fMLP or 5 μM A23187 for an additional 5 min in the presence or absence of 10 μM AA. Values are means of three experiments performed in triplicate. ± refers to presence or absence of exogenous AA. ND, nondetectable. Reproduced with permission from A. Wozniak, G. McLennan, W. H. Betts, G. Murphy, and R. Scicchitano, *Immunology* **68,** 359 (1989).

[b] Values which differ significantly from the corresponding diluent control ($p < 0.05$).

Assay Conditions

Mobile phases	
LTB_4	67% Methanol/33% H_2O/0.08% acetic acid (v/v/v) (pH adjusted to 6.2 with ammonium hydroxide)
5-HETE	77% Methanol/23% H_2O/0.08% acetic acid (v/v/v) (pH adjusted to 6.2 with ammonium hydroxide)
HPLC conditions	
Injection volume	25 μl
Wavelength	270 nm (LTB_4), 235 nm (5-HETE)
Flow rate	1 ml/min
Column and guard pack	C_{18} Nova Pak (Waters Millipore)
Chart speed	0.25 cm/min
Retention times	
LTB_4	8.8 min
Prostaglandin B_2	4.4 min
5-HETE	11.5 min
15-HETE	8.4 min

Enzyme-Linked Immunosorbent Assay (ELISA) for Quantification of Substance P

The assay used is a competitive, nonequilibrium-type ELISA that offers a number of advantages over the more commonly used radioimmunoassays (RIA). Because no radioactive ligands are used, thus eliminating the problems associated with using and disposing of radioactive material, it lends itself to automation and is relatively inexpensive compared to RIAs. Most importantly the sensitivity and reproducibility are comparable to that of RIAs (15). In our laboratory, the lower limit of detection is 5 fmol/well. Intra- and interassay variance is ≤5 and ≤7%, respectively.

Preparation of Substance P–BSA Conjugate

Substance P is a 1348-Da peptide and when it is bound directly to the ELISA plate there is inadequate exposure of antigenic sites to the antibody. To overcome this problem, SP is conjugated to BSA according to the method of Folkesson *et al.* (16).

Solutions and Materials

- 0.1 *M* Phosphate buffer: [11.5 m*M* KH_2PO_4, 81 m*M* Na_2PO_4, pH 7.4]
- 0.3% (w/w) Glutaraldehyde (Sigma)
- 0.01 *M* phosphate buffer: [1.2 m*M* KH_2PO_4, 8.1 m*M* Na_2PO_4 containing 145 m*M* NaCl, pH 7.4. Referred to as 0.01 *M* PBS]
- BSA fraction V (Sigma)
- Synthetic SP

Procedure

A total of 1.8 mg of SP and 9.8 mg of BSA are dissolved in 720 μl of 0.1 *M* phosphate buffer and cooled on ice. Then 180 μl of ice-cold 0.3% glutaraldehyde is added dropwise and stirred for 30 min at 0°C followed by 2 hr at room temperature. This mixture is then dialyzed extensively against 0.01 *M* phosphate buffer, pH 7.4. The concentration of the SP–BSA conjugate is determined by the Folin–Lowry method using BSA as standard. The SP–BSA conjugate is diluted to 1 mg/ml and stored at −20°C in 500-μl aliquots until used. This stock solution can be freeze-thawed up to nine times without loss of antigenicity.

Substance P ELISA

Buffer Solutions

1. 0.01 *M* PBS is prepared weekly and stored at 4°C.
2. 0.1 *M* phosphate buffer containing 145 m*M* NaCl and 0.05% (v/v) Tween 20, pH 7.4 (referred to as 0.1 *M* PBS/Tw), is prepared weekly and stored at 4°C.

3. Washing buffer: 0.01 *M* PBS containing 0.05% Tween 20 is prepared monthly and stored at room temperature.
4. Blocking buffer: 0.01 *M* PBS containing 1% (v/v) horse serum and 0.05% (w/v) sodium azide is prepared daily and kept on ice.
5. Primary antibody diluent: 0.1 *M* PBS/Tw containing 1% horse serum and 0.05% sodium azide is prepared daily and kept on ice.
6. Conjugate diluent containing 0.1 *M* PBS/Tw and 1% horse serum, pH 7.4, is prepared daily and kept on ice.
7. *o*-Phenylenediamine hydrochloride (Sigma) stock solution: 12.79 mg/ml methanol is prepared just before use and stored at room temperature in the dark. This is referred to as OPD stock solution.
8. Citrate–phosphate buffer pH 5 containing 40 m*M* citric acid and 2.7 m*M* Na_2PO_4 is prepared weekly and stored at 4°C. This is referred to as Cit/Phos buffer.
9. Substrate buffer: 4.152 ml OPD stock solution and 35 ml of 30% hydrogen peroxide (v/v) are mixed to 100 ml with Cit/phos buffer and prepared immediately before use.

Preparation and Storage of Anti-SP Polyclonal Antisera, Standard SP, and Quality Controls

The anti-SP antibody used is a rabbit polyclonal antiserum (Rb anti-SP) directed against the C-terminal end and may be purchased from AUSPEP (Australia). Antibody reactivities in our assay, where reactivity to SP is expressed as 100%, were ≤0.01% for SP(1–6), SP(1–7), neurokinin A, neurokinin B, and eleidosin; 0.016% to kassinin and 0.032% to physalaemin. Cross-reactivity with other tachykinins has been discussed in Morris *et al.* (18). We detected no interbatch variation in the anti-SP antibody at the dilution used. This antiserum is diluted to 1/200 stock solution in 0.1 *M* PBS/Tw containing 0.1% sodium azide (w/v) and 0.75% BSA (w/v) and may be stored at 4°C for 1 month without loss of activity. A 1/15,200 dilution in primary antibody diluent is prepared daily and stored at 4°C until used.

Synthetic SP is stored as a 1 mg/ml solution in 0.01 *M* acetic acid in 20-μl aliquots in microtubes at −70°C under nitrogen. Under these conditions the stock solution is stable for at least 1.5 years. This stock solution is diluted daily for the standard curve to a starting concentration of 20 ng/ml in primary antibody diluent (two parts) containing methanol/0.1 *M* HCl (1 part). Methanol/0.1 *M* HCl is a 1 : 1 v/v solution. This starting concentration is equivalent to 11.2 n*M* SP.

Concentrations of SP at 0.362 and 0.181 n*M* in 0.1*M* PBS/Tw containing 0.75% BSA (w/v) are prepared and stored at −70°C in 500-μl aliquots in microtubes and are used as quality control samples for the assay. We detected no loss in concentration after storage for 2 years.

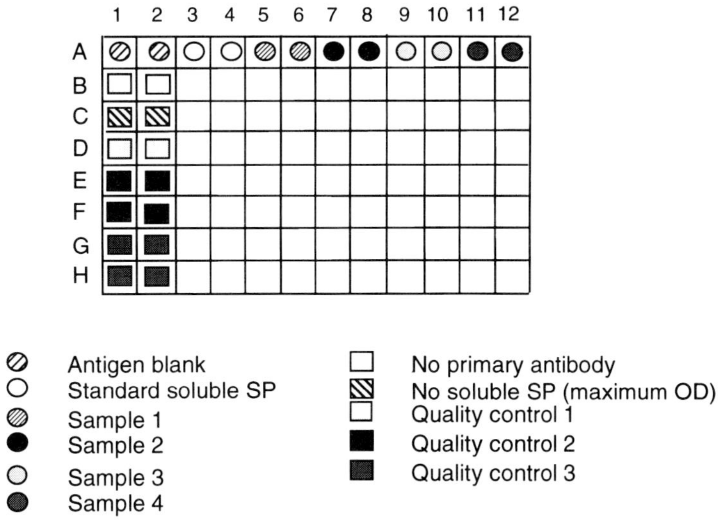

FIG. 6 Layout of the ELISA tray.

Preparation of Secondary Antibody and SP-BSA Sensitizing Solution

The secondary antibody is a swine anti-rabbit antiserum conjugated with horseradish peroxidase (Dakopatts, Denmark) (Sw anti-Rb HRP). A final dilution of 1/1500 is prepared in conjugate diluent daily and kept on ice.

The 1 mg/ml stock solution of BSA–SP is diluted to 0.5 μg/ml in 0.01 *M* PBS, in polypropylene containers, just before use. These containers have been pretreated with blocking buffer to prevent loss of conjugate by adherence to the tubes.

ELISA Procedure

All steps are performed at room temperature except where stated. The trays are kept covered to prevent evaporative losses. The layout for the plates is shown in Fig. 6. We perform the assay in duplicate.

1. Nunc Immuno Plate Maxisorb flat-bottom 96-well ELISA trays (Nunc, Denmark) are sensitized with 100 μl/well of 0.5 mg/ml SP–BSA conjugate for 4 hr. The negative control wells (A1, A2) are antigen-free and contain 100 μl of 0.01 *M* PBS.
2. Trays are washed three times with washing buffer by the flicking technique.

3. Nonspecific binding sites are blocked with 200 μl/well of blocking buffer for a minimum of 30 min.

4. Trays are washed as in step 2.

5. A total of 50 μl of the 20 ng/ml standard SP (wells A3, A4) or unknown samples (wells A5 $\rightarrow$ A12) are added and then serially titrated in doubling dilutions down the tray in primary antibody diluent. For example, 50 μl of standard SP is added to A_1, A_2 and then diluted with 50 μl diluent. Then, 50 μl is removed and added to B_3, B_4.

6. Quality controls (50 μl) are added to wells E1, E2 $\rightarrow$ H1, H2 without further dilution.

7. A total of 50 μl of a 1/15,200 dilution of Rb anti-SP is added to the wells giving a final dilution of 1/30,400. "Negative" primary antibody wells (B1, B2) contain 100 μl primary antibody diluent and act as a control for nonspecific binding of Sw anti-Rb HRP and subsequent steps. Wells C1 and C2 have primary antibody added but no soluble SP and yield the maximum OD. We aimed for a maximum OD of 1.0–1.5.

8. The trays are left overnight at 4°C in sealed containers.

9. Wash trays as in step 2.

10. A total of 100 μl of Sw anti-Rb HRP at 1/1500 dilution is added to all wells and left for 2 hr.

11. Wash trays as in step 2.

12. Substrate solution (100 μl) is added to all wells for 30 min and kept in the dark.

13. Reaction is inhibited by the addition of 100 μl of 2.5 *M* sulfuric acid to each well.

Optical density is read at 490 n*M*, blanked on air with reference, at 630 nm using an MR 7000 EIA-CALC Dynateck ELISA reader (Dynateck, Chantilly, VA). The sigmoid program used for curve fitting is based on the Rodbard four-parameter equation (16, 19). This is also described in the operating manual for the ELISA reader. The manual number is DMPL/RB/CP/8010/13/0391. This fitted curve routinely generates an *r* value of $\geq$0.99.

Comments

Some tray brands tend to give variable results. Nunc Maxisorb is reliable for consistency in results between and within trays. Storage of the BSA–SP conjugate is not stable at less than 1 mg/ml.

Polypropylene containers pretreated with blocking buffer are used to prevent loss of samples. Glass is to be avoided. Primary antibody activity is lost when stored at dilutions greater than 1/200. The OPD substrate powder is stored desiccated and in the dark to maintain maximal activity. Standard soluble SP is more stable when stored in 0.01 *M* acetic acid compared with the methanol/0.1 *M* HCl (1 : 1) (16) buffer for long periods of time. Polypropylene containers pretreated with primary antibody diluent buffer are used to minimize loss of activity of rabbit anti-SP at high dilutions.

Tissue Processing and Extraction

The tissue of interest is removed as quickly as possible and washed with ice-cold 0.01 *M* PBS. Then it is snap frozen in a methanol/dry ice bath and stored at −70°C until it is used. The samples are weighed out frozen and placed into 10 volumes of boiling 1 *M* acetic acid containing 10 m*M* 2-mercaptoethanol for 5 min, cooled on ice, and homogenized with three 10-sec bursts in a Polytron Kinematica Ag (Kinematica, Switzerland) at 10,000–11,000 rpm. The solution is then reboiled at 90°C for a further 5 min. The homogenate is left at 4°C overnight and the supernatants (containing SP) are collected in 3-ml aliquots by centrifugation at 10,000*g* (Beckman) for 15 min at 4°C. These supernatants are stored at −70°C.

For extraction of SP from biological fluids, e.g., bronchoalveolar lavage fluid, the fluid is collected into low-absorption polypropylene tubes containing the following protease inhibitors: phosphoramidon (25 μl of 1 mg/ml), chymostatin (2 μg/ml), leupeptin (4 μg/ml), and bacitracin (25 μg/ml). The fluid is spun at 2000 rpm for 15 min at 4°C to remove cells and the supernatant is recovered and stored on ice. One-tenth volume of 10 *M* acetic acid containing 100 m*M* 2-mercaptoethanol is added and the mixture is boiled for 10 min. The fluid is then cooled on ice and stored at −70°C until lyophilized as per tissue extraction.

Cartridge Preparation

Sep-Pak C_{18} reversed-phase cartridges (Waters Millipore) are prewet with 2 ml methanol and washed with 5 ml distilled water followed by 0.1% (v/v) trifluoroacetic (TFA) in distilled water. Flow rates should not exceed 5 ml/min.

Procedure

Tissue supernatants are applied to the cartridge to the equivalent of 300 mg wet weight and washed with 20 ml 0.1% TFA. Then, SP is eluted in 5 ml of methanol which is collected, cooled to −70°C, and lyophilized before ELISA. A further 10 ml of methanol is applied, collected, and stored at −70°C. If necessary this too is lyophilized and SP-quantified to ensure the column is not overloaded.

The appropraite extracts are reconstituted to 300 μl in primary antibody diluent containing methanol/0.1 *M* HCl in a 2 : 1 ratio and used in the ELISA. The methanol/0.1 *M* HCl is in a 1 : 1 ratio. The recovery rate of standard soluble SP from the cartridge is >85%.

Acknowledgments

The work described in this chapter was supported by the National Health and Medical Research Council of Australia, The Royal Adelaide Hospital Research Review Committee, and the Royal Adelaide Hospital Special Purposes Fund.

References

1. A. Wozniak, G. McLennan, W. H. Betts, G. Murphy, and R. Scicchitano, *Immunology* **68,** 359 (1989).
2. A. Wozniak, W. H. Betts, G. McLennan, and R. Scicchitano, *Immunology* **78,** 629 (1993).
3. I. Iwamoto, H. Yamazaki, N. Nakagawa, A. Kimura, and S. Yoshida, *Neuropeptides* **16,** 103 (1990).
4. C. J. Wiedermann, F. J. Wiedermann, A. Apperl, G. Kieselbach, G. Konwalinka, and H. Braunsteiner, *Naunyn-Schmiedeberg's Arch. Pharmacol.* **340,** 185 (1989).
5. M. R. Ruff, S. M. Wahl and C. B. Pert, *Peptides* **6,** 107 (1985).
6. A. Perianin, R. Snyderman, and B. Malfroy, *Biochem. Biophys. Res. Commun.* **161,** 520 (1989).
7. M. C. Serra, F. Bazzoni, V. Della Bianca, M. Greslowiak, and F. Rossi, *J. Immunol.* **141,** 2118 (1988).
8. I. Hafstrom, H. Gyllenhammar, J. Palmblad, and B. Ringertz, *J. Rheumatol.* **16,** 1033 (1989).
9. S. Brunelleschi, S. Tarli, A. Giotti, and R. Fantozzi, *Life Sci.* **48,** 1 (1991).
10. A. Wozniak and R. Scicchitano, unpublished observations, 1989.
11. S. R. McColl, W. H. Betts, G. A. Murphy, and L. G. Cleland, *J. Chromatogr.* **378,** 3047 (1986).
12. B. F. Van Gelder and E. C. Slater, *Biochim. Biophys. Acta* **58,** 593 (1962).
13. M. A. Vadas, N. A. Nicola, and D. Metcalf, *J. Immunol.* **130,** 795 (1983).
14. R. Y. Tsien, T. Pozzan, and T. J. Rink, *J. Cell Biol.* **94,** 325 (1982).
15. T. J. Rink and T. Pozzan, *Cell Calcium* **6,** 133 (1988).
16. R. Folkesson, A. Neil, and L. Terenius *J. Neurosci. Methods* **14,** 169 (1985).
17. R. Murphy, J. B. Furness, A. M. Beardsley, and M. Costa, *J. Regul. Pept.* **4,** 203 (1982).
18. J. L. Morris, L. Gibbins, G. Campbell, R. Murphy, J. B. Furness, and M. Costa, *Cell Tissue Res.* **243,** 171 (1986).
19. P. J. Munson and D. Rodbard, *Anal. Biochem.* **107,** 220 (1980).

[4] Molecular Techniques for Detection of Gene Expression in Neuroimmunology

Elliot P. Cowan and Suhayl S. Dhib-Jalbut

Introduction

Neuroimmunology is built around the ability of the immune system to recognize cells of the nervous system, on the one hand, and the remarkable observation that certain features of each system are shared. For example, a number of cytokines that play central roles in immune activation also have defined roles in the nervous system. Analysis of gene expression in the cells that make up the nervous system, as well as in the cellular infiltrates in pathologic conditions, is crucial to the understanding of cellular interactions and immune recognition. Yet, the nervous system presents us with some unique issues that have made it difficult to perform that analysis, especially with regard to human tissue. First, samples are difficult to obtain and biopsy is associated with some risk to the patient. Second, samples contain multiple cell types which must be subjected to multiple purification procedures, resulting in considerable cell loss. Third, these cells do not grow, or divide poorly, *in vitro*. These considerations point to the necessity to analyze limited numbers of cells or small amounts of tissue. A number of techniques are now available that allow the analysis of relatively small numbers of cells. This chapter describes some of these methods currently in use in our laboratories, with particular emphasis on detection of gene expression in cells derived from the human central nervous system (CNS). Detailed methods are presented for the isolation of total cellular RNA from relatively small numbers of cells and its analysis through the use of mini-Northern blots and the reverse-transcribed polymerase chain reaction (RT-PCR). The overall scheme is shown in Fig. 1, along with time considerations for each step. We also discuss additional methods available for the analysis of gene expression in individual cells.

Isolation of Total Cellular RNA

We routinely isolate total cellular RNA by a scaled-down version of the acidified guanidinium–phenol–chloroform method (1, 2). In this method, cells are solubilized in a solution of guanidine isothiocyanate that contains

Methods in Neurosciences, Volume 24

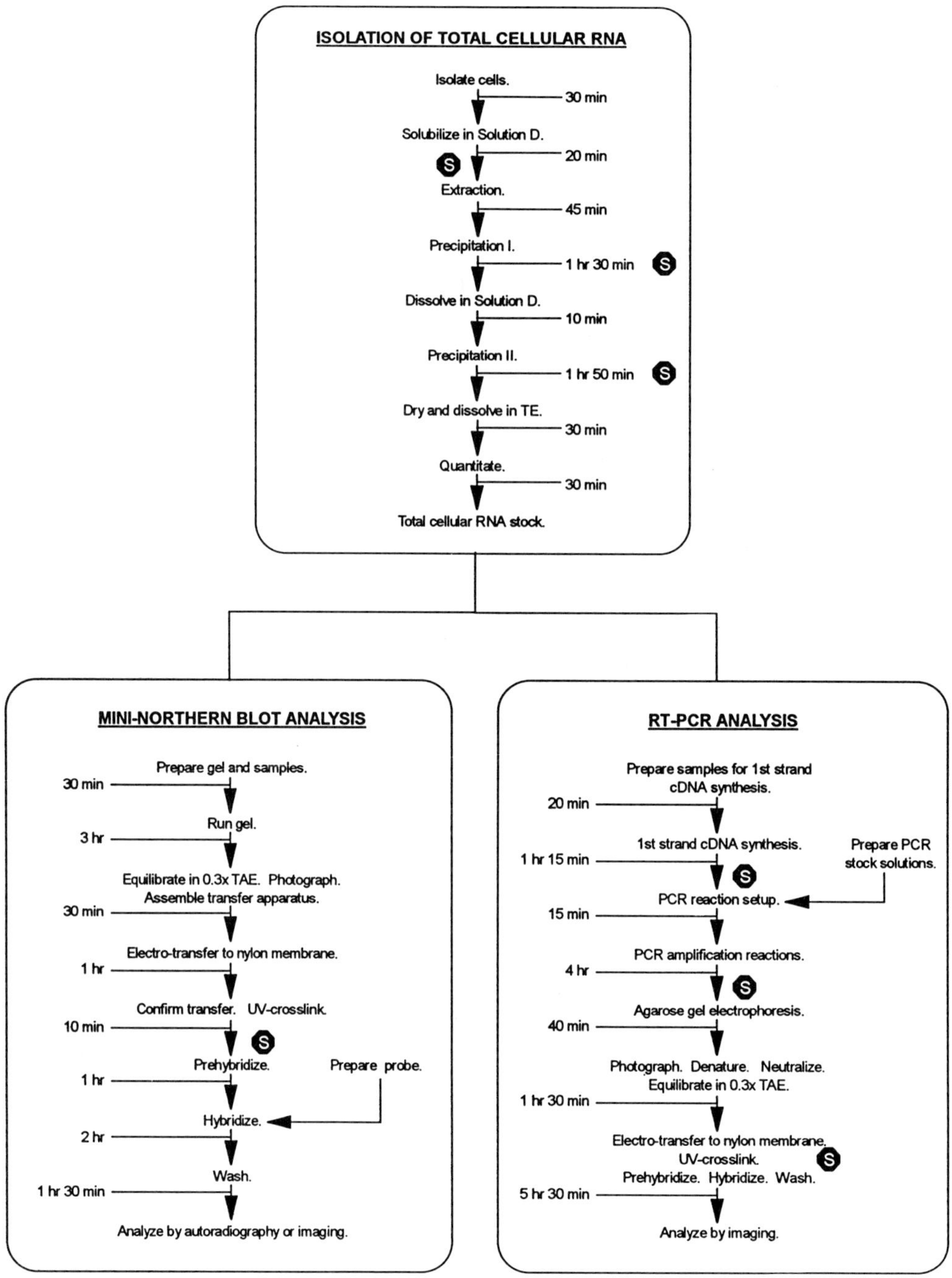
ISOLATION OF TOTAL CELLULAR RNA
Isolate cells.
30 min
Solubilize in Solution D.
20 min
S
Extraction.
45 min
Precipitation I.
1 hr 30 min
S
Dissolve in Solution D.
10 min
Precipitation II.
1 hr 50 min
S
Dry and dissolve in TE.
30 min
Quantitate.
30 min
Total cellular RNA stock.
MINI-NORTHERN BLOT ANALYSIS
Prepare gel and samples.
30 min
Run gel.
3 hr
Equilibrate in 0.3x TAE. Photograph.
Assemble transfer apparatus.
30 min
Electro-transfer to nylon membrane.
1 hr
Confirm transfer. UV-crosslink.
10 min
S
Prehybridize.
Prepare probe.
1 hr
Hybridize.
2 hr
Wash.
1 hr 30 min
Analyze by autoradiography or imaging.
RT-PCR ANALYSIS
Prepare samples for 1st strand
cDNA synthesis.
20 min
1st strand cDNA synthesis.
Prepare PCR
stock solutions.
1 hr 15 min
S
PCR reaction setup.
15 min
PCR amplification reactions.
4 hr
S
Agarose gel electrophoresis.
40 min
Photograph. Denature. Neutralize.
Equilibrate in 0.3x TAE.
1 hr 30 min
Electro-transfer to nylon membrane.
UV-crosslink.
S
Prehybridize. Hybridize. Wash.
5 hr 30 min
Analyze by imaging.

a detergent (*N*-lauroylsarcosine) and 2-mercaptoethanol. This chemical environment serves to solubilize the cells efficiently and to inactivate ribonuclease (RNase). An organic extraction is then performed at pH 4.0, during which the DNA partitions into the organic phase while the RNA remains in the aqueous phase. The RNA is then collected by two precipitations with 2-propanol, washed, dried, dissolved, and quantitated by spectrophotometry.

General Comments

In contrast to DNA, which is relatively stable, RNA is particularly susceptible to degradation. Therefore, several precautions must be followed to avoid the introduction of RNases. Detailed instructions are provided in standard molecular biology manuals (e.g., Refs. 2 and 3), but some basic points are worth mentioning here. Gloves must be worn at all times. It is wise to set aside micropipettors that are dedicated for RNA use and to use pipette tips with hydrophobic barriers to avoid cross-contamination (especially important for PCR work, see below). Similarly, stock reagents (both solid and liquid) should be labeled for RNA use only. When preparing reagents, shake or pour crystals and powders, rather than using a spatula. Use sterile disposable labware (microcentrifuge and standard tubes, pipettes, etc.) when possible, which should not require further treatment. All water should be doubly distilled and deionized and treated with diethyl pyrocarbonate (DEPC) (an inhibitor of RNase) according to standard protocols (2, 3). Finally, RNA should not be prepared in a room in which RNase is being or has been used. The inconvenience presented by these relatively simple procedures is minor compared to the time necessary to repeat an isolation.

Reagents

Guanidinium stock solution (4 *M* guanidinium thiocyanate, 25 m*M* sodium citrate, pH 7.0, 0.5% *N*-lauroylsarcosine): Dissolve 250 g guanidinium thiocyanate (Fluka, Ronkonkoma, NY, #50990) in 293 ml H_2O (can be warmed to 37°C to aid in dissolving), then add 17.6 ml of 0.75 *M* sodium citrate, pH 7.0, and 26.4 ml of 10% *N*-lauroylsarcosine, sodium salt (Sarkosyl) (Sigma, St. Louis, MO, #L-5125) (3 g *N*-

FIG. 1 Overview of protocols for detection of gene expression. Time estimates are given for each step in a protocol. Each protocol may be interrupted for a day or more, if necessary, at steps marked with a stop sign.

lauroylsarcosine and H_2O to 30 ml, dissolve at 65°C, and use 26.4 ml). Store in the dark at room temperature for up to 3 months.

Solution D (guanidinium stock solution with 0.1 *M* 2-mercaptoethanol): In a fume hood, add 0.36 ml 2-mercaptoethanol to 50 ml guanidinium stock solution. This solution can be stored for about 2 months in the dark at room temperature (a foil-covered 50-ml polypropylene centrifuge tube works well).

H_2O-saturated phenol: Place a 100-g bottle of redistilled crystalline phenol (molecular biology grade, e.g., Life Technologies, Gaithersburg, MD, #15509-011) in a water bath at 65°C until the phenol has liquefied. Swirl the bottle occasionally to assist in the melting. In a fume hood, add 100 ml H_2O and shake to mix the phases. Let stand at room temperature until the phases separate (usually overnight). The resulting H_2O-saturated phenol solution (lower phase) should be colorless. Any pink color indicates oxidation products which could damage the nucleic acid and the phenol should not be used. Store at 4°C.

2 *M* sodium acetate, pH 4.0: Dissolve 16.4 g anhydrous sodium acetate in 40 ml H_2O and 35 ml glacial acetate acid. Adjust to pH 4.0 with glacial acetic acid and add H_2O to 100 ml. Store at room temperature.

TE (10 m*M* Tris, pH 8.0, 1 m*M* EDTA): Add 1 ml of 1 *M* Tris, pH 8.0, and 0.2 ml of 0.5 *M* EDTA, pH 8.0, to 98.8 ml H_2O. Sterile filter through 0.22 μm filter. Store at room temperature.

Chloroform : isoamyl alcohol (50 : 1): Add 10 ml isoamyl alcohol to a 500-ml bottle of chloroform in a fume hood. Store at room temperature.

Procedure

Cell Collection

Harvest cells and count. When dealing with adherent cells, remove from growth surface with trypsin or other method of choice. Pellet cells by centrifugation. Washing with phosphate-buffered saline may be done, but is not necessary. Remove as much of the supernatant as possible by aspiration using a sterile pipette and scrape tube on a test tube rack grid to break up the cell pellet.

Solubilization

Add Solution D to the cells, using 0.5 ml for up to 5×10^6 cells and proportionately larger volumes for more cells. Mix by vortexing gently for a few seconds. Let stand at room temperature for 15–20 min. Transfer the solubilized cells in Solution D to 1.5-ml microcentrifuge tubes, adding no more than 0.6

ml/tube. *Note: the solution may be quite viscous due to cellular DNA. Transfer carefully.* The tubes can be stored at −70°C at this point if it is not convenient to proceed to the next step.

Extraction

In a fume hood, add the following to each tube, gently mixing by inverting a few times after each addition:

0.1 volume 2 *M* sodium acetate, pH 4.0
1 volume water-saturated phenol
0.2 volume chloroform : isoamyl alcohol (50 : 1) (this solution has a low surface tension—pipette carefully)

Note: volumes of these solutions are based on the original Solution D lysate volume. Shake vigorously for 10 sec, then let stand for 15 min on ice. Spin 10 min at top speed in a microcentrifuge (~14,000*g*) at 4°C. Collect aqueous phase (top), being careful not to disturb the interface, and transfer to a clean 1.5-ml microcentrifuge tube. It is better to leave some of the aqueous phase behind rather than risk transferring part of the interface. *Note: if two phases are not seen, it is most likely due to insufficient chloroform. Add another 50–100 μl chloroform : isoamyl alcohol, shake, cool, and spin, as above.*

Precipitation

Add 1 volume 2-propanol and mix by inverting several times. Let stand 1 hr to overnight at −20°C. Spin 30 min in a microcentrifuge at top speed at 4°C. Decant supernatant and blot excess on a paper towel. Dissolve each pellet in 200 μl Solution D (~10 min at room temperature) and mix gently with a micropipette. Pool solutions to give no more than 700 μl/tube. Add 1 volume 2-propanol and reprecipitate the RNA as above. After decanting the supernatant, add 1 ml 75% ethanol to each tube and vortex briefly to dislodge the pellets from the sides of the tubes. Let stand for 15 min at room temperature. Spin 2 min in the 4°C microcentrifuge at top speed (~14,000 *g*), decant the supernatant, and blot the excess. Dry the pellets in a vacuum centrifuge [such as a Speed-Vac (Savant, Farmingdale, NY)] for ~10 min. Dissolve in 5 μl TE at room temperature for each 1×10^6 cells of starting material. After the TE has been added, let the tubes sit for ~15–20 min at room temperature, then carefully mix with a micropipettor.

Quantitation

Transfer 1 μl of the RNA solution to 99 μl TE. The RNA aliquot is best removed using an ultramicropipettor, such as a Rainin Pipetman P-2 (Woburn, MA) and the accompanying ultramicrotips. Read OD_{260} and OD_{280} in a microcuvette capable of reading 100-μl sample volumes. The $OD_{260}:OD_{280}$ ratio should be >1.8, indicating the absence of protein and phenol (which absorb significantly at OD_{280}). Since the concentration of 1 OD_{260} unit of RNA is 40 μg/ml, the RNA concentration is calculated as follows:

$$OD_{260} \times 40 \times \text{dilution (i.e., 100)} = \mu\text{g RNA/ml}$$

Storage
Store RNA at −70°C.

Expected Results

The total cellular RNA that we obtain by this procedure usually gives an $OD_{260}:OD_{280}$ ratio of >2.0. The amount of RNA recovered varies with cell type. For example, 1×10^6 glioblastoma multiforme cell lines, human cerebral microvessel endothelial cells, or cultured primary normal adult human glial cells (astrocytes and microglia) yield 5–10 μg RNA. On the other hand, human T cells may yield fivefold less RNA.

Variations

When dealing with adherent cells, it sometimes may not be desirable to remove the cells prior to solubilization. In this case, aspirate the medium completely and add Solution D directly to the culture flask or dish. Use approximately 1 ml Solution D/25 cm^2 of culture area, rock back and forth to cover the cells, and let the culture vessel lie flat for 15 min. Tilt up for 10–15 min so that the Solution D then collects in a pool, transfer to microcentrifuge tubes, and proceed as above.

We have found that a single 2-propanol precipitation (precipitation step, above) is sufficient if the RNA is to be used for Northern blotting, but both precipitations are necessary if the RNA is to be used in RT-PCR (see below).

Mini-Northern Blot Analysis of Total Cellular RNA

Northern blotting is a procedure whereby RNA species are electrophoretically separated on a denaturing agarose gel and transferred to a membrane (typically made of nitrocellulose or nylon). The transcripts of interest are then detected by hybridization with labeled probes. We use the following procedure in our laboratories, which is a streamlined and down-sized version of traditional Northern blotting methods.

Materials

Gel Electrophoresis

MOPS buffer [2 *M* 3-(*N*-morpholino)propanesulfonic acid (MOPS), pH 7.0, 0.5 *M* sodium acetate, 10 m*M* EDTA]: Dissolve 209 g MOPS (free acid, Sigma, #M 8899) in 200 ml H_2O + 83 ml 3 *M* sodium acetate + 10 ml 0.5 *M* EDTA. Adjust pH to approximately 7.0 and bring final volume to 500 ml with H_2O. Sterile filter and store in the dark at 4°C. *Alternative:* This buffer is also available commercially, for example, Sigma, #M 5755. Note that this product is fivefold less concentrated than the buffer indicated above. Therefore, make certain to check the composition of these solutions and adjust the volumes used accordingly in the recipes listed below.

Agarose: SeaKem GTG (FMC Bioproducts, Rockland, ME).

Formaldehyde: 37% solution, reagent grade. *Always use in a chemical hood.*

Formamide: Reagent grade, available from a number of manufacturers. Store at 4°C.

Ethidium bromide; 5 mg/ml solution in H_2O. *Note: ethidium bromide is a powerful mutagen. Handle with extreme care.*

Dye solution [50% (v/v) glycerol, 1 m*M* EDTA, 0.1% (w/v) bromphenol blue, 0.1% (w/v) xylene cyanol FF]: Mix 500 μl 50% (v/v) glycerol, 5 μl 0.5 *M* EDTA, pH 8.0, 20 μl 2% (w/v) bromphenol blue, and 20 μl 2% (w/v) xylene cyanol FF. Store at room temperature.

Horizontal agarose gel electrophoresis apparatus: IBI Model QSH (available from VWR Scientific) to accommodate 5 × 7.5-cm gels, with 10-well combs (each well 2.5 mm wide × 1.5 mm thick). Other apparatus employing gels of approximately the same size with wells of similar dimensions may be used.

Transfer to Nylon Membranes

0.3× TAE transfer solution: 12 ml 50× TAE stock solution (2 *M* Tris–acetate, 50 m*M* EDTA) + 2 liter H_2O.

Nylon membrane: Nytran (Schleicher and Schuell, Keene, NH) or equivalent.

Whatman (Clifton, NJ) 3MM filter paper.

Transfer cell: Hoeffer Model TE22 minitank transfer unit (Hoeffer Scientific, San Francisco, CA)

Power supply: Capable of delivering up to 400 mA, such as the Bio-Rad Model 250/2.5 (Bio-Rad Laboratories, Richmond, CA).

Hybridization

Hybridization solution: Quik-Hyb (Stratagene, La Jolla, CA)
Hybridization oven: Robbins Scientific (Sunnyvale, CA)
Probe labeling:
^{T7}QuickPrime random hexamer oligolabeling kit (Pharmacia, Piscataway, NJ)
[α-^{32}P]dCTP (3000 Ci/mmol, 10 mCi/ml)
Probe purification: Prepacked Sepharose G-50 columns (NAP-5, Pharmacia)
Blot washing solutions:
2× SSC: prepared from 20× SSC stock (3 *M* NaCl, 0.3 *M* sodium citrate, pH 7.0).
2× SSC, 1% SDS: prepared from 20× SSC and 20% (w/v) SDS stock solutions.
0.1×SSC

Procedure

Note: All procedures involving formaldehyde should be performed in a fume hood.

1. Prepare gel for electrophoresis. Clean a 5 × 7.5-cm glass slide and a 10-well gel comb with a commercial glass cleaner (e.g., Windex, Glass Plus). Mix together 0.2 g agarose, 0.67 ml MOPS buffer, and 16 ml H_2O in a 50-ml polypropylene centrifuge tube [e.g., Falcon 2070 (Becton–Dickinson Labware, Lincoln Park, NJ)]. Microwave on high setting with loosened cap until solution just begins to boil. Stop and invert to mix. Continue carefully heating and mixing solution until the agarose is dissolved. Cool to ~60°C (but do not insert a thermometer into the tube—simply estimate temperature by feel or equilibrate for a few minutes in a 60°C H_2O bath). In the fume hood, add 1 μl 5 mg/ml ethidium bromide and 3.4 ml formaldehyde. Mix by inverting. With a 25-ml pipette, add 15 ml of the gel solution to the slide with a 10-well comb in the gel casting tray. Let set for 20–30 min.

2. Prepare sample. Prepare a denaturing gel loading solution as follows: 1 μl MOPS buffer, 4 μl formaldehyde, 10 μl formamide, and 2.5 μl dye solution. In a 0.5-ml microcentrifuge tube, mix together 5 μg of total cellular RNA and TE to give a total volume of no more than 5 μl; mix with 5 μl of

the gel loading solution. Heat to 68°C for 5 min to denature the RNA, cool on ice for a few minutes, and spin briefly in a microcentrifuge to collect condensation.

3. Run gel. Prepare running buffer in the fume hood by mixing together 500 ml H_2O, 20 ml MOPS buffer, and 15 ml formaldehyde. Carefully remove the comb from the gel to avoid tearing the bottom of the wells. Place the gel on its platform and pour in the running buffer. Load samples using a micropipettor, placing a dark piece of paper or plastic under the gel rig to facilitate visualizing the wells. Run at 35–40 V for ~3 hr in the fume hood (bromphenol blue should be approximately two-thirds down the gel).

4. Prepare sample for electroblotting. Rinse gel in H_2O to remove excess formaldehyde. *Dispose of wash and running buffer as chemical waste*. Soak gel in 0.3× TAE for 15–20 min on orbital shaker to equilibrate for electroblotting and to remove excess ethidium bromide from the gel. Photograph the gel on an ultraviolet light box (300 nm) taking appropriate precautions (2, 3). Two bands should be seen, the slower moving species at about twice the intensity as the faster moving species [representing the 28S and 18S components of ribosomal RNA (rRNA), respectively]. If this pattern is not observed, the RNA may be degraded and a new RNA preparation should be considered before proceeding.

5. Electroblot. During the running of the gel, precool 0.3× TAE in the minitransfer cell to 4°C. This is best done using a refrigerated circulating bath. Cut the nylon membrane and two pieces of Whatman 3MM paper to the same size as the gel. Mark the top side of the membrane for later orientation and soak in 0.3× TAE for ~10 min. Assemble the transfer sandwich by submersing the sandwich frame in a tray with 0.3× TAE and adding (in this order): a pad (supplied with the unit), a piece of Whatman paper, the prepared gel (face down), nylon membrane (side with markings against the gel), Whatman paper, and a pad. At each step, it is important to ensure that no bubbles are trapped which could interfere with the passage of current at that point. This can be done by gently smoothing the surface of each layer with a gloved finger. Place the assembled sandwich in the transfer unit with the nylon membrane toward the negative electrode (red). Run for 1 hr at 100 V (current will be 250–400 mA) at 4°C. Disassemble the transfer sandwich and examine nylon membrane and gel with hand-held UV light to ensure that complete transfer took place. Mark the positions of the 28S and 18S rRNA bands and the position of the wells on the membrane with a syringe needle. Rinse the membrane briefly in the transfer buffer to remove any gel pieces. Permanently fix the RNA onto the membrane by UV cross-linking (such as in a Stratalinker, Stratagene). The membrane

can be stored at 4°C in a 50-ml centrifuge tube (Falcon 2070) with some 2× SSC.

6. Prepare probes for detection of specific transcripts. Transcripts of interest are detected on the Northern blots using ^{32}P-labeled DNA probes, using all precautions associated with hard β-particle emitting isotopes (see Refs. 2 and 3). This is accomplished by incorporating [α-^{32}P]dCTP using the random hexamer primed synthesis method which has been streamlined into kit form, the Pharmacia ^{T7}QuickPrime kit in use in our laboratories. DNA fragments in purified form or embedded in low melting point agarose can be efficiently labeled using this technique, giving probes with specific activities of $>1 \times 10^9$ counts per minute (cpm)/μg following a 10-min labeling reaction. The protocol used for labeling the probes is given in detail in the literature accompanying the kit. Unincorporated [α-^{32}P]dCTP is removed by gel-filtration chromatography using a prepacked Sephadex G-50 column from Pharmacia (NAP-5) according to the manufacturer's instructions, after equilibration of the column in TE. If not used the same day, the resulting purified reaction product should be stored at -20°C in a Plexiglas safety box and used within 3 days.

7. Hybridize. All hybridization procedures are done in a hybridization oven in which tubes containing the blots and the hybridization solution are rotated continuously at a constant temperature. The advantages of such a system are that a minimal amount of hybridization solution and probe is used (thereby decreasing waste), tubes obviate the need to work with more cumbersome heat-sealable bags that are the traditional mainstays of hybridization in molecular biology, and hybridization and washes can be done in the same tube, minimizing manipulation of hazardous material. Our laboratory has been using an oven from Robbins Scientific, although others on the market are presumably equivalent. One feature of the Robbins oven is that in addition to the rotating motion, the solution is moved back and forth over the membrane to ensure even hybridization, especially critical for quantitative Northern blotting.

Prior to hybridization, the blots are prehybridized to block nonspecific binding of the probe to the membrane. Pour off excess 2× SSC from the 50-ml tube used to store the blot and add 2 ml Quik-Hyb solution (mix the stock bottle *thoroughly* by shaking before taking an aliquot). Prehybridize for ~1 hr at 68°C. During this time, it is convenient to label and prepare the probe. The probe is prepared for hybridization by mixing 2×10^6 cpm with 40 μl of 10 mg/ml sheared salmon sperm or herring testis DNA (as nonspecific carrier DNA) in a 0.5-ml microcentrifuge tube, heating for 7 min at 70°C, cooling for 10 min on ice, and briefly spinning to collect condensation. This solution is then added to the tube containing the blot and mixed gently by swirling, and the hybridization proceeds for 2 hr at 68°C in the hybridization oven.

8. Wash the blots. The conditions under which the blots are washed depends on several factors, including the degree of homology between the probe and its target sequence, the length of the probe, the G-C content, etc. Discussions of factors to consider in the establishment of hybridization and washing conditions have been described elsewhere (2–4). We present here a set of conditions that work consistently well for us using a wide variety of probes whose sequence is nearly 100% identical to the target sequence. This will usually be the case when detecting many of the molecules of interest to neuroimmunologists. Potential problems arise when dealing with polymorphic genes, such as those of the major histocompatibility complex. In this case, it is better to use probes for a relatively conserved part of the gene.

The hybridization solution is carefully poured off (*watch drips*) and ~10 ml 2× SSC is added. After the cap is replaced, the tube is rocked back and forth gently by hand and the solution is poured off. This procedure of washing with 2× SSC is repeated two more times for a total of three room temperature washes to remove the majority of the free probe. Then, 10 ml of 2× SSC, 1% SDS (prewarmed to 60°C) is added and the tubes are washed at 60°C in the hybridization oven for 30 min, after which this first wash is discarded and a second 60°C wash is performed. At this point, the blot may be analyzed or an additional "high-stringency" wash may be performed to reduce background or cross-hybridizing sequence signals. This wash is done using 10 ml 0.1× SCC for 30 min at a temperature that must be determined empirically; although for high-homology probes, 60°C seems to work well. After all of the washes are completed, the blots are rinsed briefly at room temperature in 2× SSC and placed in a heat-sealable bag with a small amount of 2× SSC (to prevent the membrane from drying and allow stripping of the probe for other hybridizations—see below) for analysis by autoradiography using intensifying screens at −70°C or by an imaging system that permits quantitation of the radioactive signal.

9. Strip the blots. The blots can be stripped and rehybridized with other probes several times (we have done up to six rehybridizations, and more may be possible). This is especially useful when the detection of multiple transcripts is necessary and to allow for normalization to a transcript that should be present at a constant level (such as actin or transferrin receptor). Stripping is performed by placing the membrane in a new 50-ml centrifuge tube and adding 10 ml 1× SSC, 50% formamide. The tube is then incubated in the hybridization oven for 1 hr at 68°C. If desired, a second round of stripping can be done. The membrane is rinsed briefly in 2× SSC and analyzed for the presence of residual activity by autoradiography or imaging. The blot

is then ready for a new round of hybridization with a different probe. We normally prehybridize before adding the new probe.

Expected Results

Signals are normally visible by autoradiography after 1–7 days of exposure. The most commonly encountered problem is that of high background. In this case, the hybridization and/or washing temperatures can be increased. It is also useful to explore the possibility of using other probes for the transcript of interest, either a probe for a different region of the transcript or a shorter probe that would eliminate troublesome cross-hybridizing sequences. If, on the other hand, no signal is seen, consider lowering the wash temperature.

Variations

Other types of probes can be used to screen for transcripts of interest, as well. RNA probes offer the advantage of a stronger signal, due to the better stability of RNA : RNA hybrids vs. DNA : RNA hybrids. Oligonucleotide probes offer the advantage of high specificity, but lack sensitivity since these probes are end-labeled and therefore contain only a single radioactive tag. In addition, there is a trend toward nonisotopic detection methods, which are available from a number of manufacturers. For details on all of these procedures, see Refs. 2 and 3.

Use of Polymerase Chain Reaction to Quantitate Specific Transcripts in the Central Nervous System

If a gene is expressed at low levels in a relatively small number of cells, it is unlikely to be detected by Northern blotting. A critical technological advance in the detection of gene expression is RT-PCR, which has the ability to detect as few as five copies of a transcript in a single cell. Many reviews have been published on this technique, in which RNA is reverse-transcribed to DNA in a single step, and this DNA serves as a template for subsequent PCR reactions using specific primers (4–6). We describe here the use of RT-PCR for the semiquantitative detection of cytokine transcripts in the adult human CNS.

Materials

cDNA Synthesis

Total cellular RNA
First-strand cDNA synthesis kit (Pharmacia, #27-9261-01)
H_2O
DNA thermal cycler (Perkin-Elmer, Norwalk, CT)

PCR Amplification

Reagents: GeneAmp kit (10× PCR buffer, 10 m*M* dNTP solutions, *Taq* DNA polymerase) (Perkin-Elmer)
Amplification primers (20 μM solutions): The primers used in these experiments were β-actin, GTGGGGCGCCCCAGGCACCA and CTCCTTAATGTCACGCACGATTTC (530 bp product); IL-1β, ATGGCAGAAGTACCTAAGCTCGC and ACACAAATTGCATGGTGAAGTCAGTT (available from Clontech, Palo Alto, CA) (802 bp product); FcR-γ-II, AGAGAATTCGCTCCCCCAAAGGCTGTGCT and AGAAAGCTTACAGCCACAATGATCCCCAT (575 bp product); and GFAP, CAGGAGGAGCGGCACGTGCGG and ACATCCTTGTGCTCCTGCTTGGAC (345 bp product)
Mineral oil
Thermal cycler reaction tubes (Perkin-Elmer GeneAmp tubes, or equivalent)

Analysis

Agarose (SeaKem GTG)
Loading dye (0.1% bromphenol blue and 30% glycerol in H_2O)
0.5× TBE [prepared from 10× TBE stock (0.9 *M* Tris–borate, 20 m*M* EDTA)] (3)
Horizontal electrophoresis apparatus
5 mg/ml ethidium bromide
Materials for electroblotting and hybridization as indicated above for Northern blotting.

Procedure

Reverse Transcription

A number of first-strand cDNA synthesis kits are commercially available; the kit from Pharmacia is used in our laboratories. One microgram of total cellular RNA solution is placed in a 0.5-ml microcentrifuge tube and DEPC-treated water is added to bring the total volume to 8 μl. In the DNA thermal cycler, the RNA is denatured at 65°C for 9 min, then cooled to 4°C. Alternatively, a heating block followed by ice may be used. The following reagents are premixed on ice to generate a stock solution [multiply these volumes by the number of tubes plus 0.5 or 1 (to allow for pipetting error)], 7 μl of which is added to the RNA solution within 5 min after preparation: 5 μl of the bulk first-strand cDNA reaction mix (containing reverse transcriptase, RNase inhibitor, BSA, dATP, dCTP, dGTP, and dTTP, and buffer); 1 μl of 0.2 mg/ml random hexadeoxynucleotides [pd(N)6 primer] in H_2O; and 1 μl of 100 m*M* DTT, all of which are supplied with the kit. The tube is *gently* vortexed for 1 to 2 sec, spun at 14,000*g* for a few seconds to remove condensation, incubated at 37°C for 1 hr, and cooled to 2°C. The tube is then spun again at 14,000*g* for a few seconds to remove condensation and stored at −20°C until PCR is performed.

PCR Amplification

The exquisite sensitivity of PCR amplification dictates that certain precautions be taken to ensure that signals are not detected as a result of contamination with target sequences. Stock reagent solutions must be strictly segregated from nucleic acids, especially amplified DNA. Gloves should be worn at all times and should be changed after handling tubes with nucleic acids. As with RNA preparation, a set of micropipettes should be designated for PCR use and tips with barriers should be used as a hedge against cross-contamination. In addition, one should physically separate work areas into those used for template preparation, stock solution preparation, and amplification and analysis.

The many parameters to be considered for PCR have been discussed extensively (4–6). A successful general set of conditions that works well for us is as follows. PCR amplification is performed in 1× PCR buffer [10 m*M* Tris–HCl, pH 8.3, 1.5 m*M* $MgCl_2$, 0.001% (w/v) gelatin], 200 μ*M* for each dNTP, 10 pmol of each specific primer (one primer pair per tube), and 1.25 units of *Taq* DNA polymerase. The mixture is overlayed with mineral oil and then amplified in the DNA thermal cycler. The following is a step-by-step description of the protocol used to detect cytokine transcripts in human cells:

1. Prepare a stock solution on ice with reagents in the following proportion:

   5 μl 10× PCR buffer
   8 μl dNTP mix (1.25 m*M* each)
   27 μl H_2O

Multiply these volumes by the number of tubes needed plus 1 to allow for pipetting error.

2. Prepare amplification mixtures by mixing the following components in 0.5-ml Perkin-Elmer thermal cycler tubes as follows:

2.5 μl cDNA solution
0.5 μl 20 μ*M* 5′ primer (10 pmol)
0.5 μl 20 μ*M* 3′ primer (10 pmol)
6.5 μl H_2O
40 μl stock solution
0.25 μl *Taq* polymerase at 5 U/μl (1.25 U)

to give a total volume of 50 μl.

3. Add two drops (~35 μl) of light mineral oil to each tube using a 200-μl micropipettor.

4. Add one or two drops of light mineral oil to the well of the heat block of the thermal cycler, load the sample tubes, and wipe excess mineral oil from the heat block.

5. Amplify the DNA sequences of interest in the thermal cycler according to the following protocol:

a. 1 cycle of 94°C for 2 min as an initial denaturation step.
b. 30 cycles of:

 Denaturation at 94°C for 1 min.
 Annealing at 60°C for 2 min.
 Extension at 72°C for 3 min.

c. 1 cycle of 72°C for 7 min to extend all products to completion.
d. Hold at 4°C, if desired, until samples are retrieved.

Agarose Gel Electrophoresis

The solution containing the PCR product (9 μl) is mixed with 1 μl of loading dye and loaded onto a 5 × 7.5-cm 2% agarose gel containing 0.5 μg ethidium bromide/ml in 0.5× TBE buffer. Markers, such as standard restriction endonuclease-digested DNA or 100-bp ladders that are available form a number of suppliers, are run in parallel to facilitate sizing of the amplification products. The samples are run in 0.5× TBE buffer for 30 min at 100 V. The resulting bands are then examined under UV light and photographed.

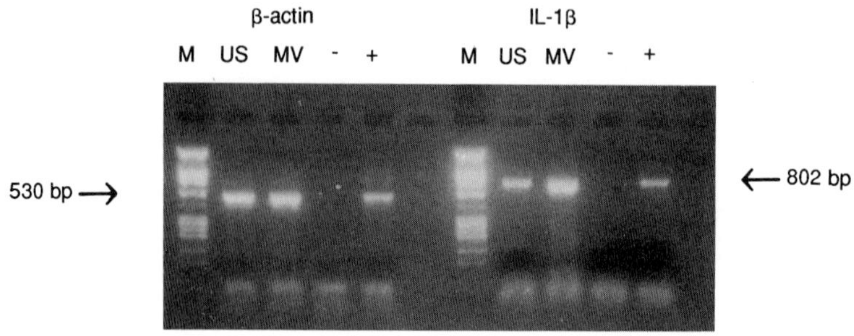

FIG. 2 RT-PCR detection of β-actin and IL-1β transcripts in adult human glial cells before and after infection with measles virus. Culture details are provided in Ref. 7. M, size markers (*Hin*dIIIλ/*Hae*III ϕX174 digested DNA); US, untreated adult human glial cells; MV, adult human glial cells infected with measles virus; −, negative control for PCR (no cDNA added to amplification reaction); +, positive control for amplification of IL-1β (cDNA from LPS-stimulated macrophages). An ethidium bromide-stained agarose gel is shown.

Southern Blot Analysis

Southern blot analysis of the PCR product using probes specific for the gene of interest is performed to confirm the specificity of the PCR product, to enhance the sensitivity of detection, and to allow quantitation of the product. The gel is prepared for transfer to nylon membranes by sequential soaking in a denaturing solution and a neutralization solution according to standard protocols (2, 3), followed by equilibration in 0.3× TAE for 30 min. The DNA is then electrotransferred to nylon membranes and hybridized with specific probes, as described above for mini-Northern blots.

Applications

One applicatioan of this technique is the quantitation of gene expression in glial cells. Figure 2 shows the results of amplification of IL-1β and β-actin transcripts from cultured human glial cells (7) that have been infected with measles virus (MV). On this ethidium bromide-stained gel, there is no obvious difference in the intensity of the amplified β-actin fragment between uninfected and MV-infected glial cells. In contrast, an increase in the intensity of the amplified IL-1β fragment is seen with MV infection. To semiquantitate this increase, PCR reactions were generated at serial cycles, to ensure that the reaction was proceeding in an exponential manner [a plateau in the accumulation of product results when 0.3 to 1 pmol of the product is present (5)]. The signals were then quantitated using a Phosphorimager (Molecular Dynamics, Sunnyvale, CA). The results of such an experiment, shown in

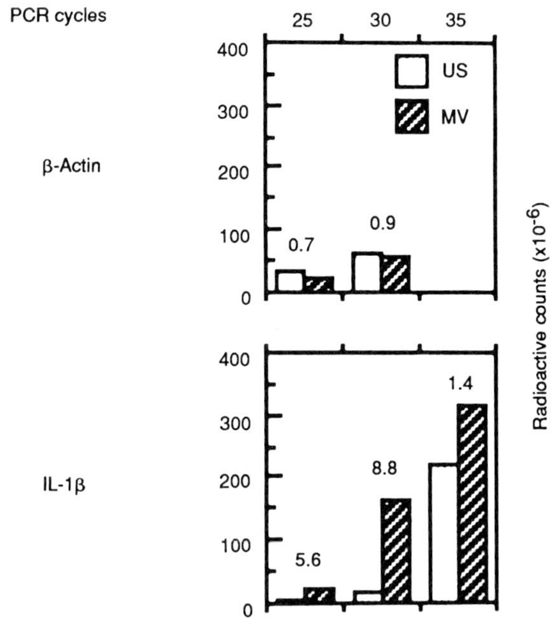

FIG. 3 Semiquantitiation of β-actin and IL-1β in uninfected and measles virus-infected adult human microglial cells by RT-PCR. cDNA was amplified for 25, 30, or 35 cycles and products were run on a 2% agarose gel and analyzed by Southern blotting using ^{32}P-labeled cDNA probes for 1L-1β or β-actin. Signals on the blots were then quantitated using a Molecular Dynamics Phosphorimager. US, uninfected; MV, measles virus infected. The numbers above the bars indicate the stimulation index (counts from infected divided by counts from uninfected cultures). The signal for β-actin at 35 cycles was too diffuse to be quantitated accurately.

Fig. 3, demonstrate that whereas the β-actin signal is relatively unaffected by infection, the IL-1β signal is increased by approximately six- to ninefold in the MV-infected glial cells. Note that this difference is dramatically reduced when the reactions are run for 35 cycles, emphasizing the necessity to determine an appropriate number of cycles for analysis. It is also possible to estimate the original number of specific transcripts in an RNA isolate. Such quantitative methods rely on the use of constructs that contain an altered version of the transcript of interest, such that the amplified product is a different size, allowing spiking of the PCR reaction with a known number of construct molecules. Details of these methods can be found elsewhere (5, 8).

Another application is the identification of cell populations present in a culture of glial cells. For example, we have used primers that detect glial

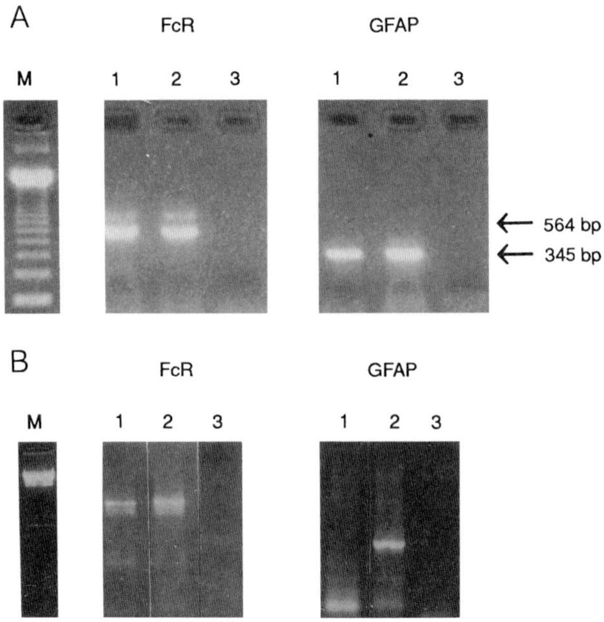

FIG. 4 Analysis of cell-specific transcripts in populations of glial cells. cDNA prepared from a population of mixed adult human glial cells (A) and from purified microglial cells (B) (7) was amplified using primers for FcR (marker for microglia) and GFAP (marker for astrocytes) for 30 cycles, as indicated in the text, and analyzed on agarose gels. M, size markers; lane 1, human glial cells; lane 2, positive control for PCR reaction; lane 3, negative control for PCR reaction. Note that in (A, lane 1) both FcR and GFAP signals were detected from the mixed glial cells whereas in (B, lane 1), a signal was only detected for FcR in the purified microglial cells.

fibrillary acidic protein (GFAP) as a marker for astrocytes and primers that detect the Fc-γ receptor II (FcR) as a marker for microglial cells. For example, Fig. 4A shows amplification of GFAP and FcR from mixed glial cells obtained from a human adult brain culture, demonstrating that this is a mixed population of astrocytes and microglia. If the microglia are then purified, the presence of an FcR signal and the absence of a GFAP signal is evidence for insignificant contamination of this population of cells with astrocytes (Fig. 4B). Such an approach could also be extended to the analysis of gene expression in other brain cells such as oligodendrocytes and neurons, using primers for myelin basic protein and neurofilaments, respectively.

Analysis of Gene Expression in Individual Cells in the Central Nervous System

The methods described in this chapter allow the analysis of gene expression in a bulk population of cells. Ultimately, however, questions will turn to the expression of genes in individual cells *in vivo,* especially with regard to the role of particular cells in immunopathological processes and the cellular tropism of viruses in the CNS. We direct the reader to two current and developing methods that make this sort of analysis possible. The technique of *in situ* hybridization essentially takes the information obtainable from Northern blotting down to the single-cell level. By doing so, one has the ability to examine the expression of a particular gene *and* identify the particular cells in which that gene is being expressed. Typically, this is done using sections of paraffin-embedded tissue that are mounted on a glass slide. Transcripts for the gene of interest are identified by hybridization with probes and cell types are identified with monoclonal antibodies directed against cell-specific markers. This technique is reviewed in Refs. 9–13. The emerging technique of *in situ* PCR, in turn, increases the sensitivity of *in situ* hybridization by amplifying the transcript from the gene of interest within the tissue section, in effect using the cell as a reaction vessel. Several laboratories have used *in situ* PCR successfully in a number of applications (4, 14–16). This technique offers tremendous potential to answer questions in neuroimmunology that previously could not be approached.

References

1. P. Chomczynski and N. Sacchi, *Anal. Biochem.* **162,** 156 (1987).
2. F. M. Ausubel, R. Brent, R. E. Kingston, D. D. Moore, J. G. Seidman, J. A. Smith, and K. Struhl, "Short Protocols in Molecular Biology." Wiley, New York, 1992.
3. J. Sambrook, E. F. Fritsch, and T. Maniatis, "Molecular Cloning: A Laboratory Manual." Cold Spring Harbor Laboratory Press, Cold Spring Harbor, NY, 1989.
4. G. J. Nuovo, "PCR *in Situ* Hybridization, Protocols and Applications." Raven Press, New York, 1992.
5. M. A. Innis, D. H. Gelfand, J. J. Sninsky, and T. J. White, "PCR Protocols: A Guide to Methods and Applications." Academic Press, San Diego, 1990.
6. R. B. Darnell, *Ann. Neurol.* **34,** 513 (1993).
7. T. Yamabe, G. Dhir, E. P. Cowan, I. L. Wolf, G. K. Bergey, A. Krumholz, E. Barry, P. M. Hoffman, and S. Dhib-Jalbut, *J. Neuroimmunol.* **49,** 171 (1994).
8. M. Piatak, Jr., K.-C. Luk, B. Williams, and J. D. Lifson, *Biotechniques* **14,** 70 (1993).

9. A. T. Haase and M. B. A. Oldstone (eds.), "Current Topics in Microbiology and Immunology," Vol. 143. Springer-Verlag, New York, 1989.
10. C. A. Jordan, *in* "*In Situ* Hybridization Histochemistry" (M.-F. Chesselet, ed.), p. 39. CRC Press, Boca Raton, FL (1990).
11. B. S. Mitchell, D. Dhami, and U. Schumacher, *Med Lab. Sci.* **49,** 107 (1992).
12. G. Mengod, E. Goudsmit, A. Proubst, and J. M. Palacios, *Prog. Brain Res.* **93,** 45 (1992).
13. P. C. Emson, *Trends Neurosci.* **16,** 9 (1993).
14. O. Bagasra, T. Seshama, and R. J. Pomerantz, *J. Immunol. Methods* **14,** 131 (1993).
15. J. Embretson, M. Zupancic, J. Beneke, M. Till, S. Wolinsky, J. L. Ribas, A. Burke, and A. T. Haase, *Proc. Natl. Acad. Sci. U.S.A.* **90,** 357 (1993).
16. B. K. Patterson, M. Till, P. Otto, C. Goolsby, M. R. Furtado, L. J. McBride, and S. M. Wolinsky, *Science* **260,** 976 (1993).

[5] Class I and Class II Major Histocompatibility Complex Molecules

William E. Winter, Richard H. Buck, and
Dorlinda A. Varga-House

Introduction

The goal of the immune system is to establish and maintain separation of self and nonself. Invasion of otherwise sterile tissues by nonself in the form of microorganisms is harmful on a local basis. Such infections can be superficial, such as cellulitis, or deep, such as osteomyelitis, septic arthritis, or pyelonephritis. When microorganisms disseminate systemically, infection can be life threatening due to bacteremia and clinical sepsis. Alternatively, infection of key organs leading to severe organ dysfunction or failure can also lead to death. Examples of this situation include viral, bacterial, fungal, or parasitic pneumonia leading to respiratory failure; carditis, endocarditis, or valvulitis producing heart failure; or encephalitis, meningoencephalitis, or meningitis leading to cerebral death.

In order to separate and identify self versus nonself, the immune system has evolved two arms: the native (nonspecific) host defense system and the adaptive (specific) immune system. The native host defenses of the immune system include the integument and its products (i.e., fatty acids), certain cells of the immune system [neutrophils, macrophages, and natural killer (NK) cells], nonspecific defensive proteins (e.g., C-reactive protein, and the plasma proteins of the alternative complement pathway), chemical barriers (e.g., low pH in the stomach), and mechanical barriers (e.g., peristalsis). Characteristic of the native immune system, there is no improvement in the immune response with reexposure to antigen. Thus, the native immune system lacks immunologic memory. On the other hand, the adaptive immune response does improve with reexposure to antigen. This is recognized in the increased vigor of secondary immune responses as compared to primary immune responses.

Adapative Immune Response

There are three phases to the adaptive immune response; (1) antigen recognition, (2) immune cell communication/amplification, and (3) the effector stage of antigen clearance. The adaptive immune response is orchestrated by lym-

Methods in Neurosciences, Volume 24

phocytes. Lymphocytes are either T cells (thymus-derived lymphocytes) or B cells (bursa-derived lymphocytes). In order to identify self versus nonself, lymphocytes carry *antigen receptors* to accomplish the first phase of the immune response: antigen recognition (Janeway, 1993). The α/β T-cell receptor (TCR) on the T-cell surface does not see intact antigen but sees only antigen–peptide fragments that are "presented" to the TCR by specialized molecules of the immune system termed major histocompatibility complex (MHC) molecules. The MHC molecules are present on the surface of cells of the body. In contrast to TCRs, the B-cell receptor (surface immunoglobulin) recognizes intact, soluble antigen. In the naive B-cell repertoire, surface immunoglobulin receptors are IgM and IgD while the antigen-driven, mature B cell can have IgG, IgA, IgE, or, less commonly, IgM on its surface as the antigen receptor. The interaction between lymphocyte receptors and antigens or antigen–peptides is a ligand–receptor interaction.

T-Cell Antigen Recognition

The manner in which T cells recognize antigen is highly specialized as compared to how B cells recognize antigen. There are two general classes of T cells: $CD4^+$ T-helper cells and $CD8^+$ T-cytotoxic (killer) cells (Nossal, 1987; Royer and Reinhertz, 1987). The $CD4^+$ T cells control the immune response and help determine whether the response will be predominantly cell-mediated or humoral, or a combination of both (the effector/antigen clearance stages of the immune response). Antibody provides "humoral" immunity. $CD8^+$ T killer cells afford "cell-mediated" immunity. The nature of the effector stage is controlled by the cytokines that the $CD4^+$ T cell produces during the amplification/cell communication (second) stage of the adaptive immune response (Miyajima *et al.*, 1988).

$CD4^+$ T-helper cells have been further classified into two subdivisions: T-helper cell type 1 cells (TH1) that produce predominantly interleukin 2 (IL-2) and γ-interferon cytokines and drive a cell-mediated immune response and TH2 T-helper cell type 2 (TH2) cells that produce the IL-4, IL-5, IL-6, and/or IL-10 cytokines that drive the humoral immune response (Street and Mosmann, 1991; Salgame *et al.*, 1991). In fact, different combinations of cytokines appear to be responsible for the specific B-cell class switching that takes place. IL-4, IL-5, and IL-2 together stimulate IgM; IL-4, IL-6, IL-2, and γ-interferon induce class switching to IgG; IL-5, IL-2, and T-cell growth factor β (TCG-β) influences class switching to IgA; and IL-4 alone causes class switching to IgE.

T cells *in vivo* do not recognize soluble antigen–peptides. Antigen-derived peptides must be bound to cell-surface molecules of other cells and presented to the TCRs of $CD4^+$ and $CD8^+$ T cells. Antigen presentation is the function of the protein products of the major histocompatibility complex (MHC) (Hoffman, 1992a). In the human, the MHC is termed the human leukocyte antigen (HLA) complex. In mice, the MHC is titled the H-2 complex. While the TCRs of $CD4^+$ T cells and $CD8^+$ T cells are organized identically (TCR-α is composed of V, J, and C regions, TCR-β is composed of V, D, J, and C regions), $CD4^+$ and $CD8^+$ T cells recognize antigen via different types of MHC molecules: class I MHC and class II MHC. $CD8^+$ T cells see antigen-derived peptides in the context of class I MHC. $CD4^+$ T cells view antigen-derived peptides in the context of class II MHC.

Thymic T-Cell Ontogeny and Major Histocompatibility Complex Molecules

Antigen–peptide recognition is a key feature of T-cell development in the thymus (Ramsdell and Fowlkes, 1990). During T-cell ontogeny, double-positive ($CD4^+$ $CD8^+$) T cells that do not rearrange a functional TCR die (von Boehmer and Kisielow, 1990). If a functional TCR is expressed, the TCR must engage either a class I MHC molecule or a class II MHC molecule to survive (positive MHC selection) (Blackman *et al.,* 1990). This ensures that TCRs can perceive self-MHC (MHC restriction). If the TCR cannot see self-MHC, the T-cell dies. Double-positive T cells that are "saved" by class I MHC interaction lose CD4 expression to become $CD8^+$ T cells. Double-positive T cells that are "saved" by class II MHC interaction lose CD8 expression to become $CD4^+$ T cells (von Boehmer, 1988). MHC restriction ensures that TCRs can see peptides in the context of self-MHC. Without self-MHC because of MHC restriction, T cells are not able to respond to specific antigen–peptides. If non-self-MHC is present, an allograft reaction occurs to foreign MHC molecules. This is the major barrier to tissue transplantation. The term "major histocompatibility complex" is derived from early experiments in transplantation where "MHC" alleles had to be matched between donor and recipient to permit successful transplantation. When the grafts are xenogeneic, the vigor of the anti-MHC response is even more intense than when allografts are placed.

In the thymus, self-peptides are presented by class I MHC and class II MHC molecules. If the affinity of the TCR for the MHC self-peptide is too great, an opportunity for autoimmunity results (Kappler *et al.,* 1989). In this case the T cell undergoes apoptosis (negative selection). Without negative selection there would be no tolerance to self that prevents autoimmunity (Nossal, 1989). Those T cells that survive these processes leave the thymus as mature T cells.

T Cells and Peripheral Tolerance

If all self-antigens were expressed in the thymus, tolerance would be complete after T cells exit the thymus. However, not all self-antigens enter the thymus during T-cell ontogeny. To prevent autoimmunity to self-antigens that never enter the thymus, peripheral tolerance has evolved. Peripheral tolerance refers to the process where T cells are inactivated if antigen–peptides are presented without all of the normal costimulatory signals (i.e., B7). We will see shortly that antigen–peptide presentation by either class I MHC or class II MHC is a complex process (Germain, 1986; Marrack, 1987). If this process is incomplete, such as absence of a key adhesion molecule interaction, anergy (tolerance) to antigen develops instead of an immune response to antigen (Marrack and Kappler, 1993). The ''anergized'' T cell may be inactivated or may undergo apoptosis. ''Inactivation'' without T-cell death could be permanent. However, if the inactivation were reversible, tolerance could be ''broken'' or abrogated with later development of autoimmunity.

Selection of the TCR repertoire in the thymus and via peripheral tolerance is the key to self–nonself discrimination (Sinha *et al.,* 1990). When self–nonself discrimination fails, infection can result from a failure to respond to the invading pathogen (Nossal, 1993). Alternatively, failure of self–nonself discrimination and an active immune response to infection could permit molecular mimicry and autoimmunity (Röcken *et al.,* 1992).

Class I Major Histocompatibility Complex Molecules

Class I MHC molecules are located on all nucleated cells of the body. Class I antigen (molecule) density can vary from tissue to tissue. Indeed, class I antigen density on neurons is very low. There are three types of human class I molecules: HLA-A, HLA-B, and HLA-C. These molecules are coded for by separate loci within the HLA complex. In the mouse, the two main types of class I MHC are H-2K and H-2D.

Class I MHC molecules are composed of an MHC-encoded α (heavy) chain (~44 kDa) and non-MHC-encoded nonpolymorphic β_2-microglobulin (~12 kDa; B2M) (Fig. 1). If B2M is not synthesized by the cell, class I molecules are not expressed.

Each class I α chain has three external domains, a transmembrane domain, and a cytoplasmic domain. Each of the three extracellular domains are composed of ~90 amino acids. The α 3 domain is Ig-like in structure with an intradomain disulfide bond. The hydrophobic transmembrane domain contains ~25 amino acids and the cytoplasmic domain is ~30 amino acids long.

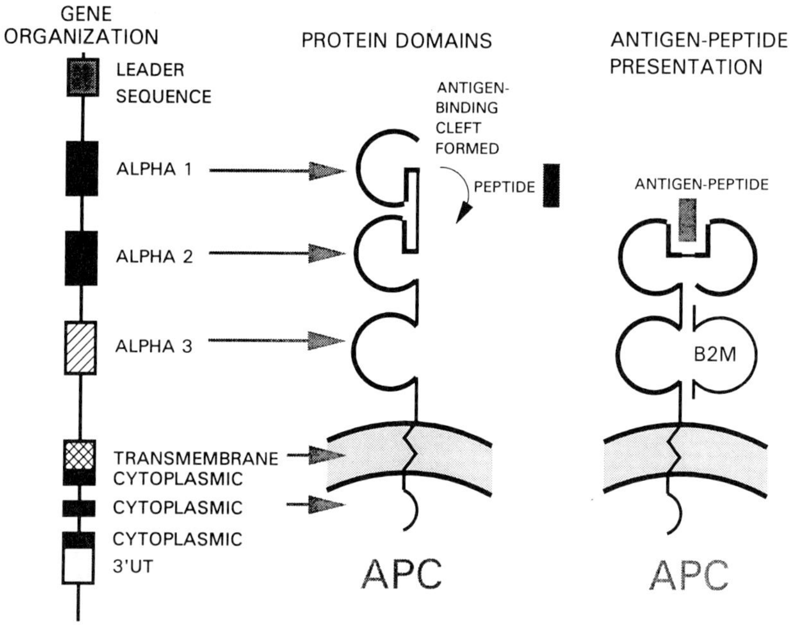

FIG. 1 Class I MHC heavy chains are composed of seven exons: leader sequence, $\alpha 1$, $\alpha 2$, $\alpha 3$, transmembrane/cytoplasmic, cytoplasmic, and cytoplasmic/3′UT. With binding of the antigen–peptide to the class I MHC heavy chain, the antigen-binding cleft is formed. Along with β_2-microglobulin expression, the class I MHC molecule is formed. The promoter sequences upstream (5′) of the class I MHC leader exon are not illustrated. 3′UT, 3′ untranslated region; APC, antigen-presenting cell.

The B2M molecule is a member of the immunoglobulin supergene family. The single B2M domain and the three external domains of the class I molecule provide a total of four extracellular domains. Two of these domains ($\alpha 1$ and $\alpha 2$ domains of the class I MHC α chain) are involved in antigen–peptide presentation.

On the genomic level, there is a leader sequence that pilots the newly synthesized class I MHC molecule to the rough endoplasmic reticulum (RER). The leader sequence, each of the external domains, and the transmembrane domain are coded for by separate exons. The cytoplasmic domain is coded for in part by the same exon as the transmembrane domain and two separate exons, the second of which contains the 3′ untranslated region of the gene.

Allelic variation among class I MHC molecules results from variations in the amino acid sequences of the $\alpha 1$ and $\alpha 2$ domains. These polymorphic

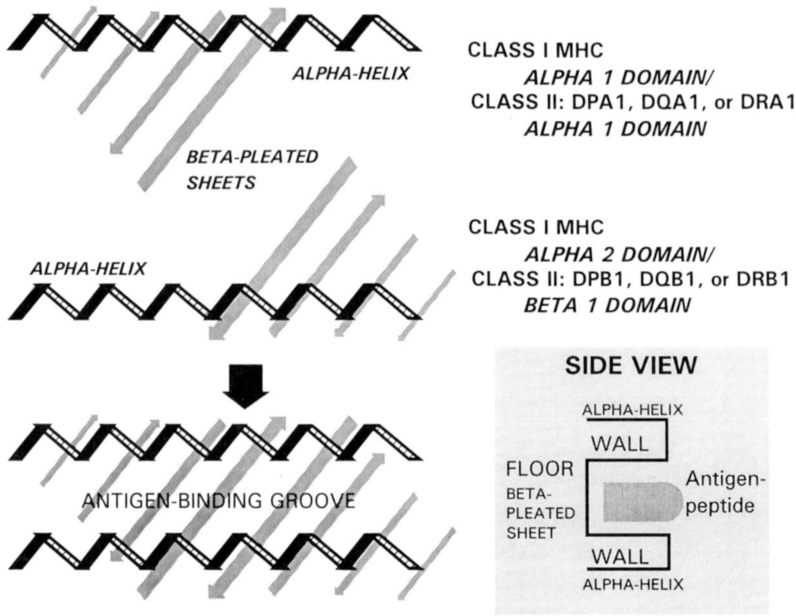

FIG. 2 MHC antigen-binding cleft. Each domain contributes an α helix and four β-pleated sheets. The antigen-binding groove is formed from two α helices and eight β-pleated sheets. The cartoon depicts the view of the cleft as seen from the perspective of the T-cell receptor. The antigen–peptide would be nestled within the cleft. This generic scheme serves as a model for class I MHC and class II MHC clefts.

sequences are those that pertain to the antigen-binding groove. The class I and class II MHC molecules display more germline variation and alleles than any other mammalian gene system. More than 40 class I MHC alleles have been described.

Antigen-Binding Groove

Crystallization of class I MHC molecules and their X-ray analysis in 1987 lead to the discovery of the structure of the antigen-binding groove (sometimes referred to as a "cleft") (Bjorkman *et al.*, 1987). The outermost two domains of the class I molecule ($\alpha 1$ and $\alpha 2$) fold together to form an antigen–peptide-binding groove (Fig. 2). Each domain provides an α helix that forms a side of the groove and four β-pleated sheets that form part of the floor of the groove. Altogether provided by the $\alpha 1$ and $\alpha 2$ domains, there are two α

helices forming the two sides of the groove and eight β-pleated sheets that form the complete floor of the groove. Peptides have been identified in the cleft and studied by crystallography (Fremont *et al.*, 1992; Barinaga, 1992). The antigen-binding pocket is approximately 25 × 10 × 11Å and is closed off at both ends limiting the size of the peptide that can be presented. An analogy between the MHC-binding groove and a baseball glove is helpful in understanding the concept of a peptide-presenting MHC molecule. The peptide contained in the groove is analogous to a baseball which is partially buried in the glove and partially exposed. TCRs see both MHC and associated antigen-derived peptide. In the thymus, the TCRs were positively selected ("educated") to be able to see self-MHC. Shortly after the paper by Bjorkman *et al.*, a model for the class II MHC cleft was published based on the class I MHC crystallographic data (Brown *et al.*, 1988).

Peptides Presented by Class I Major Histocompatibility Complex Molecules

The antigen-derived peptides presented by class I MHC are typically 9 to 10 amino acids in length and have valine (or leucine or isoleucine) at their N-terminal ends that binds to specific amino acid residues in the class I MHC groove (Falk *et al.*, 1991). Basic amino acids, either arginine or lysine, are located at the C-terminal end. The antigen–peptide is thus placed into a "bowed" configuration within the class I MHC cleft with the peptide tethered at its ends. Approximately seven amino acids are projected out of the groove to be recognized by the TCR of $CD8^+$ T cells.

TCRs have not been crystallized. Therefore, the exact nature of the TCR that binds MHC and antigen–peptide is unknown. When $CD8^+$ T cells see antigen–peptide presented by class I MHC, the CD8 molecule on the surface of the $CD8^+$ T cell noncovalently binds to a conserved portion of the $\alpha3$ domain of the class I molecule. This stabilizes the class I MHC–antigen–peptide–TCR interaction. Further stability of this interaction is afforded by noncovalent association of the LFA-1 and intercellular adhesion molecule (ICAM), LFA-2 (CD-2) and LFA-3, and CD28 and B7, respectively, on the T cells and the class I MHC-bearing cells (Fig. 3).

Cytoplasmic Peptide Transport to Class I Major Histocompatibility Complex Molecules

The peptides that are presented by class I MHC are derived from cytoplasmic proteins (Fig. 4). Class I MHC molecules thus present to the $CD8^+$ T cells of the immune system a spectrum of peptides from within the cell [shortly

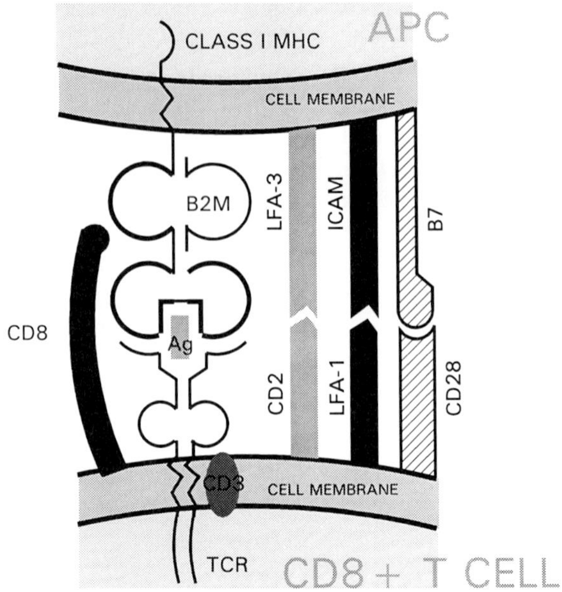

FIG. 3 The interaction of class I MHC-bearing antigen-presenting cell (APC) and CD8$^+$ T cell. Numerous accessory molecules stabilize this association as depicted. Ag, antigen–peptide.

we will see that class II MHC present peptides from outside the cell to the CD4$^+$ T cells]. Cytoplasmic proteins, either endogenous (self) proteins or proteins derived from infectious organisms like viruses (nonself), are degraded by a special cytoplasmic proteasome(s) (LMP, low molecular mass polypeptide) (Robertson, 1991; Goldberg and Rock, 1992). The resulting "antigen"–peptides are transported into the RER by the transporter of antigen–peptides (TAP) system (Monaco, 1992). The genes for the LMP proteasomes and transporters are located in the class II region of the MHC (Spies *et al.*, 1990; Glynne *et al.*, 1991; Ortiz-Navarrete *et al.*, 1991). Polymorphisms of the TAP genes have been described (Powis *et al.*, 1992). In turn, the TAP genes may influence which peptides enter the RER for eventual presentation by class I MHC molecules (Parham, 1992).

Peptides "pumped" into the RER are able to associate with the class I MHC antigen-binding clefts. Previously, the leader sequence of newly synthesized class I MHC α (heavy) chains guided these molecules into the RER. Likewise, coordinate synthesis of B2M provided B2M for assembly with the class I MHC α chain to form a complete class I MHC molecule. The transmembrane domain of the class I MHC molecule integrates into the

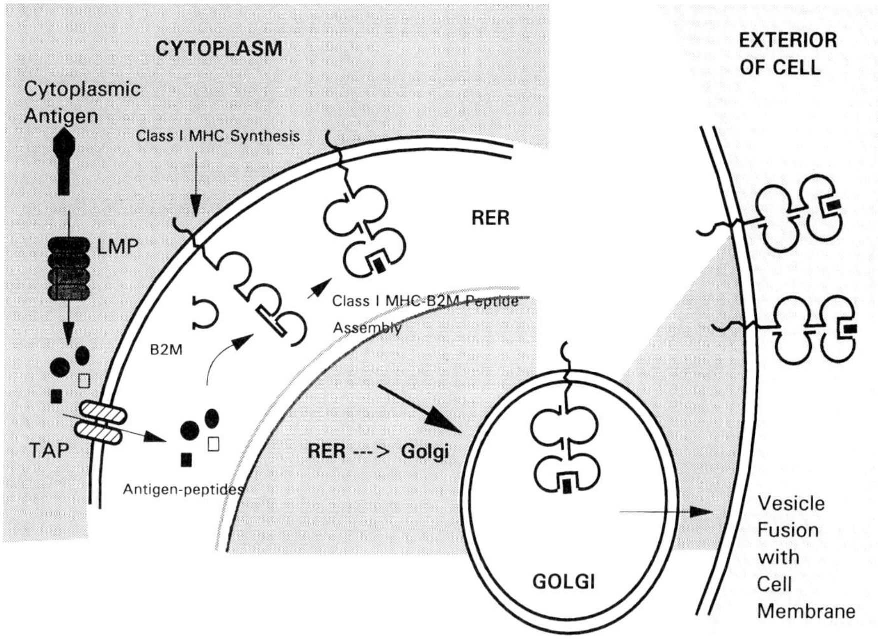

FIG. 4 Protein antigens from the cytoplasm are degraded by the LMP complex into peptides, the peptides are transported into the RER via the TAP protein, and the peptides associate with class I MHC heavy chain and β_2-microglobulin to form the class I MHC–antigen–peptide molecule. From the RER, the MHC molecule migrates to the Golgi, then to a vesicle which fuses with the cell membrane placing the class I MHC (with peptide) at the exterior of the cell for antigen–peptide presentation to $CD8^+$ T cells (see Fig. 3).

membrane of the RER. As the RER blends into the Golgi, the class I MHC molecule "travels" toward the cytoplasmic membrane with a cytoplasm-derived peptide now located in its antigen-binding groove. Vesicles containing class I MHC (α chain-B2M and antigen–peptide), derived from the Golgi, fuse with the plasma membrane to place the class I MHC–antigen–peptide complex on the outside of the cell. Peptides generated from cytoplasmic proteins are now expressed on the cell surface. TCRs of $CD8^+$ T cells search for class I MHC–antigen–peptides that they might recognize. $CD8^+$ T cells literally crawl over the surface of cells. Therefore, the immune system is surveying what is inside the cell. In the normal situation, presentation of a nonself peptide via class I MHC would alert the immune system that a cell has been infected and should be targeted to destroy the "household" that the invader has set up within the body.

T-Cell Activation

When T cells encounter an antigen–peptide (presented by MHC) that they recognize, signal transduction within the T cell occurs via the CD3 complex (Crabtree, 1989; Isakov *et al.*, 1986). CD3 is physically associated with the TCR in the endoplasmic reticulum and modification occurs in the Golgi complex. CD3 has three major subunits (γ, δ, and ε) and two smaller subunits. TCR-CD3 triggering leads to activation of phospholipase C, cleavage of phosphatidylinositol 4,5-bisphosphate (PIP_2) to diacylglycerol (DAG) and inositol 1,4,5-trisphosphate (IP_3). An influx of calcium from the endoplasmic reticulum and extracellular space acts as a second messenger. As well, there is activation of protein kinase C and protein phosphorylation. CD8 and CD4 binding to MHC molecules also contributes to T-cell activation (Julius *et al.*, 1983; O'Rourke and Mescher, 1993) and CD28 binding by B7 is an important trigger for the process (June *et al.*, 1990).

Target Cell Killing

When $CD8^+$ T cells are thus activated and receive cytokine help from $CD4^+$ T-helper cells (i.e., IL-2), $CD8^+$ T cells are able to kill cells that present nonself antigen–peptides (Dinome and Young, 1987; Marx, 1986). When foreign peptides are presented by class I MHC and recognized by the $CD8^+$ T cell receptor, the immune system will eliminate this particular cell because the cell is infected and harbors nonself proteins. The immune system eliminates "cytoplasmic" nonself by destroying the "virus factory." This protects noninfected cells from future infection and damage. The $CD8^+$ T cells (and $CD4^+$ T cells) have undergone thymic education regarding self–nonself discrimination during the development of the TCR repertoire and should not normally recognize self-peptides.

Class I Major Histocompatibility Complex Summary

Class I MHC molecules provide the window through which the immune system surveys the "inside" of self: the cellular cytoplasm. Nonself is eliminated through cell-mediated immunity accomplished by $CD8^+$ T-killer cells.

Class II Major Histocompatibility Complex Molecules

In contrast to the distribution of class I MHC molecules, class II MHC molecules are located on a select group of cells of the immune system termed "antigen-presenting cells" (APCs). Antigen-presenting cells include

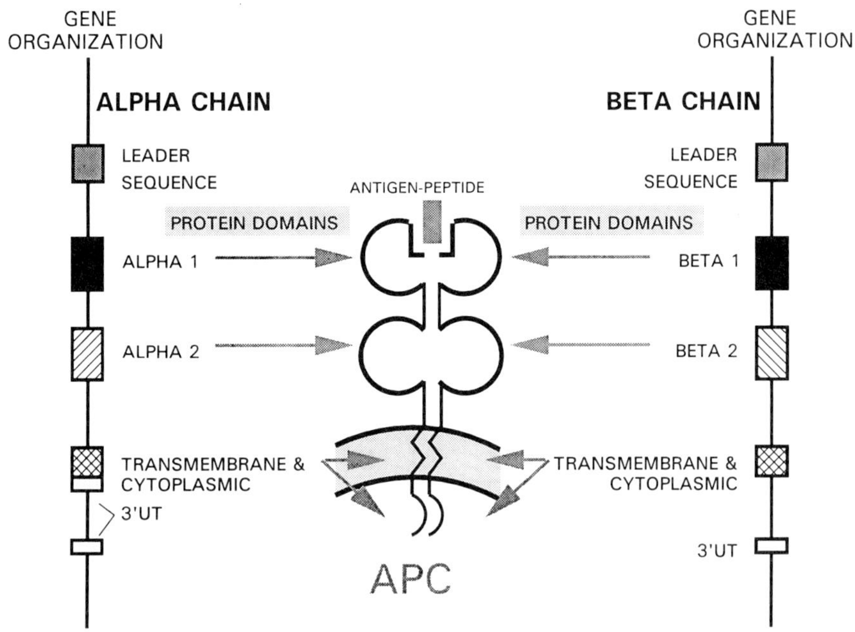

FIG. 5 Class II MHC heavy chains are composed of five exons: leader sequence, $\alpha 1/\beta 1$, $\alpha 2/\beta 2$, transmembrane/cytoplasmic (± including some 3′UT region), and 3′UT. The promoter sequences upstream (5′) of the class II MHC leader exon are not illustrated. 3′UT, 3′ untranslated region; APC, antigen-presenting cell.

monocytes in the circulation, macrophages in the tissues (i.e., intraglomerular, alveolar, serosal, splenic, and lymph node macrophages), dendritic cells, Langerhans cells of the skin, Kupffer cells in the liver, central nervous system microglia, and B cells. These cells have been termed "professional" APCs. With inflammation and γ-interferon production by $CD4^+$ T cells, class II MHC expression significantly increased on macrophages. Activated T cells may express class II molecules in humans but not in mice. Class II MHC expression can be induced on endothelial cells or fibroblasts during the immune response by γ-interferon. The cells that normally do not express class II MHC but can be induced to express class II MHC are termed "nonprofessional" APCs.

Each class II molecule is a noncovalently associated heterodimeric cell-surface molecule composed of two chains (α and β) each coded for by two separate genes within the MHC (Fig. 5). α Chains are 32–34 kDa and β chains are 29–32 kDa. Each class II α and β chain has two external domains, a transmembrane domain, and a cytoplasmic domain. Allelic variation among class II MHC α and β chains is located in the respective $\alpha1$ and $\beta1$ domains. The $\alpha2$ and $\beta2$ domains are immunoglobulin-like, similar to the class I MHC $\alpha3$ domain. Class II MHC extracellular domains are each ~90 amino acids long. The hydrophobic transmembrane domain is ~25 amino acids long and the cytoplasmic domain is of variable length.

There are three types of human class II molecules: HLA-DP, HLA-DQ, and HLA-DR. In the mouse, the class II molecules are IA (mouse homolog of the human DQ) and IE (mouse homolog of the human DR). In humans, the DPB1 and DPA1 genes code for the DPβ chain and DPα chain that form the DP molecule. Likewise, DQB1 and DQA1 code for DQβ and DQα that produce the DQ molecule and DRB1 and DRA1 code for DRβ and DRα that produce the DR molecule. In contrast to other expressed class II MHC chains, DRA1 is essentially nonpolymorphic. For both the class I and class II genes, there are several nonexpressed pseudogenes (i.e., DPB2, DPA2, DQB2, DQA2, and DRB2). Similar to class I MHC molecules, class II MHC molecules displace extreme polymorphism with over 60 alleles described.

The outermost extracellular domains of the class II MHC α and β chains, respectively, the $\alpha1$ and $\beta1$ domains, associate to form the antigen binding groove of the class II MHC molecules. This has been demonstrated by X-ray crystallography (Brown *et al.*, 1993). Each $\alpha1$ and $\beta1$ domain provides an α helix and four β-pleated sheets forming an antigen–peptide-binding groove analogous to the class I MHC groove. These data also suggested that class II MHC molecules might occur as a dimer of the α/β dimers (Ploegh and Benaroch, 1993).

Peptides Presented by Class II Major Histocompatibility Complex Molecules

While class I MHC molecules survey the cytoplasm of cells (endogenous or cytoplasmic antigens), class II MHC present antigen–peptides of proteins obtained from outside the antigen-presenting cell (exogenous or external antigens). Where class I MHC molecules present to $CD8^+$ killer T cells, class II MHC molecules present extracellular antigen-derived peptides to $CD4^+$ T-helper cells (Unanue and Allen, 1987).

APCs, either by pinocytosis or phagocytosis, take up circulating proteins, proteins secreted by cells, proteins released by damaged or dying cells, and nonself proteins (i.e., microorganisms) that have entered the sterile tissues of the host (Fig. 6). In the resulting endosome, the ingested material is degraded at low pH. Protein is broken down into peptides. The peptide-containing endosomes fuse with vesicles containing newly synthesized class II MHC molecules.

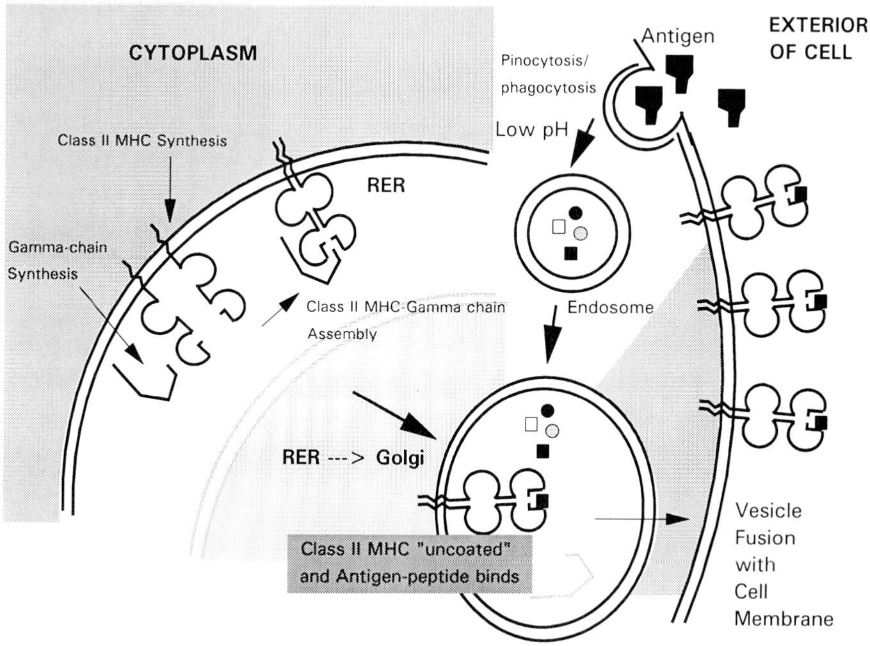

FIG. 6 Extracellular transport of class II MHC molecules. Protein antigens from the extracellular space are pinocytosed or phagocytosed by "professional" antigen-presenting cells and are degraded at low pH in endosomes (or lysosomes) into peptides; with fusion of the endosome and a Golgi-derived vesicle, and release of the γ chain, the peptides associate with class II MHC molecules. The vesicle containing class II MHC molecules with bound peptide fuses with the cell membrane placing the class II MHC (with peptide) at the exterior of the cell for antigen–peptide presentation to $CD4^+$ T cells (see Fig. 7).

Each class II MHC α and β chain is synthesized from separate genes within the MHC. In the RER, the class II MHC α and β chains associate with the γ chain (invariant chain). This has an important effect on antigen–peptide presentation from exogenous versus endogenous antigens (Teyton *et al.*, 1990). One hypothesis proposes that the γ chain protects the class II MHC molecule from binding peptides that enter the RER via the LMP proteasome/TAP transporter system (Nefjes and Ploegh, 1992). Recall that the LMP proteasome/TAP transporter system normally furnishes peptides to class I MHC molecules (Brown *et al.*, 1991). The hypothesis further suggests that the γ chain is released from the class II MHC α/β pair at low pH when the Golgi vesicle containing class II MHC has fused with the endosome as

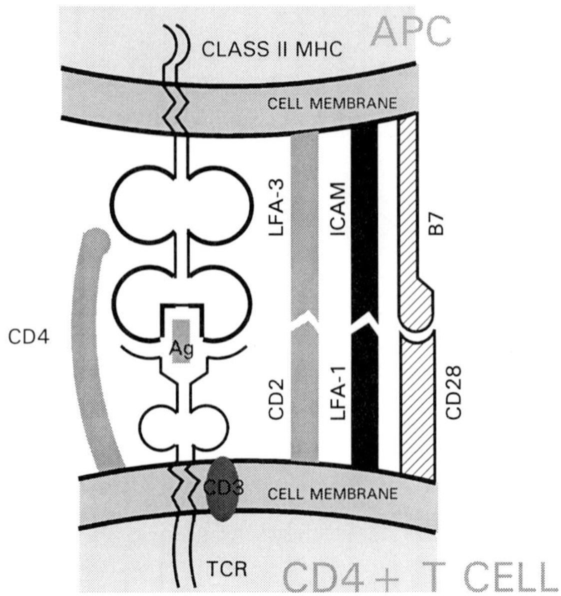

FIG. 7 The interaction of a class II MHC-bearing antigen-presenting cell (APC) and $CD4^+$ T cell. Numerous accessory molecules stabilize this association as depicted. Ag, antigen–peptide.

described above. Heat-shock proteins (or chaperones) may also assist in the assembly of the class II MHC–peptide complex (DeNagel and Pierce, 1992).

The antigen–peptides presented by class II MHC to the TCRs of $CD4^+$ T cells can be 16 to 20 amino acids in length (Rudensky *et al.,* 1991). There are fewer restrictions on the specific sequences of the peptides that can be presented because the antigen binding cleft is open at both ends. Each class I and class II MHC molecule can present a very large number of peptides, but the number of peptides presented is not infinite.

Similar to class I MHC–CD8 molecular interactions, when APCs present antigen to $CD4^+$ T cells, the CD4 molecule binds to a portion of the conserved class II MHC extracellular domain to stabilize the class II MHC–TCR interaction (Fig. 7). Further stabilizing this interaction are noncovalent affiliations of the LFA-1 and ICAM; CD28 and B7 (Cohen, 1992); and LFA-2 (CD-2) and LFA-3, respectively, on the T cells and the class II MHC bearing APCs. The CD28-B7 appears to be particularly important. B7 distribution may be limited to professional APCs and thus further define which types of cells can present antigen–peptides to $CD4^+$ T cells and $CD8^+$ T cells.

$CD4^+$ T-Helper Cell Function

Activation of $CD4^+$ T cells is afforded by the surface–surface interactions described above and cytokine stimulation by IL-1 released from macrophages acting as APCs. As with $CD8^+$ T cells, $CD4^+$ T cells have CD3 associated with their TCR. Once TCR binds MHC and peptide, CD3 transduces the signal to activate the $CD4^+$ T cell.

Activation of $CD4^+$ T cells leads to the elaboration of cytokines, expression of cell-surface receptors (the p55 IL-2 receptor), expression of class II MHC, and cell proliferation when stimulated by secreted IL-2. The p70 IL-2 receptor is present on resting T cells. Interleukin 2 induces the expression of the p55 IL-2 receptor that together with the p70 IL-2 receptor forms a high-affinity receptor [an older name for the p55 IL-2 receptor is TAC (for T activation antigen)].

Interleukin-2 acts as an autocrine and paracrine T-cell growth factor, respectively, for $CD4^+$ T cells and $CD8^+$ T cells. Interleukin 2 not only causes $CD4^+$ T-cell proliferation, but also stimulates $CD8^+$ T cells to proliferate providing increased numbers of killer (cytotoxic) cells. This fosters cell-mediated immunity as described under the discussion of class I MHC. Interleukin 2 produced by the $CD4^+$ T-helper cells stimulates NK cells augmenting nonspecific (native) immunity. Interleukin 2 also incites B-cell proliferation and antibody synthesis. γ-Interferon secretion activates macrophages to switch to oxidative metabolism and increase their production of superoxides (O_2^-). Superoxides are needed to kill ingested microorganisms. γ-Interferon causes increased class II MHC expression on APCs affording increased levels of antigen–peptide presentation with inflammation. Particular combinations of cytokines (IL-4, IL-5, IL-6, IL-2, and γ-interferon) influence immunoglobulin class switching as described above.

$CD4^+$ T-Helper Cell–B-Cell Interactions

The body has evolved an interesting mechanism to target T-cell-derived cytokines to B cells that have encountered soluble antigen (Myers, 1991; Noelle and Snow, 1991; DeFranco, 1991). We start with the premise that the $CD4^+$ T cell has been activated by antigen–peptide presentation by a professional APC and that this same antigen has been bound to surface immunoglobulin on a B cell.

APCs like macrophages are "dumb" with respect to antigen–peptide presentation: they display peptides from *all* of the antigens that they pinocytose or phagocytose. This is not the case when B cells function as APCs. B cells are "smart" regarding the antigen–peptides that they present: they only display peptides from antigens taken up via their surface immunoglobulin receptors. Since immunoglobulin binds specific antigen motifs, the B cell is highly selective in internalizing a single antigen (or a very limited number of cross-reactive antigens). In turn, these antigens are processed within the B cell to present a select number of antigen-derived peptides via the B-cell class II MHC molecules. The activated $CD4^+$ T cell can recognize antigen-peptide presented by the class II MHC molecule of the B cell. Again as with "dumb" APCs, there are CD4 molecule–class II MHC interactions and other adhesion molecule combinations that stabilize the $CD4^+$ T-cell TCR–B-cell class II MHC association. The physical attachment of the activated $CD4^+$ T cell and B cell permits the B cell to be exposed to high concentrations of T-cell-liberated cytokines (i.e., IL-4, IL-5, IL-6, γ-interferon, and IL-2). In this antigen-driven stage of the humoral immune response, the B cell is stimulated to proliferate, class switch, and undergo affinity maturation of its surface and secrete immunoglobulin.

Control of Immune Response

The direction of the effector immune response is controlled by the cytokines elaborated by the $CD4^+$ T-helper cell. In turn, the antigen–peptides that the $CD4^+$ T-helper cell responds to are a function of its TCR and the peptides presented by the class II MHC molecule. This is also true for $CD8^+$ T cells. Therefore, class I and class II MHC molecules influence which antigens the immune system responds to as well as the intensity of the response.

The question arises as to why germline class I MHC and class II MHC genes are so extremely polymorphic and why in humans there are three types of class I MHC molecules and at least three types of class II MHC molecules. Teleologically, having several different class I MHC and class II MHC alleles should provide any one individual with a wide variety of antigen-presenting molecules that can present to TCRs an extremely large number of foreign peptides. Recall, that the immune system does not develop receptors in response to infection. Receptors, such as TCRs, must be preexistent. In turn, the body must have a preexistent ability to present a wide spectrum of peptides to these TCRs. From an epidemiologic perspective, having a population of people with a variety of class I MHC and class II MHC alleles should ensure that no pathogen can evade immune recognition by an entire cohort of people. The foreign invaders that the immune system endeavors to exclude or destroy seek entrance into the sterile tissues of the body and/or cell cytoplasm or organelles to live and reproduce.

Certain alleles of class II MHC genes appear to provide inherited susceptibility to autoimmune disease (Winter *et al.,* 1991a) by influencing antigen–peptide presentation (Todd *et al.*, 1987, 1990). α and β chains, either DP, DQ, or DR, are able to complement one another and coexpress (Nepom *et al.*, 1987). This may explain why in autoimmune diabetes, a combination of alleles (DR3 and DR4) strongly predisposes to disease (Winter *et al.*, 1991b).

TCR variety is generated through germline V, (D), J variation; combinatoral V, (D), J association during receptor rearrangement; junctional diversity; N-region diversity; and α–β pairing (Robertson, 1984a,b; Strominger, 1989). In contrast, all class I MHC and class II MHC variation is present in the germline. Expressed TCR variation is orders of magnitude greater than MHC variation. To consider this further, contrast what class I MHC and class II MHC bind versus what TCRs bind. While each class I and class II MHC molecules may present millions of antigen-derived peptides to TCRs, a single TCR can recognize only a single peptide. Thus, expressed TCRs must be more polymorphic than MHC.

Class II Major Histocompatibility Complex Summary

Class II MHC molecules allow the immune system to scrutinize the "self" that is outside of the cellular cytoplasm. These spaces are the intercellular (interstitial) space, the intravascular space, and the special compartments of the body like the joints, pleura, and peritoneum. Nonself is eliminated through opsonization (via IgM and IgG and subsequent complement deposition) and phagocytosis. The $CD4^+$ T cell orchestrates these events.

Organization of Human Major Histocompatibility Complex

The human MHC (HLA complex) is located on the short arm of chromosome 6 (Fig. 8) (Steinmetz and Hood, 1983; Kaufman *et al.*, 1984; Korman *et al.*, 1985). The MHC is divided into three general regions (in order from centromeric to telomeric): class II MHC region, class III MHC region, and class I MHC region (Peter and Hawkins, 1992). Molecules not directly involved in antigen–peptide presentation but present in the MHC are located in the class III MHC region and within the class II MHC region. The class III MHC gene products include complement proteins [C4B, CBA, factor B (Bf), C2], enzymes of the P450 complex (CYPB: 21-hydroxylase B and CYPA: 21-hydroxylase A), heat-shock protein 70 (2, 1, and Hom), G7a (synthetase valyl-tRNA ligase), tumor necrosis factor-β [TNFB, lymphotoxin (LTB)], TNFα (TNFA), and many genes of unknown function (G18, G17, G16, G15, G14, G13, G12, OSG, XA, G11, G10, G9a, G9, G8, G7b, G7, G6, BAT5, G5, G4, G3, G2, G1, B144, and BAT1).

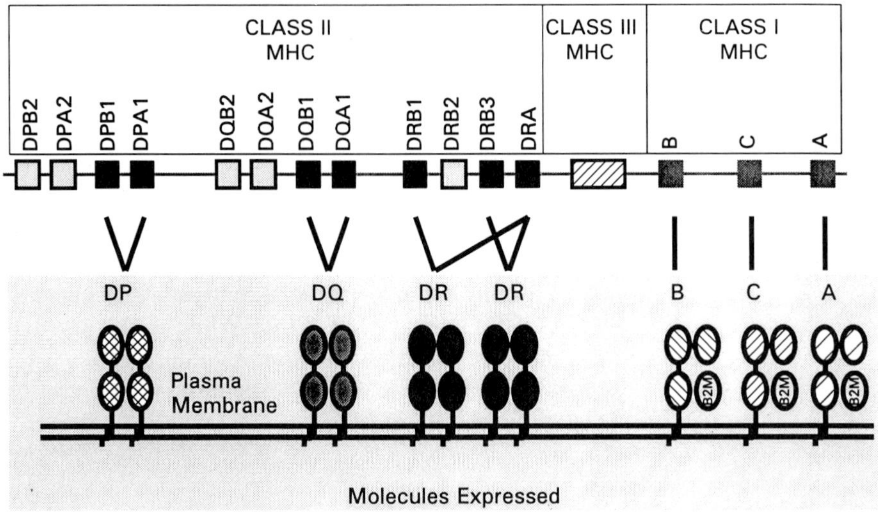

FIG. 8 The major histocompatibility complex (MHC) in humans is organized into three regions bearing class II, class III, and class I MHC genes. The expressed antigen-presenting proteins are as depicted. Numerous additional genes are located within the MHC. These are discussed in the text in detail.

Besides the DP, DQ, and DR genes, several proteasome-like genes and TAP [or ABC (ATP-binding cassette) transporter] genes are found in the class II MHC region. The proteasome-like genes include LMP2 and LMP7. The ABC (ATP-binding cassette) transporter genes include TAP1, RING9, and TAP2. Several genes in the class II MHC region have no known function as of yet (KE3, RING1, RING2, KE4, KE5, and RING3). COLIIA2 is a collagen gene. Class II genes that consist of DNA (DZα/DOα), DMA, DMB, DOB, DQB3 have been described. There can be several different DRB genes depending on the specific DR haplotype. There are also many new class I MHC genes described: 17, X, E, 30, 92, J, 21, 70, 16, H, G, 90, 75, and F. Genes in the class I MHC of unknown function encompass OCT-3, TUBB, P5-1, HSR1, VI, I, III, V, IV-2, P5-2, II-1, P5.3, IV-3, P5-4, and P5-5. Campbell and Trowsdale (1993) have supplied a summary of the organization of the MHC with extensive references.

Class I and Class II Major Histocompatibility Complex Molecules in the Nervous System

Inflammation in the central and peripheral nervous systems must be tightly regulated to avoid uncontrolled damage to neurons. For example, contrast the liver and the nervous system. Up to 80% of the liver can be destroyed during viral hepatitis and yet the liver can survive and regenerate. On the other hand, 80% destruction of the nervous system would be fatal. If a neuron is destroyed as part of the immune response to viral intracellular infection, the neuron is not replaced whereas the hepatocyte can readily be replaced by proliferation of healthy hepatocytes. Therefore, immune responses in the nervous system must be highly specific and controlled. In part, this may reflect why neurons have very low concentrations of class I MHC molecules on their surface. As a consequence, neurons have only a limited ability to present cytoplasmic (endogenous) antigen-derived peptides. This in turn restricts the degree to which $CD8^+$ T killer cells can lyse virally infected neurons. Teleologically, the body may "choose" to deal with a chronic viral infection instead of destroying nonreplicating neurons.

Extracellular (exogenous) antigen–peptide presentation is also highly regulated in the nervous system. Regardless of the mixture or doses of cytokines applied, neurons cannot be stimulated to express class II MHC molecules. Class II MHC expression is restricted to the microglial cells which are embryologically derived from monocyte/macrophage precursor cells present in the bone marrow (Theele and Streit, 1993; Flaris *et al.*, 1993; Williams *et al.*, 1992). Microglia make up ~20% of the glial cell population of the central nervous system and are ubiquitously distributed (Banati *et al.*, 1993). Microglial morphology is typically ramified or highly branched. Activated microglia can phagocytose material; produce arachidonic acid metabolites, proteases (cathepsin B/L), and reactive oxygen intermediates; release cytokines (IL-1, IL-6, TNFα); and express class I and class II MHC, CD4, and LFA-1 (Dickson *et al.*, 1991). With inflammation, microglia can transform into intrinsic brain macrophages.

Antigen–peptide presentation by class II MHC is the key step in initiating an immune response when $CD4^+$ T-helper cells are alerted to the presence of an infection in the host tissues. In the case of pathogens that take up intracellular residence (e.g., viruses, chlamydia, rickettsia, and some bacteria and parasites), the pathogen must still travel through the body to the target tissue. During this transit for a protective immune response to be initiated, the pathogen must be taken up by the body's APCs and antigen-derived peptides must be presented via class II MHC molecules to $CD4^+$ T cells. If the body develops IgM or IgG antibodies to the pathogen during the immune response, the antibodies can bind the pathogen during its journey to its cellular target. Antibody binding can prevent infection by causing the removal of the invading antigen (pathogen) prior to its binding to host target tissues. On the other hand, the cell-mediated response is necessary when the cells have been intracellularly invaded and the infected cell must be destroyed (by $CD8^+$ T killer cells) to arrest further infection of adjacent healthy cells.

Class I and class II MHC gene expression is highly regulated. In part, the body uses this mechanism to control the immune response within the nervous system. *Cis*-regulatory sequences are located 5′ of both the class I MHC and class II MHC genes. These regions are turned off and on by *trans*-acting transcriptional regulators. The class I MHC promoter has sequences that can respond to cytokines. For class II MHC genes, there are three well-defined 5′ promoter sequences: W (or H), X, and Y. In neurons, these class II MHC promoters appear to be permanently turned off and class I MHC expression is low.

When cells are induced to ectopically express class II MHC on the basis of transgenic gene placement, the class II MHC do not appear to be able to illicit an immune response. When this experiment was attempted with pancreatic β cells, antigen presentation by the β cells appeared to induce peripheral anergy (Markmann *et al.*, 1988). Ectopic class II MHC expression occurs with inflammation (Ballardini *et al.*, 1984; Malik *et al.*, 1984). This may be the natural way the body attempts to develop active peripheral tolerance as a method for controlling the immune response.

Another mechanism to control the immune response in the nervous system is to restrict immune cell entrance into the nervous system (Fig. 9). The blood–brain barrier is composed of the capillary–vascular nonfenestrated endothelium joined together by tight junctions, basement membrane (e.g., basal lamina appears to be an extension of the pia mater), and astrocyte foot processes. In contrast to other parts of the body, macrophages do not normally traffic through the central nervous system. Lymphocyte trafficking in the central nervous system appears to occur to a lesser degree than that in the tissues outside of the central nervous system. This restricts antigen presentation by limiting the APC–lymphocyte interaction. Indeed, the central nervous system and deeper portions of peripheral nerves lack lymphatics and lymph nodes. Fluid lost from the capillaries in nervous tissue flows through minute interstitial channels instead of lymphatics. In the case of peripheral nerves, the fluid is absorbed by adjacent lymphatics. In the case of the central nervous system, the fluid enters the cerebrospinal fluid (CSF) to be reabsorbed into the circulation as CSF is reabsorbed. Normally, cerebrospinal fluid is almost acellular with <5 white blood cells per mm^3.

The blood–brain barrier and blood–CSF barrier also restrict inflammation by essentially excluding IgG from the extracellular central nervous system fluids. For example, CSF IgG is normally ≤ 6 mg/dl which is far less than 1% of serum IgG.

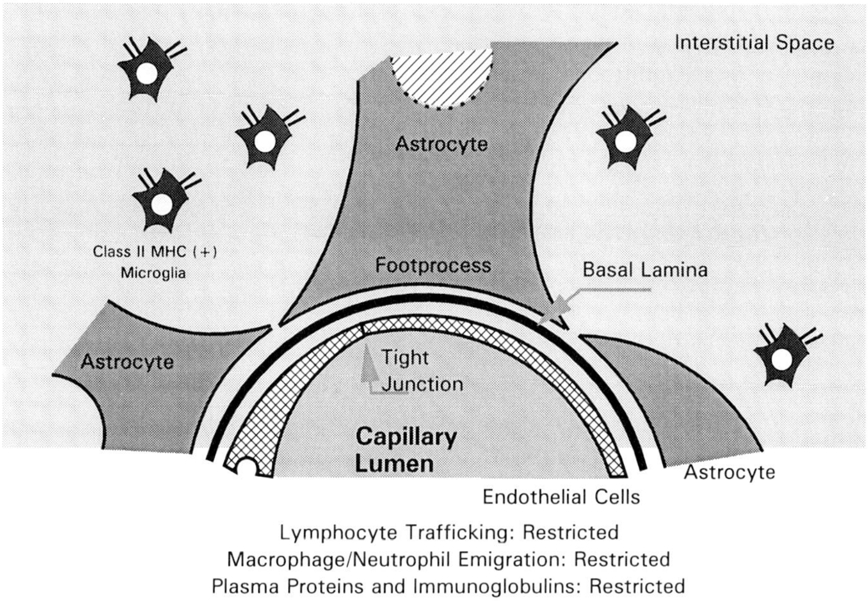

FIG. 9 The blood–brain barrier includes the capillary endothelial cells which have tight junctions between them. These cells limit or exclude passage of immune cells and plasma into the interstitial space of the central nervous system. The next component of the barrier is the basal lamina which is derived from pia mater. Adjacent to the basal lamina are foot processes from astrocytes. Microglia have class II MHC on their surface and function as antigen-presenting cells. Neurons are not depicted.

Measuring Major Histocompatibility Complex Antigen Density Using Flow Cytometry

From the previous discussion, it is obvious that control of class I MHC and class II MHC expression has a major role in regulating the immune response in the nervous system. Therefore, the ability to measure class I and class II MHC antigen (molecule) density on cells could be of great value to researchers interested in the nervous system.

To illustrate how flow cytometry can be used to determine MHC antigen density, we describe our studies of class I MHC density on lymphocytes from control mice and lymphocytes from mice that develop autoimmune diabetes. An analogy can be drawn between neurons and pancreatic β cells. Both types of cells produce chemical messengers (neurons produce neuotransmitters; β cells produce insulin), both cell types are restricted to specific tissues, and both cell types are end stage and are not replaced once destroyed. Furthermore, in autoimmune diseases of both the central nervous system (e.g., multiple sclerosis) and the β cell (e.g., insulin-dependent diabetes), lymphocytes are responsible for the destruction of target tissues.

Researchers from Harvard University published data in 1991 demonstrating decreased levels of class I MHC on splenocytes from NOD (nonobese diabetic) mice and humans with autoimmune insulin-dependent diabetes mellitus (Faustman *et al.*, 1991). Faustman and colleagues proposed that the 80% decrease in class I MHC expression was due to a faulty peptide transporter (i.e., TAP gene, transporter of antigen–peptides) termed HAM in mice, and RING4 in humans. Theoretically a defective transporter would lead to decreased cytoplasmic peptide transport into the RER. Class I molecules which were not associated with peptide would not assemble properly and would not be exported to the plasma membrane leading to the observed decrease in class I MHC expression. Furthermore, the presentation of endogenous self-antigens via class I MHC molecules may be a crucial step in the development of self-tolerance and inadequate presentation of self-peptide would permit the existence of autoreactive $CD8^+$ cytotoxic T cells with the ability to cause insulin-dependent diabetes mellitus (1). To address this controversy, we sought to examine the expression of class I MHC H-$2K^d$ antigens in lymphocytes from control and NOD mice. In murine H-2, K^d represents the *d* haplotype allele at the class I MHC *K* locus.

Splenocyte Isolation

To this end, 4-week-old female NOD, BALB/c, and C57BL/6 mice were euthanized by cervical dislocation. An incision was made in the left upper quadrant and the spleens were removed. Extraneous connective tissue was carefully dissected from the spleens which were separately extruded through a fine wire mesh using a pair of tweezers into approximately 5 ml of Hanks' buffered salt solution (HBSS) with 10% fetal calf serum (FCS) per spleen.

Percoll gradients were prepared in 50-ml polypropylene test tubes. Ten milliliters of a 40% Percoll solution was carefully layered on top of 10 ml of 75% Percoll using a pipette. When this step is done properly one should be able to see a distinct demarcation between the two solutions. The cell suspension was carefully layered on top of the gradient. All gradients were centrifuged for 30 min at 600*g*. After centrifugation the cells at the interface of the 75 and 40% Percoll were aspirated using a pipette and washed three times in HBSS with 10% FCS. After the final wash, cells were resuspended in 1 ml HBSS with 10% FCS per spleen. Viability of splenocytes was determined using a hemocytometer and trypan blue. Viability greater than 98% was calculated for all samples tested.

Splenocyte Staining

Aliquots of 2×10^6 cells were added to 5-ml polypropylene test tubes. A solution of 0.01 *M* phosphate-buffered saline (PBS), 10% newborn calf serum (NBCS), and 0.02% azide was added to bring the volume to 3 ml. Cell suspensions were centrifuged for 10 min at 1400 rpm. Supernatant was decanted and cells were resuspended in 100 μl NBCS and 5 μl of appropriate fluorescein isothiocyanate (FITC)-conjugated antibody. In our study we used SF9-9.9 (Pharmingen, San Diego, CA) that reacts with H-2K^d. This was allowed to incubate on ice in the dark for 30 min. After incubation, cells were washed two times in 0.01 *M* PBS and 0.02% azide solution and resuspended in 2 ml of 0.01 *M* PBS, 0.02% azide, and 1.0% paraformaldehyde fixative.

Flow Cytometry

Mean channel fluorescence (MCF) of class I MHC H-2K^d antigens was measured on the splenocytes as an indicator of relative antigen density (Hitchcock *et al.*, 1986). Analysis of cell samples was performed with a Becton–Dickinson FACScan flow cytometer. For each cell sample a dot-plot matrix was generated by plotting side scatter vs forward scatter. Ten thousand splenocytes were counted to generate each dot-plot. From the dot-plot, the population of cells being examined was gaited. The gaited population of cells was then plotted for each strain of mice examined with channel fluorescence on the *x* axis (log scale) and cell number on the *y* axis (Fig. 10). In our study, BALB/c (d haplotype) was used as a positive control. C57BL/6 (b haplotype) was used as a negative control. Nonobese diabetic mice are known to be H-2K^d. The boundaries for "percent positive" were determined using the positive control cell samples from BALB/c mice. Table I summarizes the results for MCF and percent of positive cells.

No significant difference in the MCF of the class I MHC antigen H-2K^d was found between 4-week-old NOD and the positive control strain BALB/c. It is important to note that the measurement MCF of H-2K^d on C57BL/6 splenocytes gives a paradoxical MCF result. This occurs because the measurement of MCF takes into account *only* the cells which fall within the percent positive range. Thus, small numbers of cells which fall in the positive range can have unusually large effects on MCF. In the case of C57BL/6, only 2.1% of gaited splenocytes fell within the positive range. The latter

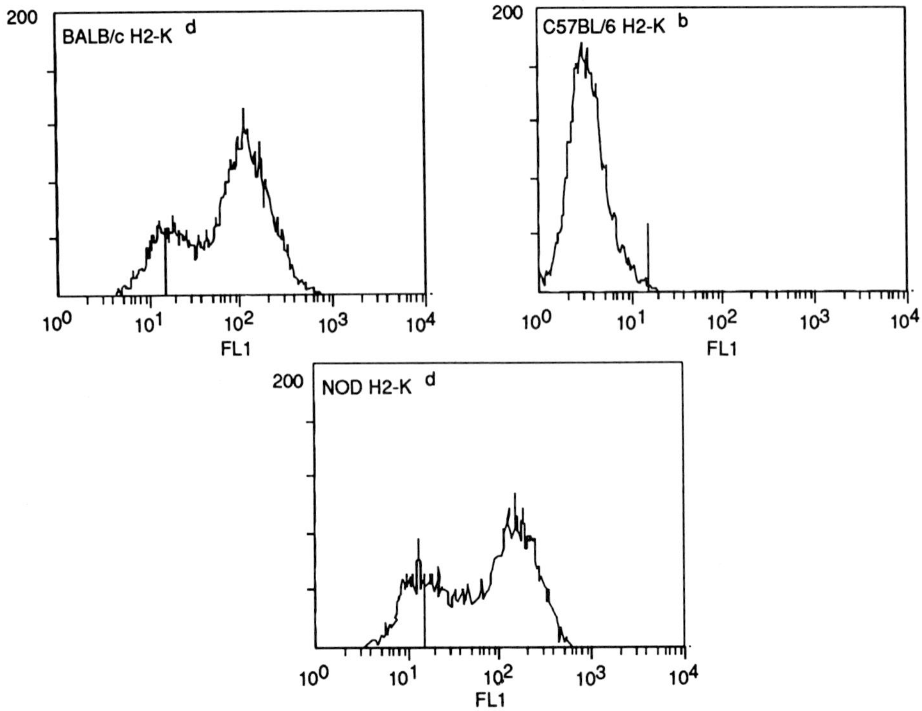

FIG. 10 For each strain of mice examined, cell number on the *y* axis was plotted against the channel fluorescence on the *x* axis (log scale). These data demonstrate that there was no difference between mean channel fluorescence in NOD and BALB/c mice for H-2K expression. The BALB/c was the positive control strain and C57BL/6 was the negative control strain.

result indicates that the anti-H-2K^d FITC-conjugated antibody used was very specific for the haplotype studied. In the case of C57BL/6, the MCF result is artifactual.

The results of our study are in contrast with those of Faustman and colleagues but are consistent with those of Wicker *et al.* (1992). This issue has

TABLE I Class I MHC H-2K^d Flow Cytometric Analysis

Strain	MCF	Percent positive
NOD	141.59	80.7
BALB/c	130.80	87.2
C57BL/6	180.66	2.1

generated considerable controversy (Hoffman, 1992a). In 1993, Faustman and colleagues extended their findings to a description of decreased class I MHC expression in a variety of autoimmune disorders (Fu *et al.*, 1993). If class I MHC expression was altered by the length of time *ex vivo* between cell isolation and flow cytometric analysis, Faustman and colleagues followed a very rapid protocol for splenocyte isolation and analysis. We used Percoll splenocyte isolation which lengthened the overall procedure to ~4 hr. According to the Harvard researchers, this problem might be exacerbated if cells were stored on ice because class I antigens that are not associated with endogenous peptide might be stabilized at low temperatures and could persist on the surface of the cell. In their view, this would cause a falsely high MCF. Extremely rapid procedures for splenocyte isolation and analysis may suffer from their limited ability to remove large amounts of cell debris producing large amounts of background signal. This may make analysis and calculation of MCF troublesome.

MHC and the Nervous System

Measuring class I MHC and/or class II MHC antigen (molecule) density on neurons and neuroglia can provide important data on the regulation of the immune response in health and disease. New frontiers to conquer concern the amelioration of autoimmune disease of the central nervous system (Steinman, 1993) and viral infection of the central nervous system with specific emphasis on control of the human immunodeficiency virus (Dickson *et al.*, 1991; Höllsberg and Hafler, 1993).

Acknowledgments

The authors thank Desmond Schatz, M.D., for advice and assistance in performing the flow cytometry studies. Mr. Buck was supported by a grant from the University of Florida College of Medicine.

References

G. Ballardini, R. Mirakian, F. B. Bianchi, E. Pisi, D. Doniach, and G. F. Bottazzo, *Lancet* **2,** 1009–1113 (1984).

R. B. Banati, J. Gehrmann, P. Schubert, and G. W. Kreutzberg, *Glia* **7,** 111–118 (1993).

M. Barinaga, *Science* **257,** 880–881 (1992).

P. J. Bjorkman, M. A. Saper, B. Samraoui, W. S. Bennet, J. L. Strominger, and D. C. Wiley, *Nature (London)* **329,** 512–518 (1987).

M. Blackman, J. Kappler, and P. Marrack, *Science* **248,** 1335–1341 (1990).

J. H. Brown, T. Jardetzky, M. A. Saper, B. Samraoui, P. J. Bjorkman, and D. C. Wiley, *Nature* (*London*) **332,** 845–850 (1988).

J. H. Brown, T. S. Jardetzky, J. C. Gorga, L. J. Stern, R. G. Urban, J. L. Strominger, and D. C. Wiley, *Nature* (*London*) **364,** 33–39 (1993).

M. G. Brown, J. Driscol, and J. J. Monaco, *Nature* (*London*) **353,** 355–357 (1991).

F. Burke, M. S. Naylor, B. Davies, and F. Balkwill, *Immunol. Today* **14,** 165–170, 1993.

R. D. Campbell and J. Trowsdale, *Immunol. Today* **14,** 349–352, 1993.

J. Cohen, *Science* **257,** 751 (1992).

G. R. Crabtree, *Science* **243,** 355–361 (1989).

A. L. DeFranco, *Nature* (*London*) **351,** 603–604 (1991).

D. C. DeNagel and S. K. Pierce, *Immunol. Today* **13,** 86–89 (1992).

D. W. Dickson, L. A. Mattiace, K. Kure, K. Hutchins, W. D. Lyman, and C. F. Brosnan, *Lab. Invest.* **64,** 135–156 (1991).

M. A. Dinome and D-E. Young, Jr., *Hosp. Practice* **22,** 59–66 (1987).

K. Falk, O. Rötzschke, S. Stevanović, G. Jung, and H.-G. Rammensee, *Nature* (*London*) **351,** 290–296 (1991).

D. Faustman, X. Li, H. Lin, Y. Fu, G. Eisenbarth, J. Avruch, and J. Guo, *Science* **254,** 1756–1761 (1991).

N. A. Flaris, T. L. Densmore, M. C. Molleston, and W. F. Hickey, *Glia* **7,** 34–40 (1993).

D. H. Fremont, M. Matsumura, E. A. Stura, P. A. Peterson, and I. A. Wilson, *Science* **257,** 919–927 (1992).

Y. Fu, D. M. Nathan, F. Li, X. Li, and D. L. Faustman, *J. Clin. Invest.* **91,** 2301–2307 (1993).

R. N. Germain, *Nature* (*London*) **322,** 687–689 (1986).

R. Glynne, S. H. Powis, S. Beck, A. Kelly, L-A. Kerr, and J. Trowsdale, *Nature* (*London*) **353,** 357–360 (1991).

A. L. Goldberg and K. L. Rock, *Nature* (*London*) **357,** 375–379 (1992).

C. L. Hitchcock, W. J. Riley, A. Alamo, R. Pyka, and N. K. Maclaren, *Diabetes* **35,** 1416–1422 (1986).

M. Hoffman, *Science* **255,** 531–534 (1992a).

M. Hoffman, *Science* **255,** 532–533 (1992b).

P. Höllsberg and D. A. Hafler, *N. Engl. J. Med.* **328,** 1173–1182 (1993).

N. Isakov, W. Scholz, and A. Altman, *Immunol. Today* **7,** 271–277 (1986).

C. A. Janeway, Jr., *Sci. Am.* **September,** 73–79 (1993).

M. Julius, C. R. Maroun, and L. Haughm, *Immunol. Today* **14,** 177–183 (1993).

C. H. June, J. A. Ledbetter, P. S. Linsley, and C. B. Thompson, *Immunol. Today* **11,** 211–216 (1990).

J. W. Kappler, U. Staerz, J. White, and P. Marrack, *Nature* (*London*) **332,** 35–45 (1989).

J. F. Kaufman, C. Auffray, A. J. Korman, D. A. Shackelford, and J. Strominger, *Cell* (*Cambridge, Mass.*) **36,** 1–13 (1984).

A. J. Korman, J. M. Boss, T. Spies, R. Sorrentino, K. Okada, and J. L. Strominger, *Immunol. Rev.* **85,** 45–86 (1985).

S. T. A. Malik, M. Raftery, Z. Varghese, P. Sweny, and J. R. Moorhead, *Lancet* **2,** 577–578 (1984).
J. Markmann, D. Lo, A. Naji, R. D. Palmiter, R. L. Brinster, and E. Heber-Katz, *Nature* (*London*) **2,** 476–479 (1988).
P. Marrack, *Science* **235,** 1311–1313 (1987).
P. Marrack and J. W. Kappler, *Sci. Am.* **September,** 81–89, 1993.
J. L. Marx, *Science* **231,** 1367–1369 (1986).
A. Miyajima, S. Miyatake, J. Schreurs, J. De Vries, N. Arai, T. Yokota, and K-I Arai, *FASEB J.* **2,** 2462–2473 (1988).
J. J. Monaco, *Immunol. Today* **13,** 173–179 (1992).
C. D. Myers, *FASEB J.* **5,** 2547–2553 (1991).
J. J. Nefjes and H. L. Ploegh, *Immunol. Today* **13,** 179–184 (1992).
B. S. Nepom, D. Schwarz, J. P. Palmer, and G. T. Nepom, *Diabetes* **36,** 114–117 (1987).
R. J. Noelle and E. C. Snow, *FASEB J.* **5,** 2770–2776 (1991).
G. J. V. Nossal, *N. Engl. J. Med.* **316,** 1320–1325 (1987).
G. J. V. Nossal, *Science* **245,** 147–153 (1989).
G. J. V. Nossal, *Sci. Am.* **September,** 53–62 (1993).
A. M. O'Rourke and M. F. Mescher, *Immunol. Today* **14,** 183–188 (1993).
V. Ortiz-Navarrete, A. Seelig, M. Gernold, S. Frentzel, P. M. Kloetzel, and G. J. Hämmerling, *Nature* (*London*) **353,** 662–664 (1991).
P. Parham, *Nature* (*London*) **357,** 193–194 (1992).
J. B. Peter and B. R. Hawkins, *Arch. Pathol. Lab. Med.* **116,** 11–15 (1992).
H. Ploegh and P. Benaroch, *Nature* (*London*) **364,** 16–17 (1993).
S. J. Powis, E. V. Deverson, W. J. Coadwell, A. Ciruela, N. S. Huskisson, H. Smith, G. W. Butcher, and J. C. Howard, *Nature* (*London*) **357,** 211–215 (1992).
F. Ramsdell and B. J. Fowlkes, *Science* **248,** 1342–1348 (1990).
M. Robertson, *Nature* (*London*) **311,** 305–306 (1984a).
M. Robertson, *Nature* (*London*) **312,** 16–17 (1984b).
M. Robertson, *Nature* (*London*) **353,** 300–301 (1991).
M. Röcken, J. F. Urban, and E. M. Shevach, *Nature* (*London*) **359,** 79–82 (1992).
H. D. Royer and E. L. Reinhertz, *N. Engl. J. Med.* **317,** 1136–1142 (1987).
A. Y. Rudensky, P. Preston-Hurlburt, S-C. Hong, A. Barlow, and C. A. Janeway Jr., *Nature* (*London*) **353,** 622–627 (1991).
P. Salgame, J. S. Abrams, C. Clayberger, H. Goldstein, J. Convit, R. L. Modlin, and B. R. Bloom, *Science* **254,** 279–282 (1991).
A. A. Sinha, M. T. Lopez, and H. O. McDevitt, *Science* **248,** 1380–1388 (1990).
T. Spies, M. Bresnahan, S. Bahram, D. Arnold, G. Blanck, E. Mellins, D. Pious, and R. DeMars, *Nature* (*London*) **348,** 744–747 (1990).
L. Steinman, *Sci. Am.* **September,** 107–114 (1993).
M. Steinmetz and L. Hood, *Science* **222,** 727–733 (1983).
N. E. Street and T. R. Mosmann, *FASEB J.* **5,** 171–176 (1991).
J. L. Strominger, *Science* **244,** 943–950 (1989).
L. Teyton, D. O'Sullivan, P. W. Dickson, V. Lotteau, A. Sette, P. Fink, P. A. Peterson, *Nature* (*London*) **348,** 39–44 (1990).

D. P. Theele and W. J. Streit, *Glia* **7,** 5–8 (1993).

J. A. Todd, J. I. Bell, and H. O. McDevitt, *Nature* (*London*) **329,** 599–604 (1987).

J. A. Todd, H. Acha-Orbea, J. I. Bell, N. Chao, Z. Fronek, C. O. Jacob, M. McDermott, A. A. Sinha, L. Timmerman, L. Steinman, and H. O. McDevitt, *Science* **240,** 1003–1008 (1990).

E. R. Unanue and P. M. Allen, *Science* **236,** 551–557 (1987).

H. von Boehmer, *Annu. Rev. Immunol.* **6,** 309–326 (1988).

H. von Boehmer and P. Kisielow, *Science* **248,** 1369–1373 (1990).

L. S. Wicker, P. L. Podolin, P. Fischer, A. Sirotino, R. C. Boltz, and L. B. Peterson, *Science* **256,** 1828–1830 (1992).

K. Williams, A. Bar-Or, E. Ulvestad, A. Olivier, J. P. Antel, and V. W. Yong, *J. Neuropathol. Exp. Neurol.* **51,** 538–549 (1992).

W. E. Winter, A. Muir, N. K. Maclaren, and M. Obata, *Growth: Genet. Hormones* **7,** 1–6 (1991a).

W. E. Winter, M. Obata, and N. K. Maclaren, *Concepts Immunopathol.* **8,** 189–221 (1991b).

[6] *In Vitro* Immunoglobulin E-Mediated and -Independent Histamine Release from Human Basophil Leukocytes

A. Miadonna, M. Palella, M. P. Di Marco, and A. Tedeschi

Introduction

Basophils are primary effector cells of immediate anaphylactic reactions. Antigen stimulation of human basophils leads to the release of inflammatory mediators such as histamine and leukotriene C_4 (LTC_4). The evaluation of antigen-induced basophil histamine release offers an *in vitro* model of an allergic reaction.

Peripheral blood basophils were first identified in 1878 by Paul Ehrlich on the basis of the metachromatic staining properties of their cytoplasmic granules. Basophils share a common precursor with other granulocytes and monocytes. They differentiate and mature in the bone marrow, circulate in the blood, and are not normally found in connective tissue. The prevalence of basophils in peripheral blood is approximately 0.5% of total leukocytes. When examined by electron microscopy basophils are 5–7 μm in size and present a segmented nucleus with a heavily condensed chromatin; a nucleolus is generally not seen. These cells contain cytoplasmic granules which may easily be visualized using toluidine blue or alcian blue staining.

Basophils express high-affinity plasma membrane receptors (Fc and RI) that specifically bind the Fc portion of immunoglobulin E (IgE) antibodies. After active or passive sensitization with a specific IgE, exposure to antigen triggers a series of biochemical and ultrastructural events which lead to degranulation and release of both preformed (granule-associated mediators such as histamine, heparin, and proteases) and newly generated mediators (LTC_4).

Activators of human basophils can be classified into IgE-dependent (antigen, anti-IgE, anti-Fcε receptor, concanavalin A) and IgE-independent (Ca^{2+} ionophore A23187, formylmethionylleucylphenylalanine peptide, hyperosmolarity, phorbol esters, interleukin 3, C5a) stimuli.

In this chapter we present the basic requirements necessary for carrying out in the laboratory histamine release from basophils. The information allows researchers to repeat successfully procedures employed in our laboratory and is presented under three headings: (A) Separation and Purification

Methods in Neurosciences, Volume 24

of Human Basophils, (B) *In vitro* Stimuli for Histamine Release from Human Basophils, and (C) Histamine Release Assay. Information regarding suppliers can be found in the appendix at the end of this chapter.

Separation and Purification Methods of Human Basophils

Solutions Utilized by Various Methods

10× Tyrode's buffer: NaCl, 80 g; KCl, 2 g; dextrose, 9.9 g; $NaHCO_3$, 10 g; NaH_2PO_4, 0.5 g; 950 ml doubly distilled H_2O.

1× Tyrode's buffer: 1/10 dilution of 10× Tyrode's buffer. For example, 1 liter = 100 ml 10× Tyrode's buffer + 900 ml doubly distilled H_2O. It is employed to wash the cells after separation (pH 7.2–7.4).

HEPES-buffered Tyrode: NaCl, 135 m*M*, KCl, 2.6 m*M*, HEPES, 10 m*M*, glucose, 5.5 m*M*, pH 7.4.

Ethylenediaminetetraacetic acid disodium salt 0.1 *M* (EDTA): 3.75 g in 100 ml of doubly distilled H_2O. This is employed as an anticoagulant and a chelating agent. Add 1 ml of EDTA to every 10 ml of blood.

EDTA (0.01 *M*): Dilute 1/10 0.1 *M* EDTA and 0.9% (w/v) NaCl. For example, 100 ml = 10 ml EDTA (0.1 *M*) + 90 ml saline solution 0.9%. This solution is used as anticoagulant for Alcian blue staining.

The solutions are stored at 4–8°C and employed within 1 week. Freezing at −25°C is suggested for longer storage.

Staining Methods

Alcian Blue

NaCl 0.9 g; cetylpyridinium chloride, 76 mg; $LaCl_3 \cdot 7H_2O$, 700 mg; Tween 20,200 μl; Alcian blue 143 mg; 98 ml doubly distilled H_2O. Vortex and warm gently for about 24 hr, then filtrate twice using a common filtrating paper (pH 7–7.5). Filtrate again every week. Basophils will appear green-blue, whereas all the other cells are not stained. This staining method is elective for evaluating basophil concentration in leukocyte suspensions.

Staining technique: 400 μl of 0.01 *M* EDTA (see above); 450 μl Alcian blue; 100 μl cell solution. Vortex and then add 50 μl 1 *N* HCl and vortex again (1).

Toluidine Blue

Toluidine blue, 75 mg; 95% ethanol, 25 ml; doubly distilled H_2O, 75 ml; pH 3.4 (to adjust pH use a few drops of acetic acid). Basophils appear red and the other cells show a blue nucleus.

Staining technique: 90 μl toluidine blue; 10 μl cell solution (2).

Total basophil count is performed in a Fuchs–Rosenthal chamber (Walter Schrenck, Hofheim am Taunus, Germany). Use the following to determine total count: Number of counted basophils × 3.13 = number of basophils/mmc (3).

Dextran Sedimentation

Dextran solution: Anhydrous glucose, 7.5 g; 6% dextran 70 in saline solution, 240 ml.

The venous blood is drawn into plastic tubes containing 0.1 *M* EDTA (see above).

Add 6% dextran solution (500 μl every 1 ml of blood). Agitate gently. Take off the top of the tube and let the solution settle for at least 60–90 min at room temperature. Take up the leukocyte-rich plasma by using Pasteur pipettes (taking care not to pick up the red zone) and then centrifuge at 400 *g* at 4°C for at least 10 min. Then the cell pellet is washed twice in 1× Tyrode's buffer (fill the plastic tubes) (4).

Dextran sedimentation is used for obtaining leukocyte-rich suspensions with contaminating cells other than basophils (monocytes, neutrophils, eosinophils, lymphocytes). Basophil concentration in the leukocyte suspensions is evaluated by staining methods (see above).

Percoll Separation

Reagents Employed

Percoll (polyvinylpyrrolidone-coated colloidal silica) solution; 10× Tyrode's buffer (see above).

Preparation of Percoll Densities

Percoll densities are necessary to obtain the separation of different cells from peripheral blood.

Isosmotic Percoll solution (IPS) contains 90% Percoll solution; 9% 10× Tyrode's buffer without Ca^{2+} or Mg^{2+}; 1% HEPES buffer, pH 7.4. Prepare isosmotic solutions of specified density by mixing the IPS with 1× Tyrode's buffer. Volume ratios of IPS to Tyrode's buffer are approximately 1.7 and 1.2 for Percoll solutions of density 1.078 and 1.070 g/liter, respectively. Layer a discontinuous gradient of Percoll (5 ml) into polystyrene conical-bottom centrifuge tubes and then layer anticoagulated blood. A steady rate of blood flow is assured by applying the tip of the pipette to the side of the tube about 5 to 10 mm above the meniscus of Percoll and controlling the flow very carefully. When run improperly, even if a small amount of blood enters the Percoll or if the pipette penetrates the Percoll layer inadvertently, the density of Percoll is affected. In such cases the procedure should be repeated. After layering blood over Percoll, the tubes are centrifuged at 600 *g* for 10 min at room temperature to obtain a clear band of mononuclear cells at the interface between plasma and Percoll and a dense band of neutrophils and eosinophils immediately above the packed red blood cells at the bottom. Basophil cells make a ring at the interface between the different densities of Percoll (1.078–1.070 g/liter). After centrifugation, the plasma layer and the mononuclear cell layer at the interface are removed together, and most of the Percoll layer is removed separately. Great care is taken to remove all of the mononuclear cell layer and to avoid disturbing the neutrophils situated beneath the Percoll layer, because admixture of even a small number of these cells in the Percoll leads to a decrease in basophil purity due to a "dilution effect." Then the cells are washed twice in 1× Tyrode's buffer and are ready to be stained and counted (see above) (5).

With this method, total basophil recovery by combining interface and Percoll layers is maximal at 1.078 g/liter.

Ficoll–Lymphoprep Separation

Ficoll is a commercially available solution for the preparation of lymphocyte suspensions. The most common technique for separating leukocytes is to collect blood into a centrifuge tube and to mix it with a compound which aggregates erythrocytes, thereby increasing their sedimentation rate (from a dilution of whole blood with 1× Hanks' balanced salt solution; ratio of dilution 1 : 2).

Carefully layer the diluted and anticoagulated blood (2/3) over Lymphoprep (1/3). Avoid mixing the blood and separation fluid.

Cap the tube to prevent the formation of aerosols. Centrifuge at 800 *g* for 20 min at room temperature. If the blood is stored for more than 2 hr, increase the centrifugation time to 30 min. Use a Pasteur pipette to remove the mononuclear cells which form a distinct band at the sample/medium interface (do not remove the upper layer).

The contamination of erythrocytes in the lymphocyte suspension is usually between 1 and 5% of the total cell number (6, 7).

Basophil Separation by Elutriation

This method is employed to obtain a high percentage of basophils (60–80%) in leukocyte suspensions. A buffy coat of 500 ml of blood is layered over a Percoll gradient, obtained using two Percoll solutions with a specific gravity of 1.079 and 1.070 g/liter, and centrifuged for 20 min at 20°C (2100 rpm). The fraction at the interface between the two Percoll solutions is injected in an elutriator centrifugation system (Beckman J2-21C centrifuge with a JE-6B elutriation rotor). The elutriation medium consists of Tyrode's buffer without Ca^{2+} and Mg^{2+} and contains 13 m*M* trisodium citrate and 5 mg/ml of human serum albumin. After cell injection, the centrifuge is started (4000 rpm at room temperature). To separate basophils, the flow rate is maintained constant at 20 ml/min, while the rotor speed is reduced progressively from 4000 to 0 rpm.

For fraction 1, a 150-ml volume is collected which contains the remainder of the platelets, between 4000 and 3700 rpm.

Fraction 2 (250 ml) is collected when the rotor speed is slowly reduced to 2600 rpm. Lymphocytes and erythrocytes are mainly contained in this fraction.

Fraction 3 (150 ml) is collected when the rotor spseed is lowered from 2600 to 1000 rpm. This fraction contains monocytes.

Fraction 4 is collected in 100 ml at 0 rpm and contains basophils but is usually contaminated with monocytes and lymphocytes. This fraction is then centrifuged at 400 *g* for 5 min at 20°C and resuspended in Ca^{2+}-free Tyrode's buffer with 13 m*M* trisodium citrate and 5 g/liter human serum albumin. The cell suspension is layered on two Percoll solutions with a specific gravity of 1.075 and 1.068 g/liter, respectively, and centrifuged at 1000 *g* for 15 min at 20°C. After centrifugation, cells are harvested from the two interfaces in each gradient. The upper interface contains monocytes; the lower interface, containing basophils, is washed and resuspended in Tyrode's buffer with Ca^{2+} and Mg^{2+} for cell counting (8).

Basophil Purification by Monoclonal Antibodies Coupled to Dynabeads

Dynabeads are uniform supermagnetic microspheres of polystyrene which are in suspension when they are not attracted by a magnetic field. If they are coated with adequate ligands, they selectively recognize and bind specific targets. In this way target cells may be isolated by exposition to a magnetic field. Cells are attracted and retained in the wall of the tubes, and supernatant is separated by aspiration or decantation.

To obtain a high percentage of basophil purification from whole blood or buffy coat, two separation methods may be used such as dextran sedimentation or Ficoll–Lymphoprep followed by centrifugation on a discontinuous Percoll gradient. In this way, the lymphocyte/basophil fraction is ready for purification with Dynabeads. We propose the following protocol:

1. Incubate leukocytes and monoclonal antibodies of choice for 30 min on ice in 3 ml of sterile PBS (phosphate-buffered saline). For basophil separation a mixture of monoclonal antibodies against the contaminating cells (CD2, CD14, and CD16 at 1 μg/ml and CD19 at 2 μg/ml) can be used. A cocktail of antibodies, reacting with several cell-surface antigens, is more efficient than separation using a single antibody. After this incubation, wash the cells in incubation medium.

TABLE I Separation of Human Basophil Leukocytes

Separation technique[a]	Time (min)	Ease[b]	Purity (%)	Cost
1. Dextran	60–90	++++	1–2	Very low
2. Ficoll–Lymphoprep	60	+++	1–8	Low
3. Percoll	120	++	1–15	Moderate
4. Elutriation	240	+	20–90	High
5. Dynabeads	60	++	70–97	Very high

[a] Best results may be obtained using the following sequences: 1–3; 1–3–4; 1–3–4–5; 1–3–5. Time multiplies accordingly.
[b] (+ + + +) Not difficult; (+ + +) some difficulties; (+ +) quite difficult; (+) very difficult.

2. Incubate cells in a head-over-head rotator (angle 10°) for 1 hr at 4°C with goat anti-mouse IgG-coated magnetic Dynabeads (ratio of beads to cells, 5 : 1).

3. Shake the bottle to resuspend beads. Centrifuge tube must be placed for 2–3 min in the magnetic rack; in this way beads adhere to the side of the tube. Without removing the tube, aspirate the supernatant with a Pasteur pipette at the opposite side of the tube (where beads are bound). Add sterile PBS (do not let the beads dry out) to the aspirated solution. Agitate by hand with care to resuspend the solution. Remove any residual beads by placing the tube in the magnetic rack and allowing the beads to adhere. Repeat this procedure twice to ensure efficient depletion. Do not let beads sit in the magnetic rack; remove from the rack after washing.

4. After addition of this supernatant to the first supernatant, wash and resuspend the cell suspension in PBS supplemented with 1 m*M* Ca^{2+}.

5. Elective staining procedures for basophils such as alcian blue or toluidine blue and May–Grunwald Giemsa stain can be used to assess the purity of basophil suspensions (9). The procedure may result in a basophil purity of more than 90%.

Advantages and disadvantages of the separation methods of human basophil leukoycytes are shown in Table I.

In Vitro Stimuli for Histamine Release from Human Basophils

There are many different secretagogues which release histamine from human basophils through IgE-dependent and IgE-independent biochemical pathways. Membrane IgE cross-linking by antigen activates a variety of membrane-associated enzymes, with mobilization of intracellular Ca^{2+} and transmembrane Ca^{2+} flux from the extracellular to the intracellular medium. Increasing intracellular Ca^{2+} leads to modulation of different biochemical pathways, such as the activation of protein kinase C (PKC), granular membrane fusion, and degranulation.

Histamine release induced by IgE-independent stimuli involves biochemical steps which may differ from one stimulus to another. The optimal dose for each stimulus must be determined by dose–response curves.

Immunoglobulin E-Dependent in Vitro Stimuli

Antigen challenge of sensitized basophils leads to histamine release. Of course, this challenge can be performed only with cells obtained from sensitized subjects, who have circulating and cell-bound antigen-specific IgE antibodies.

Human anti-IgE is a useful stimulus for experimental purposes because it induces an IgE-mediated basophil activation also in subjects without documented type 1 allergy.

Anti-IgE antiserum after reconstitution may be frozen and stored in working aliquots. Repeated freezing and thawing of anti-IgE can alter its efficiency. The optimal doses of anti-IgE antisera from different sources must be identified by dose–response curves which must be determined in every laboratory. Analysis of release kinetic indicates that anti-IgE-induced histamine release is optimal after incubation for 15 min ($t_{1/2}$ about 4 min). The optimal temperature of incubation is 37°C. Extracellular Ca^{2+} is required for anti-IgE-induced histamine release.

Concanavalin A (Con A) induces cross-linking of IgE antibodies (through the Fc portion) and then triggers basophil histamine release. Histamine release is Ca^{2+}-dependent and 45 min of incubation is required. The temperature optimum is 37°C.

Immunoglobulin E-Independent in Vitro Stimuli

The Ca^{2+} ionophore A23187 is a lipid-soluble antibiotic which carries Ca^{2+} ions across various biological membranes bypassing calcium channels. The compound must be dissolved in dimethyl sulfoxide (DMSO) and then stored at 4–8°C. The doses employed range from 0.1 to 1 μM.

Phorbol 12-myristate 13-acetate (PMA) or tetradecanoylphorbol 13-acetate (TPA) activates PKC and does not require extracellular Ca^{2+} to evoke histamine release. The histamine release induced by PMA is remarkably slow when compared for instance with anti-IgE or FMLP. After the addition of PMA a lag time of about 10 min occurs and the release reaction is completed in about 1 hr. This stimulus must be solubilized in ethanol and then stored at −20°C; the concentrations used range from 10 to 150 nM.

Interleukin 3 (IL-3) enhances histamine release from human basophils and is able to induce histamine release, in particular from basophils of allergic subjects. The dose–response range is between 0.4 and 400 ng/ml. Low concentrations of IL-3, insufficient to cause basophil histamine release, can prime cells and markedly augment their responsiveness to other secretagogues, including anti-IgE and C5a. Interleukin 3 binds to a specific membrane receptor and activates basophils. Also, IL-3 binds to a specific receptor on basophil membranes which is different from the IgE receptor. Further, IL-3 induces histamine-release peaks after 120 min and is already detectable after 2 min incubation; the effect is optimal at 37°C, although a lower histamine-releasing activity can also be detected at 4 and 20°C (15). These kinetics are different from those observed when basophils are stimulated with anti-IgE, since IgE-dependent histamine release is completed after the first 15 min. Interleukin 3 can be stored at −20°C.

The activation of serum complement with inactive zymosan, a peptide produced by *Saccharomyces cerevisiae,* generates C5a which releases histamine from human basophils. C5a can induce histamine release, but not leukotriene synthesis, and requires the presence of Ca^{2+} ions in the extracellular medium. C5a, at all concentrations, releases histamine completely in less than 2 min (more rapid than IgE-mediated reactions); the temperature optimum occurs from 17 to 37°C but histamine release does not occur at 0°C. The effect of C5a on histamine release is not enhanced by deuterium oxide; however, C5a becomes a complete agonist in the presence of D_2O because under these conditions it provokes leukotriene production. C5a can be stored at −20°C.

Formylmethionylleucylphenylalanine (FMLP) is a formylated peptide similar to bacterial products since many bacterial proteins terminate with a formylmethionine sequence. FMLP-induced histamine release requires Ca^{2+} ions in the extracellular medium and is essentially complete within 2 min ($t_{1/2}$ <30 sec) at temperatures of 25, 30, and 37°C, but does not occur at 0°C. There is no correlation in the capacity of basophils to release histamine with FMLP and their release with C5a or anti-IgE. In fact, FMLP binds to a membrane receptor which is different from IgE and C5a receptor and activates a pertussis toxin-sensitive G protein. In contrast to anti-IgE, FMLP does not cause any increase in protein kinase C (PKC) activity and activates a PKC-independent biochemical pathway. However, FMLP is a complete secretagogue in that it induces release of both histamine and leukotriene. The concentrations used range from 0.1 to 1 μM and it can be stored at −20°C.

In osmotic environments of greater than 280 mOsm/kg H_2O, human basophils are activated and secrete histamine. *In vitro* experiments indicate that hyperosmolarity is an incomplete signal since it can trigger optimal histamine release, but little leukotriene synthesis by human basophils. Hyperosmolarity may be created by mannitol, glucose, sucrose, or NaCl. Basophil histamine release starts at approximately 460 mOsm/kg and is maximal at about 770 mOsm/kg. Histamine release is partially Ca^{2+}-dependent and 45 to 60 min of incubation is required. The temperature optimum is 32°C. Osmotically activated basophils show no ultrastructural evidence of cell death. Osmotic and IgE-dependent release interact synergistically in basophils.

Histamine-Release Assay

Several methods for the determination of histamine and its metabolites are available.

Fluorometric Method

Histamine concentration in the cell supernatants may be evaluated by an automated fluorometric method, modified from Ruff *et al.* (1967).

The system can be used with a broad range of histamine concentrations and at the highest sensitivity it is capable of analyzing samples which contain 1 ng of histamine. When samples have a large amount of protein, the sensitivity is lower. This method is based on histamine extraction and fluorometric lecture as described: 6% perchloric acid is added to the sample of histamine. Then histamine is separated by isobutyl alcohol in alkaline solution (NaCl + NaOH) and then is separated again by isooctane in acid solution (H_2SO_4 0.2 *N*). Subsequently, the sample binds to the orthophthalaldehyde in alkaline solution (1.1 *N* NaOH). Fluorescence is measured in an acid medium (0.25 *N* H_3PO_4) by the fluorimeter using the UV lamp (320 nm).

Percentage of histamine release is calculated as follows: % release = $[(e - s)/(t)] \times 100$, where e is the fluorometric reading for experimental supernatant; s, spontaneous histamine release; t, total histamine content. Perchloric acid (6%) is added to some samples to obtain the total histamine content of the cell suspension (10–12).

Bioassay

The histamine concentration in leukocyte supernatants may also be evaluated by bioassay. The major problem with this method is its low sensitivity.

Pieces of terminal ileum (2-cm long), from guinea pigs weighing 300–400 g and fasted overnight, are mounted longitudinally, according to the laminar flow technique of Ferreira *et al.* (13). The ileum pieces are superfused at a flow rate of 0.2 ml/min with Krebs solution having the following composition (millimolar): NaCl (118), KCl (4.6), $CaCl_2$ (1.8), $MgCl_2$ (0.5), NaH_2PO_4 (1.0), $NaHCO_3$ (24.9), and glucose (11.1). The solution is aerated with 95% O_2/5% CO_2 (v/v).

The tissue is thermostatted at 37°C and contractions recorded using an isotonic force transducer (Basile, Comerio, Italy) connected to a two-channel recorder (Basile).

The resting tension is 2 g and after about 1 hr of equilibration, the sensitivity of the preparations to repeated bolus administration of histamine is tested. Segments of low sensitivity, high variability, and inability to maintain a steady baseline tone are discarded.

The preparations are pretreated with FPL 55712 (10 μM) and scopolamin and are standardized to respond to 1, 2, 4, 8, and 16 ng of histamine dihydrochloride until stable and reproducible responses are obtained and a dose–response curve drawn.

Aliquots of the test solutions not exceeding 0.1 ml are administered as bolus in order to produce about the same contractions as obtained with an intervening dose of histamine.

The addition of standards to the preparations causes an instantaneous and brief contraction of the same quality as those produced by test solutions.

The contactile potency of the test solutions on longitudinal strips of the guinea pig ileum is expressed as histamine dihydrochloride. Finally, in order to verify the specificity of the assay, the same histamine standards as well as the test solutions are repeated in the presence of 0.5 μM mepyramine, which fully antagonizes the contractions.

Immunoassay for Histamine

The immunoassay is sensitive and rapid. One method is based on competitive inhibition between histamine and labeled histamine conjugate for the antigen-binding sites of the antibodies. The separation step is performed by the addition of solid-phase bound anti-mouse subclass specific antibody. The sensitivity of the assay is 0.2 ng/ml for histamine.

The principle of the procedure is the following: histamine in the sample competes with a fixed amount of ^{125}I-labeled histamine–albumin complex for the binding sites of the specific monoclonal antibodies. Antibody-bound material is separated by the addition of a second antibody immunoadsorbent followed by a second incubation, centrifugation, and decanting. The radioactivity in the pellet is then measured and is inversely proportional to the quantity of histamine in the sample.

An alternative method, radioimmunoassay (RIA), utilizes monoclonal antibodies against acylated histamine (14).

Advantages and disadvantages of the histamine assays are presented in Table II.

TABLE II Histamine Assays

Method	Ease[a]	Cost	Sensitivity	Specificity
Fluorometric	+ +	Low	Good	Good
Bioassay	+	Moderate	Poor	Good
Immunoassay	+ + +	High	Very good	Very high

[a] (+++) Not difficult; (++) some difficulties; (+) quite difficult.

Appendix

A partial list of materials and suppliers is included and addresses of chemical companies are given at the end of the Appendix.

Compounds

Stimuli Methodology

Anti-human IgE: Behring Institute, Nordic Immunology Laboratories, Sigma
Calcium ionophore A23187: ICN Biochemicals, Sigma, Calbiochem
Concanavalin A: Calbiochem-Behring, ICN Biochemicals, Sigma, Aldrich
FMLP: ICN Biochemicals, Sigma
Interleukin 3: Amersham Int. plc, Boehringer-Mannheim, Genzyme Corp.
Phorbol 12-Myristate 13-Acetate: ICN Biochemicals, Sigma
Zymosan A: Sigma, ICN Biochemicals

Staining Methods

Alcian Blue and Toluidine Blue: Sigma, Aldrich, ICN Biochemicals, Merck

Separation Methods

Dextran: ICN Biochemicals, Pharmacia, Sigma, Aldrich
Dynabeads: Dynal A.S.
EDTA: ICN Biochemicals, Sigma, Aldrich
HEPES buffer: GIBCO, Sigma, Aldrich, ICN Biochemicals
Lymphoprep: Nycomed Pharma, Sigma (Histopaque)
Percoll: Pharmacia LKB Biotechnology, Sigma

Addresses of Suppliers

Aldrich
1001 West St. Paul Avenue
Milwaukee, WI 53233

Amersham International plc
Amersham Place, Little Chalfont
Bucks HP7 9NA, United Kingdom

Behring Institute
Behringwerke AG, Marburg, Germany

Boehringer-Mannheim GmbH, Biochemica
Mannheim, Germany

Calbiochem-Novabiochem
10394 Pacific Center Court
San Diego, CA 92121

Dynal A.S.
Oslo, Norway

Genzyme Corp.
50 Gibson Drive
Kent Me19 6HG, United Kingdom

GIBCO
3175 Staley Road
Grand Island, NY 14072

ICN Biomedicals, Inc.
3300 Hyland Avenue
Costa Mesa, CA 92626

Merck Frosst Laboratories D-6100
Darmstadt, Germany

NYCOMED PHARMA AS
Oslo, Norway

Nordic Immunology Laboratories
Tilburg, The Netherlands

Pharmacia Diagnostics AB
Uppsala, Sweden

Sigma Chemical Company
P.O. Box 14508
St. Louis, MO 63178

References

1. H. S. Gilbert and L. Ornstein, *Blood* **46,** 279–286 (1975).
2. J. Benveniste, *Clin. Allergy* **11,** 111 (1981).

3. J. E. Moore and G. W. James, *Proc. Soc. Exp. Biol. Med.* **82,** 601 (1953).
4. L. M. Lichtenstein and A. G. Osler, *J. Exp. Med.* **120,** 507–530 (1964).
5. E. J. Leonard, R. L. Roberts, and A. Skeel, *J. Allergy Clin. Immunol.* **76,** 556–562 (1985).
6. A. Boyum, *Nature (London)* **204,** 793 (1964).
7. A. Boyum, *Scand. J. Clin. Invest.* **21** (Suppl. 97) (1964).
8. M. De Boer and D. Ross, *J. Immunol.* **136,** 3447–3454 (1986).
9. F. P. J. Mul, E. F. Knol, and D. Roos, *J. Immunol.* **149,** 207–214 (1992).
10. F. Ruff, A. Saindelle, E. Dutripon, and J. L. Parrot, *Nature (London)* **214,** 279–281 (1967).
11. R. P. Siraganian, *J. Immunol.* **7,** 283–290 (1975).
12. R. P. Siraganian and M. J. Brodsky, *J. Allergy Clin. Immunol.* **57,** 525–539 (1976).
13. S. H. Ferreira and F. De Souza Costa, *Eur. J. Pharmacol.* **39,** 279 (1976).
14. E. Hammar, A. Berglung, A. Hedin, A. Normann, K. Rustas, U. Ytterstrom, and E. Akerblom, *J. Immunol. Methods* **128,** 51–58 (1990).
15. A. Miadonna, M. G. Roncarolo, M. Lorini, and A. Tedeschi, *Clin. Immunol. Immunopathol.* **67,** 210–215 (1993).

[7] Immunopharmacological Methods to Study Murine Allogeneic and Syngeneic Pregnancy

María Elena Sales and Enri S. Borda

Introduction

The bidirectional interaction between the neuroendorine and immune systems has been largely documented. We have specifically demonstrated that alloimmunization triggers a regulatory mechanism that modifies β-adrenergic receptor expression on uterine membranes (1). The activation of β-adrenergic receptors mediates smooth muscle relaxation in humans, as well as in experimental animals (2, 3) and, for this reason, it plays an important role in the maintenance of uterine quiescence during pregnancy and in the prevention of premature labor (4).

We have also shown that antibodies produced by alloimmunization can elicit biological effects through the activation of postsynaptic β-adrenoceptors. In this way alloantibodies inhibit the spontaneous motility of the murine oviductal tract (5).

During pregnancy, the maternal production of alloimmune antibodies against paternal antigens has been largely documented (6). In the mouse, maternal immune response to paternal antigens is restricted to certain strain combinations and it is probably associated with an immune response gene located in or close to the H-2 locus (7). Thus, we have developed experimental procedures to show that allogeneic pregnancy immunoglobulin G (IgG) interacts with C3H uterine β-adrenoceptors decreasing the spontaneous motility of IgG and increasing cAMP production. Moreover, allogeneic pregnancy IgG fixates on uterine tissue and interferes with the binding of a specific β-adrenergic radioligand behaving as a noncompetitive inhibitor.

Animals

Virgin female inbred mice from Comisión Nacional de Energía Atómica are used throughout the study. All animals are 60–90 days old. BALB/c mice (H-2^d) and C3H mice (H-2^k) are chosen for experimental procedures and their H-2 haplotypes are checked by microcytotoxicity testing using monospecific alloimmune sera as described previously (8).

Only females exhibiting a 4-day estrous cycle are selected and the stage

Methods in Neurosciences, Volume 24

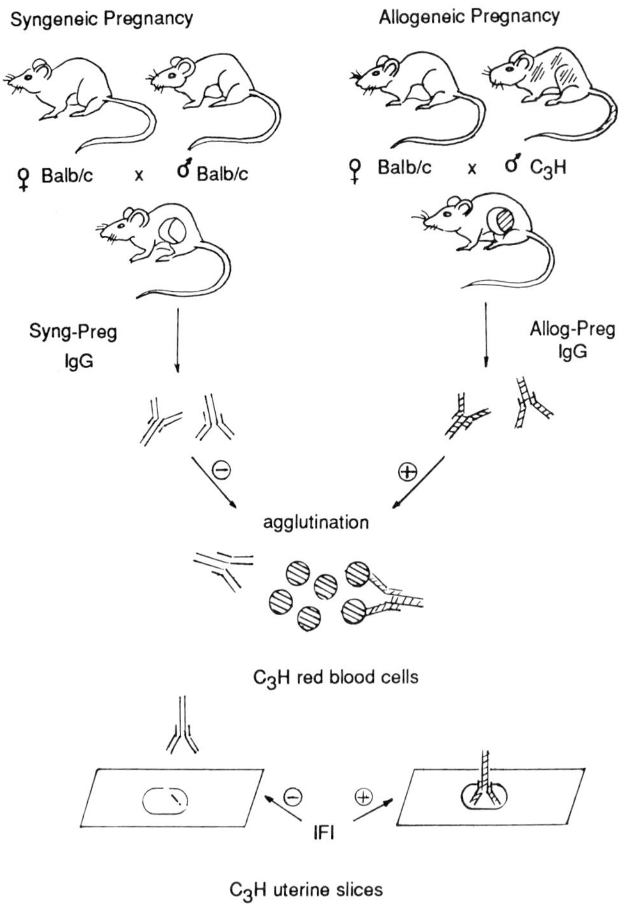

FIG. 1 Development of allogenic pregnancy (Allog-Preg) model (BALB/c × C3H) from which allogenic pregnancy IgG is obtained. Syngeneic pregnancy (Syng-Preg) (BALB/c × BALB/c) is the immunologic control of the model.

of the estrous cycle is determined on the basis of the cellular composition of vaginal fluid, which is examined daily at the same time.

In order to obtain an allogeneic pregnancy female BALB/c mice are mated with C3H male mice (Fig. 1). The mating is done in proestrus since ovulation normally occurs at the beginning of the late estrus (9). The day on which vaginal plug is found is designated as Day 1 of allogeneic pregnancy. To obtain syngeneic pregnant animals BALB/c female mice are caged in proestrus with BALB/c males and pregnancy is detected following the same procedure described above. The control group (nonpregnant animals) is composed of BALB/c and/or C3H female mice in diestrus. Animals are kept in a room with controlled temperature and illumination (14 hr light and 10 hr dark), fed Purina mouse chow, and allowed unrestricted access to water.

Production of Antibodies

Purification of Immunoglobulins

Sera from pregnant and nonpregnant female mice are obtained by ocular bleeding. Whole blood is left at 37°C for 30 min; it is centrifuged at 1500 rpm for 10 min to remove blood cells and then centrifuged, for a second time, at 4000 rpm for 15 min at 4°C to separate denaturated proteins.

Immunoglobulins are precipitated according to a previously reported procedure (10). An equal volume of 70% (w/v) saturated ammonium sulfate solution (freshly made, pH 7) is slowly mixed with the serum. After 2 hr the precipitated protein is centrifuged at 5000 rpm for 30 min. The pellet is dissolved (in deionized water) in one-half of the initial volume of serum and 1 volume of 33% (w/v) ammonium sulfate is added. This is immediately centrifuged again and the supernatant discarded. The pellet is dissolved again and the last step is repeated five times. Finally the pellet is dissolved in one-half volume of deionized water and dialyzed against 15–30 volumes of 0.01 *M* phosphate buffer solution, pH 8, at 4°C until the ammonium sulfate is totally eliminated (negative reaction of dialysis bath with barium chloride).

Purification of Immunoglobulin G Fraction

Immunoglobulin G fraction is purified by ion-exchange chromatography in DEAE-cellulose (11). About 1 g of resin is needed for 100 mg of precipitated immunoglobulins. The Ig's are loaded onto a column which has been washed and equilibrated with the same buffer. It is important that the conductivity of effluent buffer be the same as that of the initial one. The IgG fraction is eluted with 0.02 *M* phosphate buffer solution, pH 8. Fractions that correspond to the first peak of absorbance at 280 nm are pooled and concentrated by ultrafiltration (Minicon B 15 concentrator, Amicon, Danvers, MA). Protein concentration is determined by the method of Lowry (12).

Evaluation of Titer for Antibodies

Direct Hemagglutination Test

This technique is useful for mice because their red blood cells have a significant number of antigens that belong to the major H system and are involved in humoral immune response during allogeneic pregnancy (13). We use this procedure to evaluate the titer of antibodies, directed to paternal antigens, present in allogeneic pregnant animals (BALB/c × C3H). C3H erythrocytes are obtained from nonpregnant female mice and washed with phosphate-buffered saline (PBS) until hemolysis residues are no longer present. Then the erythrocytes are suspended in a 1.5% solution made up in a 50% normal C3H serum (heated to 56°C for 30 min to inactivate complement proteins) in PBS. Allogeneic pregnancy IgG is diluted in a 2% (v/v) dextran (molecular weight 70,000) solution in PBS from 1 : 40 to 1 : 1280. Equal volumes (25 μl) of the red cell suspension and allogeneic pregnancy IgG dilutions are incubated in microtiter plates of round-bottom wells for 2 hr at 37°C and then overnight at 4°C. Negative controls were one volume each of red blood cells and dextran solution, red blood cells and PBS, and red blood cells and IgG purified from syngeneic pregnant animals (BALB/c × BALB/c) or nonpregnant animals (BALB/c or C3H) diluted in dextran. We also include positive controls like IgG obtained from BALB/c female mice immunized with C3H lymphoid cells in the assay.

The results are read macroscopically: agglutinated red cells appear as a carpet spread over the entire bottom of the well, whereas nonagglutinated cells form a small tight button. Positive and negative controls are essential and doubtful results can be checked microscopically after the content of the well is placed gently onto a glass slide with a Pasteur pipette.

Indirect Immunofluorescence

We use this assay to determine if allogeneic pregnancy IgG is able to recognize and bind to antigenic structures from paternal origin present in C3H uterine tissues, which is also used to evidence the biological effects of these antibodies.

Uterine tissue from nonpregnant C3H female mice in diestrus is snap-frozen (after removing fat and peritoneal structures) by placing it in the side wall of a flask previously stored at −20°C. The flask contains absolute ethanol at −70°C. Tissue freezes rapidly and is stored at −20°C (14).

Sections from unfixed tissues are snap-frozen onto the microtome chuck by applying the smallest amount of water, with a syringe and needle, around its base to effect attachment by freezing. Sections 7 μm thick are transferred to acid-washed slides kept at room temperature by bringing the slides close to the knife surface so that the sections become attached and firmly bound to the glass. Dry the sections thoroughly with an electric fan for 10 min.

Tissue slices are incubated with allogeneic pregnancy IgG diluted in PBS from 1 : 10 to 1 : 1280 (v/v). Each dilution is applied over uterine-duplicated sections and incubated for 30 min in a wet chamber at room temperature. Then slices are washed twice with PBS for 10 min. Sections are stained with fluorescein-labeled goat anti-mouse IgG diluted 1 : 20 in PBS for 30 min in a dark wet chamber at room temperature. Then two or three washes with PBS for 1 hr are done. Finally the sections are mounted with a glycerin : PBS (9 : 1) (v/v) solution and sealed. Syngeneic pregnancy IgG and nonpregnant IgG are used as controls.

Readings are carried out in an epi-illuminated microscope.

Studies of *in Vitro* Uterine Motility

In order to investigate if uterine motility is altered in allogeneic pregnancy in comparison with syngeneic pregnancy, we have studied spontaneous uterine motility in an isolated organ bath system. Animals are killed by cervical dislocation in different stages of allogeneic and syngeneic pregnancy as well as in diestrus (control females). The entire uterus is immediately removed, trimmed of fat and peritoneal structures, and placed in gassed (95% O_2 and 5% CO_2, v/v) Krebs–Ringer–bicarbonate (KRB) solution (15):

Compound	Concentration (m*M*)
Na^+	145.00
K^+	6.02
Ca^{2+}	2.40
Mg^{2+}	1.34
Cl^-	126.00
HCO_3^-	25.00
PO_4^{3-}	1.20
SO_4^{2-}	1.33
Glucose	5.50

When uteri from pregnant mice are used, fetuses and placentas are carefully separated. Uterine horns are opened longitudinally and 0.5-cm-long strips from each one are cut between the ovarian and cervical regions. These strips are mounted in 15-ml organ baths which contain KRB solution at 37°C, pH 7.4, and are gassed with 95% O_2 and 5% CO_2. One end of the strip is attached to a fixed hook and the other is connected to a force transducer coupled to a recording oscillograph. After a resting tension of 500 mg is applied to the preparation by means of a micrometric device, the murine uterus contracts isometrically.

Tissues are allowed to equilibrate for 20 min until they present regular spontaneous contractions. The magnitude of each contraction is measured in milligrams. Tension control values are obtained by calculating the mean amplitude of all contractions recorded after the isolation period. Uterine spontaneous activity is stable during the whole experimental period (60 min) (15). In this system we evaluate the inhibition of uterine motility with cumulative concentration response curves of β-adrenergic agonists like L-(−)-isoproterenol, L-(−)-epinephrine, or L-(−)-norepinephrine. It is also possible to block β-adrenergic effects on uterine motility by using β-adrenergic antagonists like propranolol or butoxamine. In the experiments of *in vitro* uterine motility, tissue is incubated 20 min with the β-antagonist when necessary. For concentration–response curves, the tissue is incubated with each concentration of adrenergic agonist or IgG. In our experiments, the final concentration of agonists in the bath ranged from 10^{-10} to 10^{-6} *M*.

Uterine Membrane Preparations

To prepare purified membranes, uteri from allogeneic pregnant, syngeneic pregnant, and nonpregnant mice (C3H or BALB/c in diestrus) are mixed in four volumes of ice-cold buffer containing 0.25 *M* sucrose, 5 m*M* Tris–HCl, and 1 m*M* $MgCl_2$, pH 7.4, and are homogenized with Polytron PT 20 at low, medium, and high speed for 30 sec in 15-sec intervals; this procedure is repeated twice. The homogenates are filtered through four layers of gauze and spin at 700 *g* for 15 min. The supernatants are stored at 0°C. The pellets are homogenized again with one-half volume of the upper buffer and centrifuged at 10,000 *g* for 15 min; the mitochondrial fraction is discarded. Finally supernatants are combined and centrifuged at 40,000 *g* for 30 min. The pellets are resuspended in 2–3 ml of 50 m*M* Tris–HCl, 10 m*M* $MgCl_2$ (pH 7.4) and are stored at −70°C until they are used.

Membrane protein concentration is measured using a standard curve of bovine albumin (fraction V) (12).

We found 5-nucleotidase activity in our preparation, indicating the presence of the microsomal fraction (16).

Radioligand Binding to Uterine β-Adrenergic Receptors

Saturation Assay

Murine uterine β-adrenergic receptor is characterized using the tritiated β-antagonist dihydropalprenolol ([^{3}H]DHA) and purified uterine membranes from nonpregnant female mice (BALB/c or C3H). Aliquots of the membrane fraction (200 μg protein) are incubated (in duplicate) with shaking in 150 μl assay buffer (50 m*M* Tris–HCl, 10 m*M* $MgCl_2$, pH 7.4), containing increasing concentrations of the radioligand (0.3 to 3 n*M*), for 20 min at 37°C. Incubation is stopped via rapid vacuum filtration with 2 ml of ice-cold buffer through Whatman (Clifton, NJ) GF/C glass fiber filters. The filters are immediately rinsed with 10 ml of ice-cold buffer, dried, and added to 10 ml of Triton–toluene-based scintillation fluid [30% Triton X-100 in 4 g of PPO (2,5-diphenyloxazole) and 50 mg of POPOP {1,4-bis[2-(5-phenyl-2-oxazolyl]benzene} per liter of toluene]. Radioactivity is measured in a liquid scintillation β counter. Nonspecific binding is determined by filtering duplicated aliquots of membranes incubated with 10 μ*M* of the β-antagonist propranolol (DL isomer), which should not exceed 10% of specific binding. Specific binding is calculated by subtracting duplicated observations of nonspecific binding assessed separately each time the assay is run. To characterize β-adrenergic receptor in mice uterine tissue, we have chosen the ideal protein concentration, temperature, and incubation time for binding assays, from kinetics experiments (Fig. 2).

In order to obtain the amount of radioligand bound in femtomoles (fmol) from data obtained in counts per minute (cpm), we consider the efficiency (η) of the counter in the equation

$$\text{fmol } [^3\text{H}]\text{DHA} = \frac{[^3\text{H}]\text{DHA bound (cpm)} \times 10^{12}\ \text{fmol/mol}}{\eta\ (\text{cpm/dpm}) \times 2.22 \times 10^{12}\ \text{dpm/Ci} \times \text{SA (Ci/mmol)}},$$

where SA is the specific activity of the radioligand and dpm is disintegrations per minute.

Femtomoles are then normalized per milligram of protein in each assay. The equilibrium dissociation constant (K_d) and the maximal number of binding sites (B_{max}) are calculated by Scatchard analysis of the saturation curves (17):

$$\text{Bound/Free: } B_{max}(1/K_d) - 1/K_d\ (\text{Bound}).$$

Competition Binding Experiments

In order to determine the subtype of β-adrenergic receptor which is predominant in murine uteri, competition assays are done using 200 μg of uterine

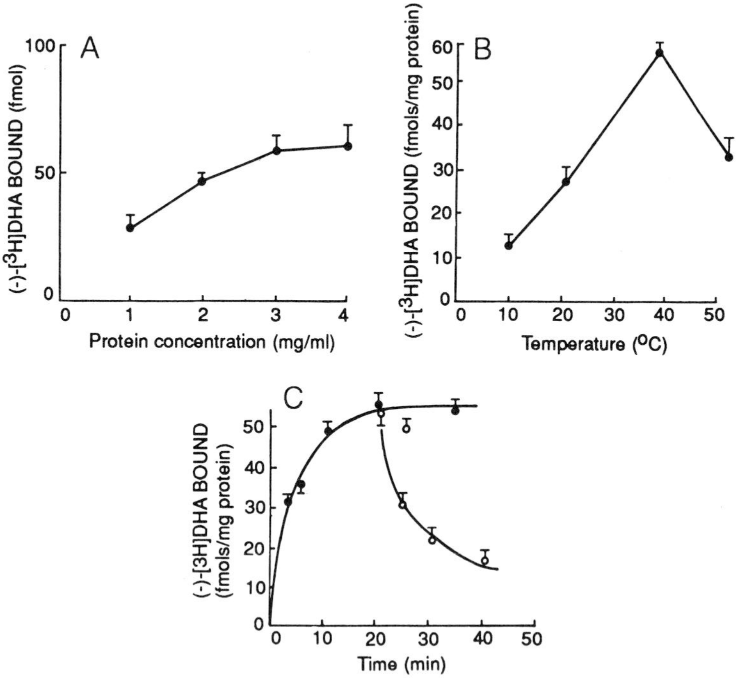

FIG. 2 [^{3}H]DHA binding to uterine membranes. (A) Membrane protein concentration dependence of [^{3}H]DHA binding. (B) Effect of temperature on [^{3}H]DHA specific binding. Uterine membranes (2 mg/ml) were incubated with 1.5 n*M* of [^{3}H]DHA for 20 min at different temperatures. (C) Time course of the association reaction (●) and the dissociation reaction (○). For the association reaction, uterine membranes (2 mg/ml) and 1.5 n*M* of [^{3}H]DHA were incubated at 37°C for different times and the specific binding was determined in the presence of 10 μM propranolol. For the dissociation reaction, at 20 min 10 μM propranolol was added and the specific binding was determined at the different times shown.

membrane per tube and increasing concentrations of adrenergic agonists (L-isoproterenol, L-epinephrine, and L-norepinephrine prepared in 0.1% ascorbic acid to prevent drug oxidation) in the presence of 1.2 n*M* [^{3}H]DHA. Table I shows the K_d values for the agonists that were calculated using the Cheng and Prussoff equation. The order of potency of the agonists (isoproterenol > epinephrine > norepinephrine) indicates that β_2-adrenoceptors are predominant in murine uterine tissue.

In this type of experiment we can also evaluate the ability of allogeneic pregnancy IgG to interact with β-adrenergic receptors present in C3H uteri. Uterine membranes are incubated with increasing concentrations of alloge-

TABLE I Inhibition of [^{3}H]DHA Binding by β-Agonists to Control Uteri

Adrenergic agent	$K_d{}^a$ (μM)
(−)-Isoproterenol	5.4
(−)-Epinephrine	26.5
(−)-Norepinephrine	92.3

[a] The K_d for the interaction of competing ligands is calculated using the equation of Cheng and Prussoff: $K_d = IC_{50}/1 + [L]/K_d$, where IC_{50} is the competing ligand concentration which half-maximally inhibits the specific binding of the radioligand at a concentration (L). IC_{50} values were obtained from competition experiments performed in duplicate at several concentrations of each agent.

neic pregnancy IgG, syngeneic pregnancy IgG, and control IgG (from nonpregnant animals) for 30 min at 30°C in buffer binding. After incubation time is completed, membranes are centrifuged at 40,000 *g* for 30 min at 4°C. The pellet is resuspended in the same buffer and used in competition assays that follow the same procedure described above.

Results are expressed as percent of the ratio of [^{3}H]DHA specifically bound in the presence of IgG/[^{3}H]DHA specifically bound in the absence of IgG (Fig. 3).

Cyclic AMP Assay

In order to evaluate whether the activation of uterine β-adrenergic receptors produced by agonists or antibodies was transducted to the intracellular compartment, we measure cAMP production by a radioimmunoassay-like procedure.

Uteri from allogeneic and syngeneic pregnant mice and nonpregnant mice are immediately removed after sacrifice and the fetuses and placentas are separated from uterine tissue as well as uterine implantation zones. Uteri are weighed and left with spontaneous activity in 1 ml of KRB with 1 mM 3-isobutyl-1-methylxanthine (MIX) (an inhibitor of phosphodiesterase activity) gassed with 5% CO_2 and 95% O_2 (v/v) with shaking at 37°C for 30 min. When agonists or antagonists of β-adrenoceptors are used to modify cAMP production, they are added 3 and 15 min before incubation time is over, respectively. Tissues are then homogenized with an Ultraturrax T 18/10 disperser at maximal speed for 30 sec, three times, in 15-sec intervals, in

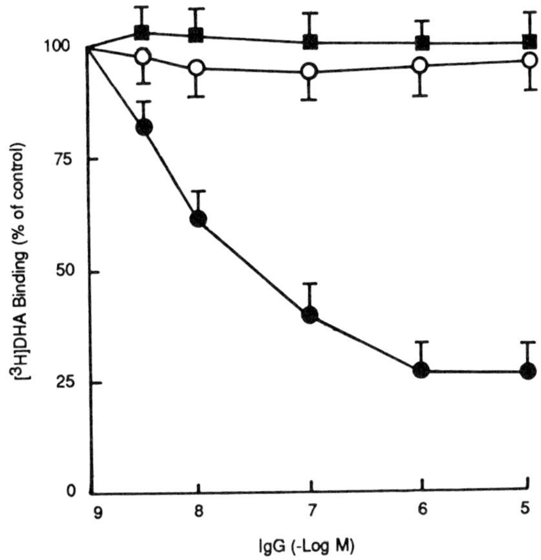

FIG. 3 Inhibition of binding of [^{3}H]DHA by increasing concentrations of allogeneic pregnancy IgG (●), control IgG (○), and syngeneic pregnancy IgG (■). C3H uterine membranes were preincubated with different concentrations of IgG for 30 min at 30°C and then with 1.2 nM of [^{3}H]DHA at 37°C for 15 min. Control binding of 100% refers to the radioactivity bound to uterine membranes in the absence of IgG. Means ± SEM of five independent experiments are plotted.

2 ml of absolute ethanol, and centrifuged at 2500 g for 15 min at 4°C. The supernatants are collected and pellets are homogenized in 1 ml of ethanol : water (2 : 1, v/v) and centrifuged. Supernatants are combined and evaporated at 55°C under a nitrogen stream.

cAMP residues are dissolved in 2 ml of assay buffer (50 mM Tris–HCl, 8 mM theophylline, 6 mM 2-mercaptoethanol, 0.45 mM EDTA, pH 7.4) and stored at −20°C until the assay is carried out.

Aliquots of 100 μl are taken for the nucleotide determination using the procedure outlined in Table II.

Protocol

1. In glass tubes add 100 μl of standard solutions, samples, or buffer.
2. Add 50 μl of tritiated radioactive tracer diluted in assay buffer.
3. Vortex the tubes.

TABLE II Procedure for cAMP Assay

Parameter	Tube	Assay buffer (μl)	cAMP (μl)	[^{3}H]cAMP[a] (μl)	Protein kinase[b] (μl)
Total counts	1	350	—	50	—
	2	350	—	50	—
	3	350	—	50	—
B_0	4	100	—	50	50
	5	100	—	50	50
	6	100	—	50	50
Nonspecific binding	7	150	—	50	—
	8	150	—	50	—
	9	150	—	50	—
Standard curve[c]	10	—	100	50	50
	11	—	100	50	50
	12	—	100	50	50

[a] [^{3}H]cAMP (specific activity, 31 Ci/mmol), 7 fmol/tube.
[b] Protein kinase was purified following Brown's method (18).
[c] Standard solutions of cAMP: 20, 10, 5, 2.5, 1.25, 0.625, 0.315, and 0.156 pmol/100 μl.

4. Add 50 μl of protein kinase diluted (1 : 7) in assay buffer.
5. Vortex the tubes.
6. Incubate for 90 min at 4°C.
7. Rapidly add 200 μl of charcoal–albumin solution (except total counts tubes) (5% charcoal and 1% albumin in assay buffer) to each tube.
8. Vortex the tubes.
9. Incubate for 10 min at 0°C in ice–water.
10. Centrifuge at 2000 *g* for 15 min at 4°C.
11. Decant the supernatant from each tube in a vial containing 10 ml of scintillation cocktail. Touch the rim of the test tube onto the surface of the scintillation fluid to "draw-off" the last drop from each tube.
12. Determine the amount of radioactivity present in a β counter.

Mathematical Calculation of Results

The concentration of cAMP in unknown samples may be calculated mathematically after constructing the calibration curve as follows:

1. Determine the nonspecific binding in counts per minute for the assay by averaging the cpm for tubes 7 to 9.

2. Determine B_0 (the cpm bound in the absence of unlabeled cAMP) by averaging cpm for tubes 4 to 6 and subtracting the nonspecific binding.
3. Determine B (the cpm bound in the presence of standard or unknown cAMP) by averaging the cpm for the remaining triplicated tubes and subtracting the nonspecific binding.
4. Calculate B/B_0 for each level of standard cAMP and for the unknowns.
5. Calculate logit B/B_0 (ln $B/B_0/1 - B/B_0$) for the standard curve and for the unknowns.
6. Calculate log c (c is picomoles of unlabeled cAMP in each tube of standard curve).
7. Plot logit B/B_0 against log c on logit–log paper.
8. From the logit B/B_0 values for the unknown samples read the number of log c of inactive cAMP from the standard curve.
9. Calculate c from log c.

The within-assay (intrassay) variation is estimated for different amounts of cAMP and the mean is 9.3%. The interassay variation for 43 duplicated determinations is 13.6%.

Acknowledgment

This work has been supported by Grant BID-PID 0352 from the National Research Council from Argentina CONICET.

References

1. M. E. Sales, L. Sterin-Borda, and E. S. Borda, *Int. J. Immunopharmacol.* **8,** 947 (1989).
2. G. Berg, R. G. G. Anderson, and G. Ryden, *Am. J. Obstet. Gynecol.* **151,** 392 (1985).
3. E. M. M. Chow and J. M. Marshall, *Eur. J. Pharmacol.* **68,** 1377 (1981).
4. M. H. Litime, G. Pointis, M. Breuiller, D. Cabrol, and F. Ferre, *J. Clin. Endocrinol. Metab.* **68,** 1 (1989).
5. E. S. Borda, A. M. Genaro, G. A. Cremaschi, M. E. Sales, and L. Sterin-Borda, *Eur. J. Pharmacol.* **100,** 195 (1984).
6. C. Cunningham, D. A. Power, A. Innes, T. Lind, and G. R. D. Catto, *Hum. Immunol.* **19,** 716 (1987).
7. N. Kaliss, *in* "Immunology of Reproduction" (K. Bratanov, ed.), p. 495. Bulgarian Academic of Sciences, Sofia, 1973.
8. G. A. Cremaschi, L. Sterin-Borda, A. M. Genaro, E. Borda, and M. Braun, *J. Immunol.* **133,** 2681 (1984).

9. T. Nicol, D. L. J. Bilbey, L. M. Charles, J. L. Codingley, and B. Vernon-Roberts, *J. Endocrinol.* **30,** 277 (1964).
10. R. A. Margni, *in* "Inmunologia e Inmunoquimica" (Panamericana, ed.), p. 481. Buenos Aires, Argentina, 1982.
11. R. A. Margni, *in* "Inmunologia e Inmunoquimica" (Panamericana, ed.), p. 673. Buenos Aires, Argentina, 1982.
12. O. H. Lowry, N. J. Rosenbrough, A. L. Farr, and R. J. Randall, *J. Biol. Chem.* **193,** 265 (1951).
13. K. I. Welsh and J. R. Batchelor, *in* "Handbook of Experimental Immunology" (D. M. Weir, ed.), Vol. 2, p. 35.6. Blackwell Scientific Publications, London, 1978.
14. G. D. Johnson, E. J. Holborow, and J. Dorling, *in* "Handbook of Experimental Immunology" (D. M. Weir, ed.), Vol. 1, p. 15.1. Blackwell Scientific Publications, London, 1978.
15. E. S. Borda, J. Sauvage, L. Sterin-Borda, M. F. Gimeno, and A. L. Gimeno, *Eur. J. Pharmacol.* **56,** 61 (1979).
16. R. W. Lerner, G. D. Lopaschuk, and P. M. Olley. *Can. J. Physiol. Pharmacol.* **68,** 1574 (1990).
17. G. Scatchard, *Ann. N.Y. Acad. Sci.* **51,** 660 (1949).
18. B. L. Brown, J. D. M. Albano, R. P. Ekins, and A. M. Sgherzi. *Biochem. J.* **121,** 561 (1971).

[8] Preparation, Characterization, and Use of Human and Rodent Lymphocytes, Monocytes, and Neutrophils

L. H. Elliott, S. L. Carlson, L. A. Morford, and J. P. McGillis

Introduction

The model systems used to examine the role of the nervous and endocrine systems in degenerative and inflammatory disease processes have ranged from simple *in vitro* proliferative assays to complex *in vivo* systems (reviewed in 1, 2). Much of the progress that has been made in understanding the mechanisms of neuroimmunomodulation has come from *in vitro* studies using primary cultures of leukocytes. This chapter describes methods which can be used to prepare leukocytes for *in vitro* studies, as well as methods for lymphocyte activation and analysis of second-messenger production.

Several factors should be considered when designing a set of experiments. One of the most important is context. Is the mediator present in the physiological microenvironment represented by the model system? For example, if examining the effect of neurotransmitter or neuropeptide on lymphocyte activation, is it found in nerve endings in spleen or in lymph nodes, or, if examining the effect of an agent on B-cell differentiation, is it found in bone marrow? Thus if one wished to examine the effect of one of the "brain–gut" neuropeptides on lymphocyte function, it would be more appropriate to use lymphocytes isolated from Peyer's patch or mesenteric lymph nodes rather than from spleen. In the rodent system, effects in local microenvironments can be easily addressed *in vitro*. In the human system, this becomes more problematic. While it is possible to obtain surgical and autopsy specimens, most investigators use peripheral blood leukocytes which are easy to obtain. The use of human peripheral blood leukocytes as a model system must be considered carefully because there can be a number of functional and phenotypic differences between circulating and tissue leukocytes.

A second important consideration is the limitations of the model system. For example, while the effect of a neural or endocrine mediator on a mitogen-induced proliferative response may be an initial starting point, it tells little in terms of the current understanding of lymphocyte function. In fact, a neural or endocrine mediator could have little or no effect on lymphocyte proliferation, but could have a major effect on differentiation, cytokine production, adhesion, etc. An important corollary to the appropriate choice of

Methods in Neurosciences, Volume 24

model system is interpretation of the results in the context of other aspects of the system. Several investigators have begun to address the role of neural and endocrine agents on more specific cell functions. An emphasis is now being placed on interpreting the role of nonimmune system-derived signals in the context of closed-loop signals within the immune system. Thus, when designing a set of experiments with the goal of defining neural/endocrine–immune/inflammatory interactions, it is important to consider the context and the limitations and to consider the results in the context of what is being recognized as an increasingly complex system.

The goal of this chapter is to provide some simple, concise protocols for the preparation, characterization, and use of leukocytes. The reader is referred to several volumes devoted to immunological analysis for more specialized procedures (3–5). The procedures described here are ones with which the authors have had experience, and the reader will find that there are many variations. The specific ways in which to use these cells in unraveling neural/endocrine–immune/inflammatory communication is left to the researcher.

Preparation of Human Lymphocytes, Monocytes, and Neutrophils

Human Peripheral Blood Leukocytes

In humans, peripheral blood obtained by venipuncture is the most accessible source of lymphocytes and monocytes. Human blood contains $5–10 \times 10^6$ leukocytes/ml, of these 30% are lymphocytes, 1–3% are monocytes, and the remainder are granulocytes. Although peripheral blood lymphocytes (PBL) represent only 2% of the entire lymphocyte population in the normal, adult human body, it has been estimated that most of the lymphocyte repertoire of the body transits through the blood in a 24-hr period. Thus, it is generally assumed that PBLs are representative of the entire lymphocyte population in the human body. There are, however, a number of factors or disease states which may alter lymphocyte migration or life span resulting in decreased numbers of lymphocytes in the blood and it has been suggested that in these circumstances PBLs may not be representative of the entire repertoire (6).

Isolation of Peripheral Blood Mononuclear Leukocytes by Ficoll–Hypaque Density Centrifugation

Decant 10 to 15 ml of heparinized blood into a polystyrene or clear polypropylene 50-ml conical centrifuge tube, dilute to 35 ml with Hanks' balanced salt solution (HBSS, GIBCO, Grand Island, NY), and mix by inversion.

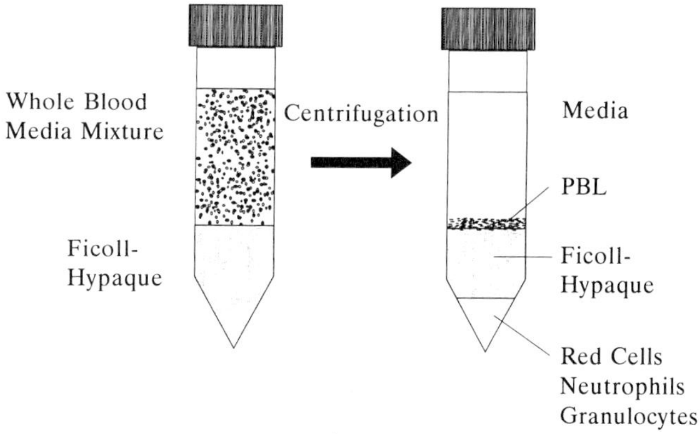

FIG. 1 Purification of human peripheral blood mononuclear cells by centrifugation of Ficoll–Hypaque. Ten to fifteen milliliters of heparinized blood is diluted to 35 ml with HBSS and is carefully underlaid with 12 ml of Ficoll–Hypaque. After centrifugation at 500 *g* for 35 min the mononuclear cells are present at the interface and the granulocytes and erythrocytes are in the pellet.

Carefully underlay 12 ml of Ficoll–Hypaque solution* and centrifuge at 500 *g* for 35 min at room temperature. Granulocytes and red cells are contained in the pellet, while mononuclear cells are at the interface as shown in Fig. 1. Aspirate off the supernatant to just about the interface. Carefully remove the interface and transfer the cells to a new 50-ml conical centrifuge tube. Dilute the cells at least fourfold with medium and centrifuge at 400 *g* for 8 min. Cell recoveries for normal adult humans range between 1.5 and 3×10^6 cells/ml of blood. Monocytes may be removed by adherence to plastic. T cells which make up the majority of the PBL (70%) can be enriched by a variety of techniques including rosetting, nylon wool columns, and positive and negative immunoselection.

Purification of Human Monocytes by Adherence to Plastic

Adjust PBLs to 5×10^6 cells/ml in RPMI 1640 containing 10% heat-inactivated fetal calf serum (FCS)† and dispsense in 10-ml aliquots into 100-mm

* Ficoll–Hypaque is prepared by mixing 100 ml of 9% Ficoll (Pharmacia, Piscataway, NJ) with 41.7 ml of 34% Hypaque [prepared by diluting 50% Hypaque (Winthrop Pharmaceutical, New York) with water at a ratio of 2.13 : 1]. Ficoll–Hypaque solutions can be filter-sterilized and should be stored in dark or foil-wrapped bottles at 4°C. Warm the Ficoll–Hypaque to room temperature before use.

† All FCS used in lymphocyte and monocyte media should be heat-inactivated by incubating for 30 min at 56°C.

plastic petri dishes (Corning, 25020). Incubate the cells overnight at 37°C in a humidified 5% CO_2 incubator. Remove the nonadherent cells and rinse the plates at least four times with 5 ml of RPMI 1640/1% FCS. Incubate the plates for 10 min at 4°C in 5 ml of 0.02% EDTA in PBS supplemented with 1% FCS. Remove adherent monocytes by vigorous pipetting and transfer to a centrifuge tube. Wash the plates twice with 5 ml of RPMI medium containing 1% FCS and remove any remaining monocytes with vigorous pipetting. Pool the washes and centrifuge at 400 *g* for 8 min. Purity of the monocytes may be quantitated by esterase staining. To avoid activation of monocytes use media and FCS which have low levels of endotoxin.

Isolation of Peripheral Blood Neutrophils

Isolation of neutrophils from human peripheral blood involves the addition of an adsorption step with dextran T70 to remove red blood cells (RBC) prior to centrifugation over Ficoll–Hypaque. Prior to venipuncture, 10 ml of 6% dextran T70 (Pharmacia, Piscataway, NJ) in saline (0.9% NaCl) and 1 ml of heparin (1000 U/ml) are drawn into a 60-ml syringe. Fifty milliliters of venous blood is collected directly into the syringe, usually by attachment to a 19-gauge butterfly. After the blood has been collected, it is mixed with the dextran solution by gently inverting the syringe five to six times. The syringe is then stored upright in a test tube rack. Over a period of about 1 hr, the dextran-absorbed RBCs will sediment. The upper white cell layer ($\frac{2}{3}$ to $\frac{3}{4}$ the volume of the syringe) can then be removed by attaching a fresh butterfly needle and then pressing the plunger upward. The leukocyte fraction is collected into a fresh tube, diluted at least fivefold with HBSS with 1% FCS, and centrifuged at 200 *g* for 10 min. After an additional wash with HBSS/1% FCS, the pellet is resuspended in HBSS or an appropriate buffer and centrifuged over Ficoll–Hypaque as described above. Following centrifugation, the lymphocytes and monocytes will be present in the interface, and the neutrophils will be present in the pellet. After the upper layers are removed, the neutrophil pellet is resuspended in a small volume of HBSS, transferred to a separate tube, washed two to three times, and resuspended in the appropriate buffer system. Yields of cells which are greater than 95–99% neutrophils are typical. The purity of the neutrophil population can be ascertained by staining with Wright's stain (Fisher Scientific).

Purification of Human Lymphocyte Subsets

The majority of lymphocytes isolated from peripheral blood by Ficoll–Hypaque density gradient centrifugation are small lymphocytes which are mature and thus immunocompetent. Peripheral blood lymphocytes are divided into two major subclasses, T cells which mature and gain immunocompetence in the thymus and B cells which mature primarily in the bone marrow. These subclasses can be distinguished functionally and by the expression of distinct cell-surface markers. B cells which are characterized by the expression of surface immunoglobulin (sIg) secrete specific antibody in response to immune stimulus (foreign antigen) and thus are involved primarily in the humoral immune response to foreign antigen. T cells which represent the majority (70%) of the small lymphocytes found in the blood are characterized by the expression of the T-cell receptor(TCR)/CD3 complex. The TCR/CD3$^+$ T cells are further divided into two nonoverlapping subsets which express two distinct cell-surface markers; CD4 which represent approximately 60% and CD8 which represent approximately 40% of the TCR/CD3+ T cells. CD4$^+$ T cells act primarily as helper T cells which secrete important cytokines required for the induction of B cells and T cells. CD8$^+$ T cells, with help from CD4$^+$ T cells, function primarily as cytotoxic T cells in the cell-mediated immune response. There is some functional overlap between CD4$^+$ and CD8$^+$ cells as CD4$^+$ cytotoxic and CD8$^+$ helper T cells have been demonstrated.

Separation of T and B Cells by Sheep Erythrocyte Rosetting

Because human T cells express a receptor (CD2) which binds to an unknown ligand on sheep erythrocytes, T cells are easily separated from B cells and monocytes in PBL by a simple rosetting technique. Adjust PBLs isolated by Ficoll–Hypaque to 2×10^7 cell/ml in HBSS. Add $4–10 \times 10^7$ cells (2–5 ml) to a 50-ml conical centrifuge tube and mix with an equal volume of neuraminidase-treated* sheep erythrocytes (SRBC) diluted to 5% in HBSS (final concentration 1×10^7 cells/ml and 2.5% SRBC). Incubate the mixture for 15 min at 37°C, centrifuge at 250 *g* for 5 min, and incubate at 4°C for 2 hr. Gently resuspend the rosetted cells by rolling the centrifuge tube and underlay with 12 ml of Ficoll–Hypaque. Centrifuge at 500 *g* at 4°C for 35 min. Nonrosetted cells, containing primarily B cells and monocytes, are concentrated at the interface. Carefully remove and transfer the cells at the interface to a new centrifuge tube and wash twice with medium. B cells may be further purified by panning (see below) and monocytes by adherence to plastic (see above). Rosetted T cells are contained in the pellet. After harvesting of the interface cells, carefully aspirate the remaining Ficoll–Hypaque.

* Wash SRBC twice with HBSS and mix 1 ml of packed SRBC with 18 ml of calcium saline buffer (0.154 *M* NaCl, 3 m*M* Ca_2Cl, 4 m*M* $NaCO_3$, pH 7.3) and 1 ml neuraminidase (Calbiochem, 480717, La Jolla, CA). Incubate 30 min at 37°C and wash twice with HBSS. Resuspend to 5% (v/v) in HBSS (20 ml).

Vigorously resuspend the rosettes in 5–8 ml of lysis buffer† and incubate on ice for 5 min or until the sheep erythrocytes are completely lysed (media will turn clear). Dilute the cells to 40 ml with medium and centrifuge at 400 *g* for 8 min. Pool the T-cell pellets into one 50-ml conical tube and wash once more in 25 ml of medium. This procedure routinely results in a 50% cell recovery containing 95 to 98% $CD3^+$, $CD2^+$ T cells. The purity of the various cell populations should be determined by fluorescence-activated cell sorter (FACS) analysis. One drawback to the use of rosetting for the enrichment of T cells is that these cells are positively selected via the CD2 marker expressed on the cell surface. Since this glycoprotein has been implicated in the activation of T cells, selection utilizing the CD2 marker may result in preactivation of the cells. This problem can be avoided by using a negative immunoselection to enrich specific lymphocyte populations.

Lymphocyte Purification by Positive and Negative Immunoselection

The availability of monoclonal antibodies (MAb) specific for glycoprotein membrane "markers" which characterize subpopulations of T cells and B cells has facilitated the development of immunoselection techniques that result in the isolation of pure subpopulations of lymphocytes based on the expression of a specific marker. When using the indirect method, lymphocytes are allowed to react with antibody directed to an antigen marker (or markers) which characterize a specific subpopulation. The antibody-coated cells are then allowed to react with a second antibody (bound to plastic or magnetic beads), directed to the immunoglobulin isotype of the first antibody. Alternatively, if a highly specific MAb is available, a subpopulation of cells may be targeted by directly absorbing the cells to plastic or magnetic beads which are coated with the specific MAb. The results obtained using antibody bound to plastic or magnetic beads appear to be equivalent. However, due to the high cost of antibody-coated magnetic beads, this technique may be cost prohibitive when large numbers of cells are needed. Thus, only the panning method for immunoselection of lymphocyte subpopulations is described here.

Purification of Lymphocyte Subpopulations by Panning

The technique of panning is based on the observation that immunoglobulin can be bound to plastic petri dishes without affecting the antigen-binding ability of the antibodies. Panning was first described by Wysocki and Sato

† 0.15 *M* NH_4Cl, 0.1 m*M* EDTA, 1.0 m*M* $KHCO_3$, pH 7.4.

(7). The desired subpopulation of cells may be isolated by negative immunoselection if all other contaminating subpopulations of cells are targeted with a cocktail of antibodies and removed by adherence either directly or indirectly (using a second antibody as described above). The desired subpopulation of cells enriched by this method are easily obtained by removing the nonadherent cells from the plate. The major drawback to negative immunoselection is that it is sometimes difficult to obtain antibodies that specifically target all other contaminating subpopulations of cells. A subpopulation of lymphocytes may also be purified by targeting an antigenic marker on that cell population with specific antibody (positive selection) and isolating these cells by indirect or direct adherence to plastic. Generally, greater purity is achieved with positive immunoselection, but cell recovery may be lower because of the difficulty in dissociating the cells from the antibody. Moreover, if the MAb recognizes an accessory molecule there is the added risk of inducing costimulatory signaling events which might result in preactivation of the cells.

Purification of Human B Cells by Positive Selection Using Direct Method

Tissue culture-grade culture dishes increase the level of nonspecific cell adherence, thus bacteriological-grade polystyrene petri dishes (100 × 15 mm) should be used for all procedures. To coat the petri dishes with antibody, incubate them with 10 ml of anti-human immunoglobulin (10 μg/ml diluted in 0.05 *M* Tris–HCl, pH 9.5) for 1 hr at room temperature or at 4°C. Decant the antibody solution and wash the dishes three times with Dulbecco's phosphate-buffered saline (PBS, GIBCO, Grand Island, NY), pH 5.4, containing 1% FCS and once with PBS/1% FCS, pH 7.4. Set aside at least 30 min before adding the cells to allow time for the FCS to saturate all protein-binding sites on the dishes, thus decreasing nonspecific cell adherence. Decant the PBS/1% FCS and add 3–5 × 10^7 monocyte-depleted PBLs per dish in 4 ml of PBS/5% FCS and incubate at 4°C for 1 hr. After 30 min gently rock the plates to dislodge stacked cells. Transfer the nonadherent cells to a 50-ml conical centrifuge tube, wash the dishes four times with 5 ml of PBS/1% FCS, and pool the washes. The nonadherent cells will be enriched for T cells and can be used to isolate subpopulations of T cells. Remove the adherent B cells by forcefully pipetting parallel to the dish surface using 40 ml of cold PBS/1% FCS. It should be noted that the recovery of B cells will be dependent on the avidity of the antibody used. If low yields are obtained (less than 50%), add nonimmune IgG at a ratio of 10 : 1 (nonimmune : specific antibody) to the antibody solution used to coat the dish (8). Another method to remove adherent cells is to incubate them with xylocaine (4 mg/ml) for 15 min at room temperature (8).

Purification of T-Lymphocyte Subpopulations by Negative Selection Using Indirect Method

Prepare antibody-coated plates as described above using affinity-purified anti-Ig directed against the species of origin and the isotype of the T-cell reactive antibody. For example, if the T-cell reactive antibody is a mouse IgG, coat the dishes with affinity-purified anti-mouse IgG. Incubate 3×10^7 purified T cells for 20 min at room temperature with 2 ml of supernatant from a hybridoma-producing MAb which targets the subpopulation of T cell to be depleted. Alternatively, 10 μg of purified MAb diluted in 3 ml of PBS/5% FCS may also be used if the hybridoma is not available. For example, to purify $CD4^+$ T cells incubate the T cells with anti-CD8. Wash the MAb-coated lymphocytes twice with PBS/5% FCS, resuspend the cells in 3 ml of the same solution, add them to a petri dish coated with the second antibody, and incubate for 2 hr at 4°C. Carefully aspirate off the nonadherent lymphocytes. Gently wash the dishes four times with PBS/1% FCS to remove any remaining nonadherent cells and pool all the washes. Assuming that anti-CD8 MAb was the targeting antibody, the nonadherent cells will be enriched for the $CD4^+$ T-cell subset. If $CD8^+$ T cells are desired, use anti-CD4 MAb as the targeting antibody. Cell recoveries range from 30 to 40% with greater than 94% purity. T-cell subsets also may be purified by negative selection onto dishes coated with anti-CD4 or anti-CD8 MAb (direct panning).

Enrichment of Human T Cells and B Cells by Separation on Nylon Wool Columns

Pack 0.6 to 0.7 g of combed, scrubbed nylon wool (Robbins Scientific, Sunnyvale, CA) to the 10 ml mark of a 10-ml sterile syringe fitted with a three-way stopcock. Equilibrate the column by washing with 50 ml of PBS, pH 7.4, followed by 50 ml of HBSS/5% FCS. Preincubate the column for 1 hr in a 37°C CO_2 incubator. Resuspend PBLs in 1.5 ml of HBSS/5% FCS (do not exceed 1×10^8 cells/column), apply to the top of the column, allow the cells to enter the column, and follow with an additional 2 ml of HBSS/FCS to ensure that the cells are well into the column. Stop the flow and incubate the column for 1 hr at 37°C in a CO_2 incubator. Slowly elute nonadherent (T-cell-enriched) cells with 30 ml of Hanks'/5% FCS. After the nonadherent cells are eluted, remove the adherent cells (B-enriched) by filling the column with HBSS/5% FCS and use the sterile plunger from the syringe to force the media through the nylon wool. Rinse the column with 20 ml of HBSS/5% FCS and pool with the adherent cell (B-cell-enriched) fraction. The adherent cell fraction will also contain monocytes if these cells have not previously been removed.

Preparation of Rodent Lymphocytes and Monocytes

The preparation of lymphocytes from spleen, thymus, and lymph nodes is essentially the same with some minor variations. The choice of which tissue to use depends on the goals of the experiment. The spleen is the easiest tissue to dissect and has a large number of lymphocytes (up to 15×10^7 per mouse spleen), with approximately 40% being T cells and 60% B cells. The spleen also contains a large number of red blood cells which should be removed for most applications. The peripheral lymph nodes (see Fig. 2) yield approximately 1×10^6 cells/lymph node with up to 70% T cells. The mesenteric lymph nodes are found at the root of the intestinal mesentery as a chain of lymph nodes near the posterior abdominal wall. The thymus is composed of two lobes that are found just above the heart. Since this is the tissue where T cells mature, the majority of thymocytes are immature T cells. The thymus is large in prepubertal animals and regresses in size with age.

To obtain the tissues using the sterile technique, the mice are euthanized and the fur is thoroughly wetted down with 70% ethanol. All instruments are kept in a beaker containing 70% ethanol, and flamed prior to use. To remove spleens an incision is made in the left lateral abdominal wall just below the rib cage. The spleen is retracted with a forceps and blood vessels and connective tissue cut with a fine scissors. The spleen is immediately placed in a small petri dish containing 5 ml sterile washing medium (HBSS supplemented with 0.5% BSA and 20 m*M* HEPES, pH 7.3). The cells can be dispersed by pressing them through a wire mesh screen into a petri dish or by mashing the spleen between the frosted ends of two sterile glass slides. Care must be taken to keep the cells on the screens or slides moist. The cells are drawn up into a syringe fitted with a 25-gauge needle to break up clumps of cells and are transferred to a 15-ml tube. Wash the plate with an additional 5 ml of washing medium and add this to the cell suspension. Centrifuge the cells at 200 *g* for 10 min. Resuspend the pellet in 10 ml washing medium, and wash two additional times. If the removal of red blood cells or dead cells is necessary, additional steps can be carried out just after the initial isolation of the lymphocytes.

Pellet the cells in a 15-ml tube and discard the supernatant. Resuspend

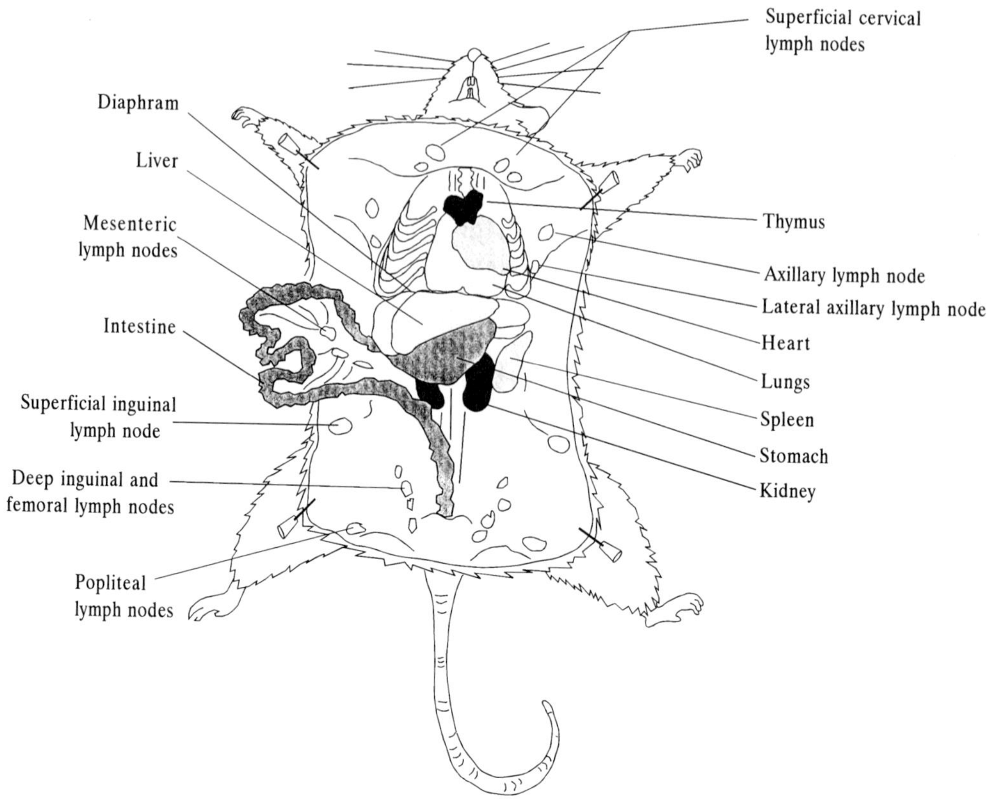

FIG. 2 Location of rodent lymphoid tissue. Courtesy of Lori Ann Morford.

the pellet in 5 ml of lysis buffer and incubate for 5 min at room temperature. If the cells must be kept cold, chilled lysis buffer can be used, and the cell suspension is incubated for 10 min on ice. After incubation fill the tube with washing medium and centrifuge at 200 *g* for 10 min. Wash the cells two additional times in washing medium. Dead lymphocytes and RBCs have a higher density than viable lymphocytes and can be removed with commercially available density separation medium (Lympholyte-M, Accurate Chemical Co., Westbury, NY). The density of rodent lymphocytes is slightly different than that of human lymphocytes, so an appropriate medium must be used. Adjust the lymphocyte suspension to a concentration of 1×10^7/ml in washing medium. Dispense up to 5×10^7 cells per 15-ml tube, and carefully underlay with 5 ml of density separation medium. Centrifuge the tubes at 500 *g* at 20°C for 20 min. The viable lymphocytes will be present at the

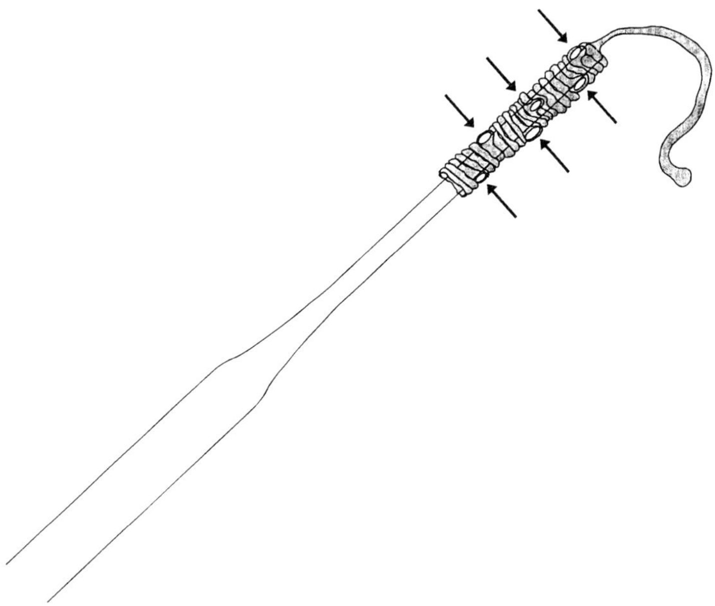

FIG. 3 Isolation of Peyer's patch lymphocytes. After dissection and thorough flushing the small intestine is threaded over a 9-inch glass Pasteur pipette. Peyer's patches will appear as small whitish nodules. Courtesy of Lorri Ann Morford.

interface between the medium and the Lympholyte-M. Aspirate off most of the media layer, and carefully transfer the lymphocyte layer to a new tube. Fill the tube with washing medium and centrifuge at 400 *g* for 10 min, then wash two additional times at 200 *g* for 10 min.

Preparation of Peyer's Patch Lymphocytes

Peyer's patches are diffuse patches of lymphocytes found in the wall of the small intestine. Unlike lymph nodes, they lack a capsule and the structural components characteristic of lymph nodes. To collect Peyer's patches, the small intestine is cut at each end, and the lumen is flushed extensively with sterile saline. If the cells are to be placed into culture, care should be taken to prevent lumenal contents from getting on the outside of the intestine. The washed intestine is then carefully threaded onto a 9-inch glass Pasteur pipette (Fig. 3). During this process the intestine will "accordion," and the Peyer's patches will be visible as small white nodules. The patches are carefully cut off with a pair of fine forceps and placed in a tube containing HBSS. The patches are washed several times by allowing them to settle and then aspirating off the HBSS. This process is repeated until the medium remains clear. The lymphocytes are then dispersed as described above and washed extensively. If the cells are to be placed into culture, we frequently double the concentration of antibiotic in the growth media.

Bone Marrow Cells

Bone marrow cells can be isolated from the hind limbs of mice. Following removal of the limbs, muscle tissue is carefully dissected off the long bones. The ends of the bones are cut off, and the bone marrow is gently forced out with a 25-gauge needle. The cells are collected in petri dishes containing 10 ml of HBSS/20 m*M* HEPES, pH 7.3, and 2% FCS. Clumps of cells are dispersed by aspiration through a 25-gauge needle. The cells are washed once by centrifugation at 200 *g* for 10 min at 4°C and then filtered through a sterile stainless steel mesh to remove any tissue. The cells are subsequently washed twice in medium, counted, and resuspended to the appropriate concentration. Cell viability can be determined by trypan blue exclusion. A typical yield from five mice is approximately $2–5 \times 10^8$ cells.

Purification of Rodent Lymphocytes and Monocytes

With the exception of sheep red blood cell rosetting, all of the methods described for enrichment of human T and B cells and monocytes can be adapted for enrichment of rodent lymphocytes and monocytes. In addition, large numbers of rodent macrophages can be collected from the peritoneal cavity. After carefully pealing back the hide, the perineum is carefully lifted and 5 ml of sterile PBS is carefully injected into the peritoneal cavity using a 22- to 25-gauge needle. The animal is then massaged gently to help dislodge the cells. After the PBS is removed, the cells are pelleted and macrophages are adhered to plastic dishes as described above. An additional technique that is useful for enrichment of rodent T and B cells is panning in the presence of high concentrations of BSA.

Separation of Rodent B Cells on Bovine Serum Albumin-Coated Dishes

Rat B cells can be purified using a modification of the BSA panning protocol described by Severson *et al.* (9, 10). This procedure can also be used for purification of mouse B cells by substituting the appropriate anti-mouse Ig antibodies. Following lysis of red blood cells splenocytes are washed in HBSS with 20 m*M* HEPES, pH 7.3, and 0.1% BSA [radioimmunoassay (RIA) grade, Sigma, St. Louis, MO]. After the final wash the cells are resuspended at a concentration of 1.5×10^7 cells/ml in HBSS/HEPES with 3.0% BSA and 3 ml is added to 25-cm^2 tissue culture flasks. After the cells are allowed to adhere for 60 min, the T-cell-enriched nonadherent cells are decanted and the B-cell-enriched adherent cells are removed by vigorous washing. The T- and B-enriched populations can be further purified by negative selection using a two-step panning procedure (7, 10). Adherent (B-enriched) and nonadherent (T-enriched) cells are washed three times in HBSS/HEPES with 0.3% BSA. The cells are resuspended at a concentration of 10^7 cells/ml and T- or B-enriched cells are incubated for 1 hr at 4°C with mouse anti-rat IgM and anti-rat IgD (MARM-4, MARD-3; BPS, Indianapolis, IN) or mouse anti-rat CD2 (OX-34; BPS) and mouse anti-rat CD5 (OX-19; BPS), respectively. The cells are washed to remove unbound antibody and resuspended at a concentration of 6.6×10^6 cells/ml in HBSS/HEPES with 0.1% BSA. Three milliliters are added to 10-cm petri plates which have been precoated with rat absorbed donkey anti-mouse IgG (Jackson Immunoresearch Laboratories, Inc., West Grove, PA) and allowed to adhere for 1 hr at 4°C. The nonadherent T- and B-enriched cells are removed and washed three to five times in HBSS/HEPES with 0.1% BSA. Following BSA panning the B cells are greater than 80% sIg positive and T cells are 80–90% CD-2/CD-5 positive. Following the antibody-panning step, the cell populations are 96 to 98% enriched for T- and B-cell markers.

Characterization of Monocyte and Lymphocyte Subsets

When doing experiments with purified lymphocyte subsets, it is important to have some measure of the degree of purity of the cells being used. This is especially important when a new or untested enrichment procedure is being set up. Depending on the question being asked, it can be critical to know what cell types are present. For example, if the effect of an agent on T-cell activation is being studied, it is important to know whether there are macrophages present. A few macrophages in a single well in a 96-well microtiter plate can produce sufficient interleukin 1 (IL-1) to stimulate the T cells in that well. Thus, if an effect on T-cell activation is observed when there are significant numbers of macrophages, it would be difficult to rule out an indirect effect mediated by macrophages. However, even under the best of conditions it is difficult to obtain absolutely pure cell populations. Thus, it is important to design experiments that provide corroborating evidence for a direct effect on any cell population.

The two most common methods for assessing cell populations are FACS analysis and the response to mitogens. The use of specific mitogens has been used for many years, but can be imprecise. For this analysis one would set up a proliferation assay in which the purified cells are treated with T-cell-specific mitogens [phytohemagglutinin (PHA) or concanavalin A (Con A)] and a B-cell-specific mitogen (LPS). Purified T cells should only respond to pHA or Con A, and not to LPS, and vice versa for B cells. The disadvantages to this type of analysis is that it may fail to detect low levels of contaminating cells and that it takes a minimum of 48 hr. The former is not a trivial problem in that a low level of contaminating cells can have significant effects in many assay systems. For these reasons FACS analysis is currently the method of choice.

Fluorescence-Activated Cell Sorter Analysis of Lymphocytes

Analysis of cells by FACS is the most precise method for phenotypic characterization of lymphocytes. This type of analysis requires access to a cell sorter facility. Most research universities and hospitals have a core FACS facility. The capabilities vary widely, depending on the specific FACS equipment and on the abilities of the operators. In general, FACS machines are run by full time technical staff. FACS applications range from simple tasks like analysis of the expression of specific cell-surface proteins to more complex tasks like the measurement of intracellular Ca^{2+} or cell-cycle analysis. In addition, some cell sorters can be used to purify specific subsets of cells. The discussion here is limited to phenotypic analysis.

When using purified populations of leukocytes, especially lymphocytes, it is important to know the degree of enrichment. While there is no universal rule for the degree of enrichment necessary, the general rule is that the cell populations being used should be as pure as possible. This is critically important in some assays. Once cells have been purified for particular studies, it is a simple matter to analyze a small portion to determine the purity of the population. The analysis can be direct by using a primary antibody with a fluorescent tag, or can be indirect by first using an unlabeled primary antibody followed by a fluorescently tagged secondary antibody directed against the primary antibody. An alternative indirect method is to use a biotinylated second antibody followed by fluorescently labeled avidin. The advantage to the indirect methods is that they give a much greater degree of amplification of the signal, whereas the disadvantage is that they are prone to higher levels of background staining.

The procedure described here is one which is used to assess the purity of rat B and T cells; however, it can be adapted to the analysis of other cell types. Each analysis requires at least three tubes: unstained blank cells, cells stained with the second antibody only, and cells stained with the primary and secondary antibodies. To assess the degree of purity and contamination we generally stain the cells with both T- and B-cell-specific antibodies. T or B cells which have been purified as described above are suspended at a concentration of 10^6 cells/0.1 ml in HBSS/1% FCS with 0.2% azide (azide is added to prevent capping). One microliter (approximately 1 μg) of anti-rat CD2 (OX-34, BPI, ascites, final dilution 1 : 100) or 1 μl each of anti-rat IgD and IgM (MARD-3 and MARM-4, BPI, final dilutions of 1 : 200) is added to the tubes which receive the primary antibody and the tubes are incubated on ice for 1 hr. The volume is brought to 1 ml with HBSS/1% FCS and the cells are centrifuged at 200 *g* for 5 min at 4°C. The cells are resuspended in 0.1 ml HBSS/1% FCS and 2.5 μl of goat anti-mouse FITC (GAM-FITC, anti-mouse IgG H+L Rat abs, Caltag, South San Francisco, CA) is added to the primary antibody and secondary antibody controls. After an additional incubation on ice for 30 min the cells are pelleted and resuspended in HBSS/0.1% FCS and are analyzed by FACS. To determine cell viability, propidium iodide is added to a final concentration of 2.5 μg/ml 10 min prior to the final wash. The FACS operator can then determine the percent viability and can gate out dead cells. The cells also can be washed once with PBS (no BSA or FCS) and resuspended in 1 ml PBS with 2% paraformaldehyde for later analysis (do not add propidium iodide if the cells are to be fixed). We have found that fixed stained cells can be kept at 4°C for up to 5 days with little loss in the fluorescent signal. Using the procedures outlined above we routinely find that purified T-cell populations are 95–99% $CD2^+$ and IgD^-, IgM^-, and purified B-cell populations are 96–99% IgD^+, IgM^+, and are $CD2^-$. When analyzing the cells, the unstained cells are used to determine autofluorescence. Ideally, the cells stained with second antibody only should be no different than unstained cells.

The method used above can be modified for analysis for other species and other cell types by using the appropriate antibody combinations. Prior to use, both primary and secondary antibodies should be titered to attain the highest level of specific staining by primary antibodies, with the lowest level of background staining by the secondary antibodies. FACS analysis also can be useful for experimental analysis of functional changes. We have routinely used FACS analysis to measure the effect of neuropeptides on sIg expression in B cells (11).

Histochemical Analysis of Purified Monocytes and Macrophages

The histochemical method for identifying monocytes and macrophages takes advantage of the high concentrations of nonspecific esterases contained in the lysosomes of these cells. The methods for staining human and rodent monocytes and macrophages differ slightly and both methods are described here (12, 13).

Adjust the human monocyte/macrophage preparation to 5–10 × 10^6 cells/ml in RPMI containing 5–10% FCS and apply two drops onto a slide. Spread the drop with the tip of a Pasteur pipette and allow it to air-dry. In Coplin jars, fix the slides for 30 sec in cold fixative (20 mg Na_2HPO_4, 100 mg KH_2PO_4, 30 ml distilled water, 45 ml acetone, 25 ml 30% formaldehyde). Rinse by transferring the slides through four jars of distilled water and air-dry for 30 min. While the slides are drying, filter 1 ml of pararosaniline solution (1 g pararosaniline hydrochloride, Sigma, 25 ml warm 2 *N* HCl; store 4°C). Mix the filtered solution with an equal volume of freshly prepared 4% sodium nitrite and allow to stand before use until the mixture is an amber color (about 1 min). Mix together in the following sequence: 44.5 ml M/15 Sorenson's phosphate buffer (2.128 g Na_2HPO_4, 6.984 g KH_2PO_4, 1000 ml distilled water, pH 6.3), 0.25 ml pararosaniline, and 3 ml of α-naphthyl butyrate solution [1 g α-naphthyl butyrate (Sigma), 50 ml dimethyl formamide (Sigma), store at −20° C in an amber glass bottle]. Filter this solution (use only once) into a Coplin jar and stain the slides for 45 min in a 37°C water bath. Rinse with distilled water as previously described, drain the slides, and counterstain for 15 sec with 0.5% methyl green (w/v in distilled water, store at 4°C and filter before use). Rinse with distilled water, air-dry for 30 min and coverslip with Permount. The esterase-containing cells are distinguished by the presence of multiple intensely dark red-stained granules in the cytoplasm compared with the blue-green-stained esterase-negative cells.

For rodent monocytes or macrophages prepare slide as described above. Fix the slides in a Coplin jar at 4°C for 10 min with ice-cold Baker's fixative (10 ml of 4% formaldehyde, 10 ml of 10% calcium chloride, 80 ml distilled water, pH 6.7; this solution is stable at 4°C, but should only be used three or four times). Rinse the slides as described previously and air-dry. Prepare pararosaniline as described above. Prepare the incubation mixture as follows: 80 ml 0.07 *M* phosphate buffer, pH 5.7, 4.8 ml pararosaniline, 0.8 ml freshly prepared α-naphthyl acetate (20 mg α-naphthyl acetate in 0.8 ml acetone). Adjust the pH of the incubation mixture to 5.8 with NaOH and stain the slides in a Coplin jar at room temperature for 17–18 hr. Keep the reaction in the dark by covering the jar with foil. Rinse the slides in distilled water and counterstain for 10–15 sec with 1% methyl green in 0.1 *M* acetate buffer, pH 5.0. Rinse and coverslip as above.

Cell Lines

As an alternative to using primary cultures of leukocytes, there are a host of cell lines available which can be used for many applications. However, before deciding to use a cell line careful consideration must be given as to the appropriateness of the model system and to limitations in interpreting the results. One of the major limitations with leukocyte cell lines is that they are transformed cells (primary cultures of most leukocytes have short life spans). The primary criterion to consider when using a cell line is whether the cell line accurately reflects the normal physiologic process. This can be especially problematic in some situations. For example, human IM-9 B lymphoblasts express SP receptors (14). Unfortunately, there is no evidence that normal human B lymphoblasts express SP receptors. Thus, experiments on the effect of SP on IgG secretion by IM-9 cells would not be meaningful in terms of a role for SP in regulating IgG secretion by normal B lymphoblasts. However, IM-9 cells have been very useful for studies on the biochemical characterization of the SP receptor and on the effects of SP on second-messenger systems (14–18). Another common use of cell lines is in bioassay systems. Several cell lines are available which are dependent on specific factors for growth, differentiation, or specific functions. An example is the use of CTLL-2 cells for the bioassay of IL-2 (described below).

The largest supplier of cell lines and hybridomas is the American Type Culture Collection (ATCC, Rockville, MD). This agency maintains a repository of hundreds of cell lines which can be obtained very inexpensively. In addition, most investigators using a specific cell line will willingly share them. The specific requirements (media, supplements, etc.) for culturing specific cell lines are generally provided by ATCC or by the investigator supplying them. In addition, there are several excellent manuals with in-depth discussions of tissue culture techniques and media and growth requirements.

Functional Studies

T-Cell Activation

The activation of resting T cells can be divided into two stages, competence and progression, which are diagramed in Fig. 4 (reviewed in 19). The competence stage is initiated *in vivo* when the TCR binds antigen. Perturbation of the TCR initiates, via CD3, a complex signal transduction cascade that ultimately results in the induction of transcription of specific genes that encode proteins which make the cell competent to enter the next stage of

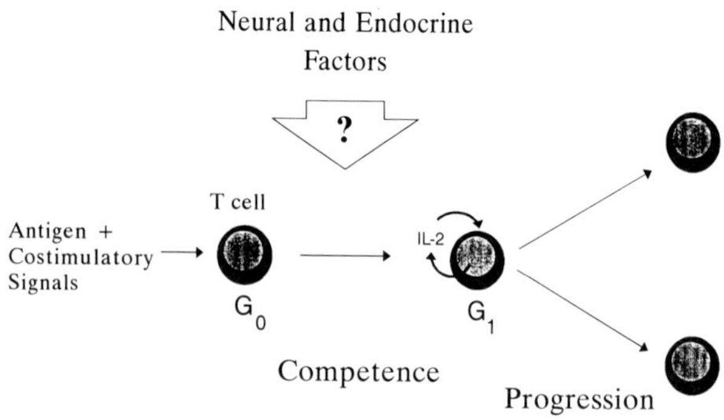

FIG. 4 T-lymphocyte activation. T-lymphocyte activation consists of two distinct temporal phases, competence and progression. On encounter with antigen and co-stimulatory signals the T cells progress from G_0 to G_1. During this period IL-2 and the IL-2 receptor are upregulated, which drives the cell from the competence phase into the progression phase. Signals derived from the neural and endocrine system have the potential to influence T lymphocytes during both of these phases.

T-cell activation. Two of these proteins are IL-2 and the α chain of the high-affinity IL-2 receptor(IL-2R). Thus, two very important events which occur during the competence stage are the secretion of IL-2 and the upregulation in surface expression of the high-affinity IL-2R. The progression stage is initiated when IL-2 binds to the IL-2R which mediates the induction of a distinct signal transduction cascade that ultimately results in the entry of the T cell into the proliferative stage of the cell cycle, clonal expansion, and differentiation into effector T cells.

The functional capacity of T cells is directly correlated with the proliferative response of these cells to specific antigen and can be measured *in vitro* by the uptake of [^{3}H]thymidine into DNA. However, since there are very few clones of T cells which can react to a given antigen it is difficult to quantitate an antigen response *in vitro*. This can be overcome with the use of T-cell-specific mitogens or with antibodies directed against CD3. These agents mimic the signals induced by specific antigen but result in the polyclonal activation of all T cells. For this reason, T-cell mitogens or MAb directed to CD3 are convenient and commonly used tools for measuring the functional capacity of T cells.

Polyclonal Activation of T Cells with Mitogens or Anti-CD3 Monoclonal Antibodies

There are a number of mitogens commonly used to polyclonally activate T cells. These include PHA, Con A, and pokeweed mitogen (PWM). Phytohemagglutinin and Con A are specific for T cells, while PWM activates both T cells and B cells. Phytohemagglutinin and Con A bind to glycoprotein subunits of the TCR and thus mimic signaling events elicited through the TCR. However, it should be noted that mitogenic effects of these lectins represent the summation of the effects induced by the binding of these lectins to a number of distinct costimulatory molecules in addition to the TCR.

The use of MAb directed to CD3 of the TCR complex to polyclonally activate T cells is more specific in that only those signaling events mediated by the TCR are induced. Thus, in studies pertaining to TCR/CD3-mediated early transmembrane signaling events this method of T-cell activation is the best choice. However, since T cells require costimulatory signals to progress into proliferation certain modifications must be made if the proliferative capacity of purified T cells to anti-CD3 MAb is to be quantitated. This is usually accomplished by immobilizing the MAb onto a solid surface and culturing the cells at a high cell density. Culturing of T cells at a high cell density increases cell–cell contact which results in homotypic interactions between accessory molecules and their ligands on adjacent T cells (20). The signals induced by these interactions replace costimulatory signals usually provided by antigen-presenting cells. In addition, immobilization of anti-CD3 MAb onto a solid surface prevents the internalization of the CD3 molecule and thus prolongs the activation signals (20).

Mitogen Stimulation of Human T Cells in 96-Well Culture Plates

Adjust the cell concentration of PBL or purified T cells to 2×10^6 cell/ml (2×10^5 cells/well) in complete* RPMI 1640 supplemented with 10% FCS. To each well add 100 μl of cells followed by the appropriate mitogen, any other treatments, and medium to bring the final volume to 200 μl. Mitogens and other treatments are generally made up as 10× stocks. The final concentration of mitogens which stimulate an optimal proliferative response in human T cells are 5 μg/ml of Con A and 25–50 μg/ml of PHA. However, it should be noted that dose–response curves should be determined for each system studied. Incubate the cultures for 72 hr in a humidified 5% CO_2 incubator. Add 2.5 μCi of [^{3}H]thymidine/50 μl during the last 6 hr of culture and harvest the cells with a multiple-sample harvester. Radioactivity incorporated into each sample is determined by liquid scintillation counting.

* RPMI 1640, 50 μM 2-mercaptoethanol, 10 mM HEPES, pH 7.4, 2 mM L-glutamine, 1× nonessential amino acids (GIBCO), 100 U/ml penicillin, and 100 μg/ml streptomycin.

Stimulation of Purified T Cells with Monoclonal Antibody Directed to CD3

Immobilize anti-CD3 MAb onto 96-well culture plates by incubating the plates at room temperature for 40 min with 50 μl/well of anti-CD3 MAb (OKT3 clone, ATCC, Rockville, MD) diluted to 10 μg/ml in 0.5 *M* Tris–HCl, pH 9.5. Wash the plate three times with 150 μl/well PBS, pH 5.2, followed by one wash with PBS, pH 7.4, supplemented with 1% FCS or 1% BSA. The plates may be stored at 4°C in this solution until needed. Adjust the T cells to 10^6 cells/ml in complete RPMI with 10% FCS, aliquot 200-μl volumes into the wells, and incubate for 72 hr as described above with [^{3}H]thymidine added during the last 6 hr of culture. Harvest and determine the radioactivity incorporated as described above. It should be noted that soluble anti-CD3 MAb (not immobilized to plastic) can be used to stimulate effectively T cells in PBL preparations which normally contain sufficient numbers of accessory cells to deliver the required costimulatory signals. Generally antibody at a final concentration of 1 ng/well is sufficient to stimulate T cells cultured at 2×10^5 cells/well, but a dose–response curve should be determined for each system studied.

B-Cell Activation

Like the T cell, B-cell activation can be divided into distinct phases (Fig. 5). During the cognitive phase, the binding of specific antigen to sIg on B cells initiates a complex cascade of biochemical events which stimulate the entry of the B cell into cell cycle and prepare it for the next phase of B-cell activation. The next phase (activation phase) is initiated when the T-helper cell delivers cell contact as well as cytokine-mediated signals to the B cell which induces proliferation (clonal expansion) and differentiation into Ig-secreting cells. In most cases antigen stimulation of B cells is T-helper cell-dependent. However, there is one class of antigens (TI-1) which is considered to be entirely T-cell-independent, but most of these are also mitogenic at high concentrations. The mechanism by which these TI-1 antigens stimulate B cells is poorly understood, but it has been postulated that a portion of the antigen molecule may possess the ability to directly stimulate the B cell and thus bypass signaling events provided by T-helper cells. The most noted example of a TI-1 antigen is lipopolysaccharide (LPS or endotoxin), which is a carbohydrate component of the cell walls of several gram-negative bacteria. LPS is frequently used as a mitogen to polyclonally activate murine B cells, but is not effective with human B cells. The most commonly used mitogen

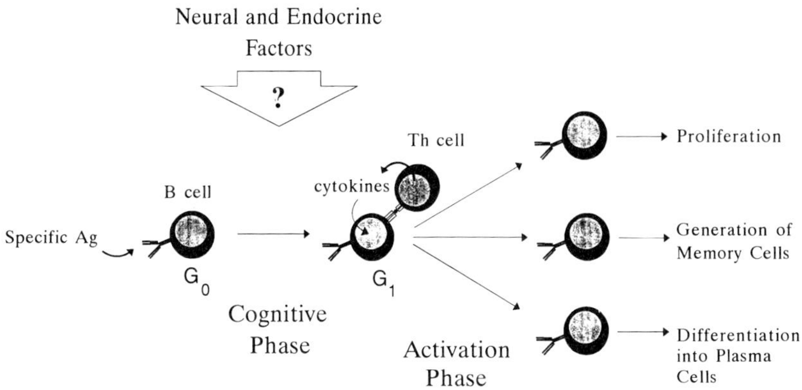

FIG. 5 B-lymphocyte activation. B-lymphocyte activation can be divided into a cognitive and an activation phase. Progression through the cognitive phase is initiated by antigen binding. For most antigens further progression requires cell–cell interaction between B cells and T helper (Th) cells and costimulatory signals, resulting in the expansion of B-cell clones. Neural and endocrine factors have the potential to modulate B-cell function during the cognitive, activation, and subsequent phases.

for human B cells is *Staphylococcus* protein A from *Staphylococcus aureus* Cowan I strain.

Activation by Calcium Ionophores and Phorbol Esters

Both T and B cells can be polyclonally activated by pharmacologic agents which mimic early transmembrane signaling events mediated by the antigen-binding receptor. These include a combination of calcium ionophores such as A23187 or ionomycin and phorbol esters such as phorbol 12-myristate 13-acetate (PMA). This combination acts synergistically to induce many of the gene activation events required for proliferation of lymphocytes. Calcium ionophores act by increasing intracellular concentrations of calcium, while phorbol esters directly activate protein kinase C. Both these events are required for optimal T- or B-cell activation and proliferation. Stock solutions of ionomycin (1 m*M*) and PMA (10 mg/ml) should be prepared in ethanol and stored at −20°C. Before use dilute the ionomycin and PMA in complete RPMI to 4 times the final concentration required per well. Dispense 50 μl of the desired concentration of ionomycin or PMA, individually and together, to triplicate wells of a 96-well culture plate. Bring the wells to 100 μl with complete RPMI and add 100 μl of purified T or B cells at a concentration of 2×10^6 cells/ml. Incubate the cultures at 37°C in a humidified 5% CO_2

incubator for 72 hr with 2.5 μCi of [^{3}H]thymidine added during the last 5 hr of culture. Harvest the cells with a multiwell cell harvester and determine the amount of radioactivity incorporated by liquid scintillation counting. Generally, final concentrations per well of ionomycin ranging from 1 to 10 μM and PMA from 5 to 20 ng/ml are used. However, as with any experimental protocol a complete dose–response should be done to determine the concentrations of these compounds which result in the optimal synergistic response.

Measurement of Cytokines

Autoregulation of the immune system relies on cell–cell contact and on a wide array of cytokines. One of the major mechanisms by which neural factors might influence immune and inflammatory responses is by the modulation of cytokine synthesis and secretion. One neuropeptide, SP, is known to influence the expression of IL-1 and IL-6 production by macrophages (21). In contrast to neurotransmitters and neuropeptides, most cytokines are not produced and stored in secretory granules, but are induced in response to appropriate stimuli. In most cases, cytokine gene induction can be measured by Northern blot or ribonuclease protection assay (RPA), and cytokine protein production can be assessed by ELISA or bioassay. The number of known cytokines involved in leukocyte regulation has grown from 3 or 4 to at least 30 to 40. Standard bioassays have been defined for many of these cytokines and cDNA probes and ELISA kits are available for most of them. One of the most critical lymphokines for T-cell activation is IL-2. Procedures outlined in this section describe an RPA and a bioassay for the measurement of IL-2 mRNA and protein, respectively. Many cytokine mRNAs can be easily detected by Northern blot analysis. However, some such as IL-2 are more difficult to detect and require a more sensitive assay such as the RPA. While ELISAs have been described for the detection of IL-2 of protein, the costs of the antibodies or of commercial ELISA kits can be prohibitive. In contrast, the major drawback to a bioassay is the specificity. Many bioassays initially described for a specific cytokine were later found to respond to other cytokines as well. For this reason it is best to correlate changes in cytokine expression detected in bioassays with some other measure such as changes in cytokine mRNA expression.

Measurement of Interleukin 2 and Interleukin 4 by Bioassay

Interleukin 2 is a 15,000 molecular weight protein produced by T cells which acts as a major progression factor for T-cell growth (22). Interleukin 2 synthesis is induced by a number of complex cellular and molecular signaling events (competence events) which include T-cell receptor activation and the action of costimulatory signals provided by accessory cells (19, 23). Without IL-2 secretion and the subsequent binding of IL-2 to the IL-2 receptor on T cells, a T cell will not enter the cell cycle and may become anergized. The production of IL-2 is controlled at several levels. Interleukin 2 gene activation is regulated by the binding of a number of specific and ubiquitous transcription factors to the enhancer region of the IL-2 gene (24, 25). Once produced, an AU-rich sequence in the 3′ untranslated region of the IL-2 message acts as a target for message degrading factors (26, 27). Thus, the levels of IL-2 mRNA and subsequent synthesis of IL-2 protein are dependent on both the level of gene induction and message stability. Interleukin 2 mRNA has a short half-life (approximately 1–2 hr) in both T-cell lines and activated peripheral blood lymphocytes (28).

CTLL-2 cells (ATCC, Rockville, MD) are a T-cell factor-dependent murine cell line which can be utilized to quantitate levels of murine and human IL-2 and murine IL-4. They are mitogen insensitive and have retained a dependence for exogenous T-cell growth factors (29–31). This basic protocol works optimally when measuring murine IL-2/IL-4 containing supernatants or human sera or culture supernatant samples. Recombinant IL-2 and/or IL-4 are used to generate a dose–response curve. Antireceptor MAb which block IL-2 or IL-4 activity are used to distinguish between the two activities in the murine system. For example, the inclusion of antibodies which block IL-4 activity will generate a bioassay specific for measuring IL-2. The inclusion of both an IL-2 and an IL-4 blocking antibody in assay wells is useful in determining whether there are any unidentified lymphokines present which can induce CTLL-2 proliferation. The CTLL-2 cells do not respond to human IL-4.

CTLL-2 cells are maintained in complete RPMI 1640 containing 10% FCS and supplemented with a source of IL-2. Interleukin 2 supplements can be obtained commercially (Delectinated IL-2, Cellular Products, Buffalo, NY) or can be prepared by stimulating rat or mouse spleen cells with Con A for 48 hr. Interleukin 2 containing supernatants should be filtered to remove debris and can be stored in aliquots at −70°C. Regardless of the source, the IL-2 supplement must be titered to determine optimal concentrations for growth and maintenance. For use in the bioassay, the cells should be collected in the log phase of growth. Wash the cells with IL-2/IL-4-free media and resuspend the cells at a concentration of 10^5 cells/ml. If blocking Ab to the IL-2 or IL-4 receptors are to be used, they should be added at this point. Controls should include cells without blocking antibodies. Incubate the cells at 37°C and 5% CO_2 for 1–3 hr to starve the cells of both IL-2 and IL-4. While the cells are preincubating set up serial dilutions of test samples (standards or unknowns) which will bracket the linear portion of the response curve. Typically, 200 μl is added to the first well in each row and a twofold serial dilution series is made by transferring 100 μl to each subsequent well. Each dilution series should be done in triplicate. Native or recombinant forms of IL-2 and IL-4 are available from a number of commercial sources for use as standards. Eight to ten 2-fold dilutions of rIL-2 beginning with 10 units/ml and of rIL-4 beginning with 100 units/ml are typically used as standards. Human serum or culture supernatant samples should be tested undiluted as the levels of IL-2 in these samples are generally very low. Preliminary assays will be necessary to determine the optimal dilution ranges for other samples. Finally, add 100 μl of preincubated cells (10^5 cells/ml) to each well. Incubate at 37°C for 24–28 hr for human IL-2 samples and 48–72 hours for murine IL-2/IL-4 samples. Label the cells by adding 2.5 μCi/50 μl of [^{3}H]thymidine for the last 5 to 6 hr of culture. Harvest the cells with a sample harvester and count by liquid scintillation. Samples containing IL-2 and/or IL-4 should give a dose-dependent rise in [^{3}H]thymidine incorporation. The concentration of unknown is determined by comparison to the standards. One unit of activity is equal to the concentration of IL-2 or IL-4 required for $\frac{1}{2}$ maximal proliferation. The results are normally expressed as units per milliliter of media/serum or units per 10^6 cells.

Measurement of IL-2 mRNA by RNase Protection

While the procedures below are described in the context of IL-2 mRNA analysis, it should be understood that the RPA can be utilized to measure the levels of a large variety mRNAs (32). One advantage of RPA is that it is several times more sensitive than either Northern blotting or S1 nuclease protection. In this assay, single-stranded (ss) antisense radiolabeled RNA probes are synthesized *in vitro*. The labeled probes are then allowed to hybridize in solution with cellular RNA to form RNA : RNA hybrids with the specific mRNA. The solutions are then treated with RNases which degrade only the single-stranded RNAs. The nondegraded RNA : RNA hybrids are then separated on denaturing polyacrylamide gels and quantitated by autoradiography. The advantages to the RPA are that: (1) high specific activity probes can be generated by *in vitro* transcription, (2) samples are not partially lost during a membrane transfer step, (3) solution hybridization occurs more readily than hybridization to membrane-immobilized RNA, (4) radiolabeled ssRNA can be produced with greater efficiency than ssDNA, (5) RNA : RNA hybrids are more stable than RNA : DNA hybrids, and (6) unhybridized RNA is removed, hence reducing the nonspecific background.

Internal and external RNA controls are used in the RPA protection assay to correct for RNA loading differences and/or to calculate absolute amounts of a specific protected RNA message. Ideally, messages which are chosen as internal RNA standards should be present in tissue at similar levels during all stages of an organisms development. Since no single gene is transcribed at a constant level in all cells under all possible conditions, one must find an appropriate RNA control for the samples being analyzed. "Housekeeping genes" which are constitutively expressed tend to be ideal internal RNA standards. Examples of internal controls commonly used in this assay include β-actin, 18S rRNA, 28S rRNA, 16S mitochondrial rRNA, and glyceraldehyde-3-phosphate dehydrogenase. External RNA controls are commonly synthesized by *in vitro* transcription and are used to spike an RNA sample. The external RNA standard chosen for an experiment should not be found naturally in the cells being examined. For example, X-Gal RNA (sense strand) would be a good external standard for use in human T-cell RNA samples. One could then use a labeled antisense X-Gal RNA for detection. Since a known amount of external RNA standard can be added to a sample, external standards are commonly used to calculate the absolute amount of RNA in a given band.

The procedure for isolating RNA is based on the method described by Chirgwin *et al.* (33). Alternative methods for extracting RNA also may be used, such as the rapid method described by Chomzynski *et al.* (34). However, in our hands the use of CsCl extracted RNA has given very consistent results and recoveries (yields of approximately 10–15 μg RNA/10^7 cells). Detectable levels of IL-2 mRNA are present in human T-cells from 4 to 18 hr after mitogen or anti-CD3 stimulation. Peak IL-2 mRNA levels occur approximately 6 hr after stimulation. PHA or PMA + Con A are more potent stimulators of IL-2 mRNA production in human T cells than immobilized anti-CD3. To isolate RNA, first pellet cells by centrifugation for 10 min at 200 *g* at 4°C. Lyse the cells by adding 2 ml of 4 *M* guanidine lysis buffer (4 *M* guanidine thiocyanate, 0.5% *N*-laurylsarcosine, 25 m*M* sodium citrate, pH 7.0, 0.1 m*M* 2-mercaptoethanol) to each sample. With a 3-ml syringe fitted to a 22-gauge $1\frac{1}{2}$ inch needle, break up the cell pellet by pulling the solution into the syringe and expelling it, three to five times while keeping foaming at a minimum. It is critical that the chromosomal DNA is sheared in this step to reduce viscosity and to allow for complete removal of DNA during the ultracentrifugation. In addition, the shearing process prevents the formation of an impenetrable DNA mat at the top of the CsCl layer, which could block the sedimentation of RNA.

The guanidinium cell lysate can be quickly frozen in dry ice/ethanol and stored at −70°C or may be stored at room temperature for up to 24 hr before ultracentrifugation. Rinse out Beckman ultracentrifuge tubes with 95% ethanol followed by DEPC-treated water, invert the tubes, and allow all liquids to drain out. Add 2 ml of 5.7 *M* CsCl solution to each ultracentrifuge tube. Carefully layer disrupted cells on top of the CsCl samples. Using a Beckman SW50.1, SW55Ti or SW60 rotor (or equivalent), centrifuge at 36,000 rpm for 16–18 hr at room temperature (20–24°C) with the brake off. After centrifugation, remove DNA at the interface of the guanidine/CsCl solutions and discard. Carefully pipette the solution out of the tube until only 0.5–1 ml of CsCl is left in the bottom of the tube. Carefully cut off the top half of the tube to get rid of any DNA and protein which may be stuck to the tube walls and invert the tube gently to remove the remaining guanidine/CsCl solution. Let stand for 15 min to drain completely. RNA pellets are translucent and may not be visible until all liquid is removed from the tubes. If only the minimum number of cells (10^7 cells) are used, the RNA is usually not visible after the guanidine/CsCl solution is removed. Resuspend the RNA pellet in 400 μl of DEPC-treated H_2O, cover the tubes with parafilm, and place on ice for 30 min. Transfer samples to RNase-free microcentrifuge tubes. Add 20 μl of DEPC-treated 5 *M* NaCl (1/20th volume) and 1 ml of cold 100% ethanol (2.5 volumes) to each sample and mix. Place samples in a −70°C freezer for a minimum of 4 hr to precipitate the RNA. Centrifuge the samples in the cold for 30 min at top speed (12,000–14,000 *g*). Wash the RNA pellets with cold 70% ethanol and vacuum-dry. Do not dry the RNA pellet to total dryness, however, or it will become difficult to resuspend the RNA. Resuspend RNA in a minimal volume of DEPC-treated H_2O (20–50 μl). To obtain a concentration and purity reading on the RNA, prepare a 1 : 100 dilution of each RNA sample in H_2O. Determine the optical density of the samples at both 260 and 280 nm. The ratio of A_{260}/A_{280} should be 1.9–2.0 for pure RNA. An OD_{260} reading of 1 corresponds to approximately 40 μg/ml of RNA. If the RNA is not pure, RNA can be extracted with buffer-equilibrated phenol : chloroform and ethanol precipitated.

Single-stranded RNA probes are produced from cDNA templates which have been subcloned into a plasmid vector containing an SP6, T7, or T3 RNA polymerase in an antisense orientation to the cDNA. To generate IL-2-specific probes a 250-bp *Pst*I/*Xba*I fragment of an IL-2 cDNA from pTCGF11 (ATCC, 39673) is subcloned into pGEM-2. For an internal standard, a 593-bp *Hin*dIII/*Sal*I fragment of β-actin from pHFβA1 (35) is subcloned into the *Sal*I/*Hin*dIII-digested pGEM-2. Once the cDNA has been subcloned into the appropriate vector, the plasmid is linearized at a suitable restriction site so that the *in vitro* transcription reaction will produce "run off" transcripts. The IL-2 and β-actin constructs we use are linearized with *Hin*dIII which results in the production of a 285-nucleotide probe for IL-2 and 633 nucleotide probe for β-actin. Ideally, the restriction digest should leave a 5′ overhang or a blunt end. Digestion with enzymes which create a 3′ overhang should be avoided since they can yield extraneous transcripts.

If it is necessary to linearize a plasmid with one of these enzymes, convert the 3′ overhang into a blunt end with Klenow prior to utilization in an *in vitro* transcription reaction. The restriction digest must be complete before the template is used in an *in vitro* transcription reaction. Even a small amount of undigested plasmid can give rise to long transcripts which encode plasmid sequence and incorporate a substantial amount of labeled nucleotide. To prevent circular plasmid contamination, purify the linearized plasmid by agarose gel electrophoresis after the digestion is complete. Several methods are available commercially (Gene Clean, Biolabs 101, San Diego, CA) which aid in the removal of DNA from agarose.

Single-stranded RNA probes are produced using the linearized plasmid as a template. To a sterile RNase-free microcentrifuge tube add the following solutions at room temperature:

Volume (μl)	Solution
4.0	5× transcription buffer (200 m*M* Tris, pH 7.5, 30 m*M* $MgCl_2$, 10 m*M* spermidine, 50 m*M* NaCl)
2.0	100 m*M* dithiothreitol (DTT)
0.5	rRNasin RNase inhibitor (40 units/μl stock)
4.0	Mixture of 2.5 m*M* rATP, rGTP, and rUTP
2.4	100 μ*M* rCTP
0.5–1.5	Linear DNA template in water or TE buffer (10–50 μg/ml final)
5.0	[α-^{32}P]rCTP (50 μCi, 400–800 Ci/mmol)
1.0	SP6 RNA polymerase* (at 15–20 units/ml, Promega, Madison, WI)
0–1.0	H_2O (to a final volume of 20 μl)

Incubate for 60 min at 37°C. Following the incubation, add 1 unit rRNasin/μl reaction mix and RQ1 RNase-free DNase (Promega) to a final concentration of 1 unit/μg DNA and incubate for 10–15 min at 37°C. Unincorporated nucleotides are removed by size exclusion chromatography using Bio-Gel A-1.5M, 100–200 MESH (prepared according to manufacturer's instructions and sterilized by autoclaving, Bio-Rad, Richmond, CA). Plug a 5-inch Plasteur pipette with glass wool, rinse the pipette with DEPC-treated H_2O, and add Bio-Gel A-1.5 *M* until the packed column level is just above the notch in the pipette. Wash the column 3–4 times with DEPC-treated H_2O. When the DNase treatment is complete, add tRNA (1–2 μl, 10 mg/ml) as a carrier and add the reaction mixture to the top of the gel. After the sample has entered the column add 400 μl of DEPC-treated water and begin collecting fractions. After collection of the first fraction is complete (400 μl), add 100 μl of DEPC-treated H_2O to the column and collect fraction No. 2 (100 μl). Repeat this procedure using 100-μl additions until 10–15 fractions have been

* If T3 or T7 polymerase are being used, the buffers should be adjusted according to the supplier's instructions.

collected and count the radioactivity in 1 μl of each fraction by liquid scintillation. The earliest fraction with the highest level of radioactive incorporation will be used in the RPA. Probes should have a specific activity of at least 1–3 × 10^8 cpm/μg and should be used the same day they are made.

Set up the hybridization by adding the test RNA (5–100 μg) and the radioactively labeled probe(s) (1–5 × 10^5 cpm of each probe) to a microcentrifuge tube. Use 5–10 μg of total RNA for the detection of abundant messages and 20–100 μg for rare messages. For the IL-2 RPA we add at least 20 μg of T-cell RNA. Add 1/9th volume of 3 *M* NaOAc (pH 5.2) to each tube for a final concentration of 0.3 *M* NaOAc followed by 2.5 volumes of cold 100% ethanol. Place samples at −20°C for at least 2 hr, then centrifuge for 15 min at 12,000–14,000 rpm at 4°C. Rinse the RNA pellets with 0.5 ml of cold 70% ethanol. Centrifuge at 12,000–14,000 rpm at 4°C for 5 min. Vacuum-dry the RNA pellets to near dryness. Prepare the hybridization buffer by mixing one part 5× hybridization buffer (200 m*M* PIPES, pH 6.7, 2.0 *M* NaCl, and 5 m*M* EDTA) with four parts of deionized formamide and resuspend each RNA pellet in 30 μl of hybridization solution. Heat the samples at 85°C for 5 min to denature the RNA and rapidly transfer the samples to the optimum hybridization temperature for the probe being used (30–60°C; 45°C may be a good starting point if the optimum hybridization temperature for a probe is unknown). The optimal temperature for the IL-2 probe described here is 48–50°C. Hybridize the samples for at least 12 hr. Add 300 μl of freshly prepared ssRNA digestion solution (300 m*M* NaCl, 10 m*M* Tris–HCl, pH 7.0, 5 m*M* EDTA, 40 μg/ml RNase A, and 200 units/ml or 2 μg/RNase T_1) to each sample and incubate at 37°C for 1–2 hr. To terminate the digestion reaction add 20 μl of 10% SDS and 50 μg proteinase K (5 μl of a 20 mg/ml stock solution) and incubate at 37°C for 15 min. Extract each sample with an equal volume of buffer-equilibrated phenol : chloroform : isoamyl alcohol (25 : 24 : 1) and centrifuge the samples for 5 min at room temperature. Transfer the aqueous layer to a new tube and add 2 μl tRNA (10 mg/ml). Add 2.5 volumes of cold 100% ethanol to each tube and mix well. Place the tubes at −20°C for at least 1 hr. Centrifuge for 30 min at 14,000 rpm at 4°C. Wash the pellet with cold 70% ethanol followed by a wash with cold 95% ethanol and vacuum-dry RNA (to near dryness). Resuspend each RNA pellet in 10 μl of RPA gel-loading buffer. Prepare "probe only" samples by mixing 10 μl of gel-loading dye* with 1 μl of labeled probe in a separate tube. Heat the samples for 5 min at 95°C and chill on ice for 5 min.

The samples are resolved on a 7 *M* urea denaturing 6% acrylamide gel using 1× TBE (36) as the tank buffer. We typically use an 18 × 20-cm gel. Before the sample is loaded, the gel is prerun at 40–45 V/cm for 30 min.

* Gel-loading dye is 80% formamide, 10 m*M* EDTA, 0.1% bromophenol blue, and 0.1% xylene cyanol.

Before loading the samples, flush the urea out of the bottom of the wells. Run the gel for 1–1.5 hr at 40–45 V/cm. The exact voltage may vary; however the glass plates on the gel should be hot to the touch (this is an indication that the gel is hot enough to keep the RNA samples denatured). The gel is placed on 3MM paper and the radioactivity in the protected bands can be quantified in a number of ways depending on the equipment available. The standard method is to produce autoradiographs by exposing the gel to X-ray film. The relative radioactivity in the bands can then be assessed by densitometric analysis. An alternative method that is gaining popularity is the use of phosphor imaging systems. Once the protected bands have been quantitated, the amount of mRNA of interest is normalized by comparison to an internal standard such as actin in order to compensate for differences in recovery from individual samples. The IL-2 probe described above yields a 250-nucleotide protected fragment. The β-actin internal standard yields a 69-nucleotide fragment which is used to normalize for RNA recovery, and the results are reported as a ratio of IL-2 : β-actin optical density.

Assessment of Interleukin 2 Receptor Expression as Indicator of T-Cell Activation

The high-affinity IL-2 receptor is composed of at least three polypeptide subunits (19). Two of these subunits, the α chain (p55 or TAC) and the β chain (p75), are transmembrane glycoproteins which are involved in the direct binding of the IL-2 molecule. The β chain is constituitively expressed on resting T cells and only moderately upregulated after T-cell stimulation. The α chain which binds IL-2 with a low affinity is not expressed on resting T cells but is upregulated to at least 10-fold that of the β chain and functions primarily to keep the biologically functional p75 complexed in a high-affinity IL-2 receptor. Thus, the upregulation of surface expression of p55 after T-cell stimulation has traditionally been correlated with the appearance of the high-affinity IL-2 receptor. Upregulation of p55 can be assessed by indirect immunofluorescence and FACS analysis or by the specific binding of radiolabeled IL-2 (35). Immunofluorescence is the easier of the two methods but does not yield any information on the number of sites per cell nor the affinity of the receptor. This is accomplished by performing Scatchard analysis of saturation binding assays.

Assessment of Interleukin 2 Receptor Expression on Activated T Cells by Indirect Immunofluorescence

Dilute 10^6 mitogen or anit-CD3 MAb-stimulated T cells to 200 μl in ice-cold PBS with 0.02% sodium azide (PBS/azide) in 12 × 75-mm culture tubes

(Falcon, 2054). Add 5 μl of anti-p55 MAb [1 mg/ml; anti-p55 hybridomas are available from ATCC (Rockville, MD) or from several commercial sources]. To assess background fluorescence, to a separate tube add 5 μl of an irrelevant MAb (1 mg/ml) of the same isotype. Incubate the cells on ice for 30 min and wash twice with 1 ml of PBS/azide. Resuspend the cell pellets in 100 μl of a 1 : 10 dilution (diluted in PBS/azide) of FITC-labeled $F(Ab')_2$ goat or rabbit anti-mouse IgG. The FITC-labeled second antibody should be centrifuged at a high speed in a microcentrifuge for 15 min to remove any aggregated material. Incubate the cells on ice for 15 to 30 min and wash twice with PBS/azide. Resuspend the cells in 1 ml of 1% paraformaldehyde in PBS to fix the cells prior to FACS analysis. The upregulation of the IL-2 receptor as measured by this technique is evident at 24 hr after stimulation and peaks between 48–72 hr.

Assessment of Interleukin 2 Expression by Specific Binding of Radiolabeled Interleukin 2

Harvest activated PBL 48 hr after stimulation with PHA or anti-CD3 MAb and incubate at 37°C in 50 ml of RPMI medium for two 1-hr periods to remove endogenous IL-2. After extensive washing with RPMI, resuspend the cells in binding medium (RPMI supplemented with 10% FCS and 25 m*M* HEPES, pH 7.3) and add 80 μl containing 3×10^5 cells to microcentrifuge tubes. Duplicate total binding and nonspecific binding (NSB) tubes are set up for each concentration of hot ligand. Add 10 μl of 10 μM unlabeled rIL-2 to the NSB tubes and 10 μl of binding medium to the total binding tubes. Preincubate the tubes after the addition of the cold rIL-2 for 10 min in a 37°C water bath. Serially dilute [^{125}I]rIL-2 (sp act, 20–40 μCi/mg) in binding medium to yield final incubation concentrations ranging from 2.0 to 600 p*M*/tube. After preincubation add 10 μl of the appropriate dilution of [^{125}I]rIL-2 to the replicate total and NSB tubes and incubate the tubes for 25 min at 37°C. Stop the reaction by adding 1 ml of ice-cold binding medium and centrifuge in a microcentrifuge at 13,000 rpm for 2 min. Carefully remove the supernatant from each tube and count on a gamma counter to determine the free cpm. Count the pellets in a gamma counter to determine the total cpm bound to the cells. Specific binding is determined by subtraction of CPM in the NSB tubes from the CPM in the total binding tubes for each hot ligand concentration. Once the specific bound CPM and the free CPM are determined there are a number of computer programs (Lundon-1; LIGAND) which can be used to estimate the number of sites/cell and relative affinity of the receptors.

Analysis of Cell Signaling and Measurement of Second Messengers in Leukocytes

The earliest events in cells in response to signals such as cell–cell contact or receptor stimulation is the generation of second messengers. These second-messenger signals include the adenylyl cyclase–cAMP pathway, the phosphatidylinositol pathway, tyrosine kinase and phosphatase pathways, and the guanylyl cyclase–cGMP pathway. The generation of the second messengers occurs within seconds to minutes, initiating cascades of events that may be manifest over a period of days. Thus, it is important in planning studies of second messengers that the measurements be taken at appropriate time points to avoid missing the flux in second messengers that has occurred in response to a stimulus. The following are a few examples of well-characterized receptor-linked second-messenger systems present in T cells. The TCR complex is linked to the phosphatidyl-inositol pathway by tyrosine kinases (19). Activation of T cells through mitogen stimulation or cross-linking the TCR with antibody results in the rapid generation of IP_3 and diacylglycerol (DAG). The IP_3 stimulates the release of intracellular calcium, which together with DAG stimulates protein kinase C. Activation of T cells also can be accomplished by using a calcium ionophore and phorbol ester to stimulate a calcium flux and activate protein kinase C, thus bypassing stimulations through the TCR. Examples of receptors linked to cAMP production in lymphocytes include the β-adrenergic receptor, the CGRP receptor, and prostaglandin receptors. The binding of the ligand to the receptor stimulates the receptor–Gs protein complex. The α subunit of Gs then stimulates adenylyl cyclase to convert ATP to cAMP, which in turn activates protein kinase A.

Measurement of Intracellular cAMP by Radioimmunoassay (RIA)

Lymphocytes are isolated and resuspended at 2.2×10^6/ml in modified RPMI 1640 containing 100 μM isobutylmethylxanthine (IBMX). Preincubation of the samples with IBMX blocks the breakdown of cAMP by phosphodiesterases, thus the total accumulation of intracellular cAMP is measured in the RIA. IBMX is made as a 10 mM stock in 50 mM sodium hydroxide and is diluted 1 : 100 in the modified RPMI. Aliquots of 225 μl of cells are placed into microcentrifuge tubes and incubated 10 min at 37°C. Stimulants are added in 25 μl from 10× stock solutions and incubated for the desired length of time, usually 1–30 min. To stop the incubation, the cells are placed in an ice bath. The cells are then rapidly pelleted by spinning in a microcentrifuge for 15–30 sec and the medium is removed and replaced with 250 μl of

0.05 *M* sodium acetate buffer (mix 246.5 ml of 0.2 *M* sodium acetate with 3.5 ml of 0.2 *M* acetic acid, adjust pH to 6.5, and dilute to 1 liter with H_2O; store at 4°C up to 4 weeks). The samples are boiled for 3 min to stop enzyme activity and to lyse the cells. The lysates are kept frozen until assayed for cAMP.

The levels of cAMP are determined by RIA (37). The frozen samples are thawed, diluted to 1.25 ml total with sodium acetate buffer, and then centrifuged 10 min at 13,000 *g* in a microcentrifuge. One milliliter of the supernatant is transferred to new microcentrifuge tube. Samples and RIA standards are acetylated by the addition of 5 μl of freshly prepared triethylamine/acetic anhydride (2 : 1, v/v) and vortexing. The acetylation of the samples greatly increases the sensitivity of the assay and should be done unless very high levels of cAMP are expected. The RIA for cAMP can be done with commercially available kits which use [^{125}I]cAMP and specific anti-cAMP antiserum (Amersham; Dupont). In our assay system, 10–50 μl of sample supernatant was needed to assay cAMP. The results are adjusted to represent the pmol cAMP/10^6 lymphocytes. When using mouse lymphocytes, it may be necessary to increase the cell concentration to 5–10 $\times$ 10^6/ml in order to have measurable levels of cAMP. For many ligands such as CGRP, isoproterenol, or prostaglandins, maximal cAMP levels are reached in the cells within 5–10 min. If forskolin is used as a positive control for adenylate cyclase activity, a 30-min incubation is needed in lymphocytes to obtain a good response.

Measurement of Intracellular Calcium Mobilization

Changes in the levels of free intracellular calcium can be measured using fluorescent calcium indicators such as Indo-1 and Fura-2 (Molecular Probes, Eugene, OR). Depending on the equipment available, the analysis can be done on cells in suspension in a cuvette, by cell sorter, or by microscopy. The greatest difficulty with microscopy is the small amount of cytoplasm relative to the size of the nucleus in lymphocytes, thus limiting this approach. The protocol for loading lymphocytes with the dyes is the same for the various methods, except that the choice of dye will depend on the instrumentation. Indo-1 is the preferred dye for cell sortér analysis because a single excitation wavelength is used, while the calcium-free and calcium-bound forms of the dye emit at different wavelengths. In contrast, Fura-2 has different maximal excitation wavelengths for the calcium-free and calcium-bound forms, but the emission wavelength is the same. In addition, other dyes have been developed that provide additional options for calcium studies. The Molecular Probes catalog is an invaluable resource for references and applications. The calcium indicators are supplied as cell-permeable acetoxymethyl (AM) esters. Once the indicator is in the cell, esterases cleave the molecule such that it is now impermeant and is trapped in the cytoplasm. To load lymphocytes with Fura-2 or Indo-1, resuspend the lymphocytes at 1×10^7/ml in HEPES-buffered HBSS with 2 μM Fura-2 or 1 μM Indo-1. Incubate the cells for 30 min at 37°C and wash twice with HEPES-buffered HBSS. If the calcium measurements will be made using a fluorimeter, the cells are resuspended (5×10^6/ml) in HEPES-buffered HBSS without phenol red, as the phenol red will interfere with the calcium measurements. The cells are placed in a cuvette and maintained in solution at 37°C with continual stirring using a micro stir bar. Care must be taken not to stir too vigorously as the basal levels of calcium will change. The data are expressed as the ratio of the fluorescence intensities at the appropriate wavelengths for the calcium-free and the calcium-bound forms of the dye. Stimulants are added to the cell suspension from 100× stock solutions. For complete discussion of the methods for calibration of calcium concentrations, see Grynkiewicz *et al.* (38). The Molecular Probes catalog also includes a helpful discussion of the various dyes and provides many references. For flow cytometry, the lymphocytes are loaded with Indo-1, washed with HEPES-buffered HBSS, and resuspended at 1×10^6/ml in RPMI. The cells are maintained at 37°C in a water bath until they can be run through the cell sorter. Depending on the software available, it is possible to continuously monitor the baseline calcium and calcium fluxes in response to a stimulus. If this is not possible, samples of a specified number of events are taken at short time intervals (15–30 sec), and the average fluorescence ratio for each interval is plotted.

Quantitation of Inositol Triphosphate (IP_3) in Stimulated T Cells

The following method is for the quantitation of IP_3 in purified T cells stimulated through the TCR/CD3, but may be modified for T-cell subpopulations as well as B cells stimulated through the Ig receptor. Since soluble anti-CD3 MAb is used in this assay, it must be cross-linked on the surface of the T cells to induce an optimal response. This is easily accomplished by either cross-linking the anti-CD3 MAb with a second antibody directed to the isotype of the anti-CD3 MAb or by first biotinylating the anti-CD3 MAb and cross-linking with streptavidin. We have found that cross-linking with a second antibody is more efficient. Inositol triphosphate should be measured at no fewer than five time points in duplicate samples. Add 5×10^6 cells in 0.5 ml into 13×100 glass culture tubes and preincubate with 10 μg of anti-CD3 MAb (OKT3 clone) in a 37°C water bath for 4 min. After preincubation add 10 μg of goat anti-mouse IgG to each tube and incubate for 0.5, 1, 2, 4, and 10 min. Stop the reaction by adding 0.5 ml of ice-cold 15% trichloroacetic acid (TCA) and place the tubes in an ice bath. After the last time point is collected incubate on ice for 10 min, centrifuge the tubes at 500 *g* for 15 min, and transfer the supernatants to new tubes. Extract the supernatants three times with 3 ml of water-saturated ether. Transfer the aqueous fraction to a new 13 × 100 glass tube. After the last extraction transfer the aqueous fraction to a microcentrifuge tube and add 10 μl of 1 *M* sodium bicarbonate to each sample. The samples may be stored at −20°C. The level of IP_3 in 100 μl of each sample is measured using an IP_3 assay system kit (Amersham, Arlington Heights, IL). The results are expressed in p*M* IP_3 per 5×10^6 cells.

Tyrosine Phosphorylation of Substrate Proteins in Stimulated T Cells

Following T-cell or B-cell activation, a number of substrate proteins are phosphorylated on tyrosines (19). Proteins which are phosphorylated on tyrosine can be detected by immunoblot analysis using antiphosphotyrosine antibodies. Although this assay is described for T cells stimulated through the TCR/CD3 complex, it may be modified for T-cell subsets as well as B cells stimulated through the IgG receptor. Add 5×10^6 cells in 250 μl of RPMI 1640 to microcentrifuge tubes and preincubate the cells with 10 μg of anti-CD3 MAb for 4 min in a 37°C water bath. Add 10 μg of goat anti-mouse Ig to each tube at 10-sec intervals and incubate the tubes for the desired times. The suggested times are 0.5, 1, 1.5, 2, 5, 10, and 20 min. The baseline control is T cells without stimulus. The reaction is stopped with the addition of 25 μl of 10× lysis buffer* and incubation in an ice bath for 15 min. Centrifuge at maximum speed in a cold microcentrifuge and transfer the postnuclear lysate to a new microcentrifuge tube. Separate the proteins by SDS–PAGE (10% acrylamide) and transfer to nitrocellulose by electroblotting. After being bound by antiphosphotyrosine antibodies, the tyrosine phosphorylated proteins may be visualized by a variety of methods. The most sensitive assay currently available is enhanced chemiluminescence (ECL, Amersham, Arlington Heights). There are several sources available for MAb directed to tyrosine residues. We have found that horseradish peroxidase-labeled recombinant antiphosphotyrosine MAb (RC-20, Transduction Laboratories, Lexington, KY) consistently results in greater sensitivity with less background staining. Described below is a modification of the ECL staining protocol using RC-20 which in our hands gives us the best results.

After separation on SDS–PAGE and transfer to nitrocellulose, incubate

* 10× lysis buffer is 5% Triton X-100, 100 μg/ml leupeptin, 100 μg/ml aprotinin, 250 μg/ml phenylmethylsulfonyl fluoride, 100 m*M* iodoacetamide, 10 m*M* sodium orthovanadate, and 50 m*M* EDTA.

the blots for at least 1 hr with blocking buffer (20 m*M* Tris–HCl, pH 7.6, 137 m*M* NaCl, 0.3% Tween 20, 3% BSA). Rinse the blot with two quick changes of wash buffer (blocking buffer without BSA) followed by two 10-min washes and one 20-min, with rocking, in 200 to 300 ml of wash buffer. After washing, seal the blot in a bag with 30 to 40 ml of RC-20 MAb diluted 1:2500 in diluent buffer and incubate at room temperature with rocking for 12–18 hr. Remove the blot and rinse with two quick changes of wash buffer followed by two 10-min washes, four 5-min washes, and one 1-hr wash (with rocking) in 200–300 ml of wash buffer. Expose the blot for 1 min on each side (with gentle swirling to completely coat the blot) to 30–40 ml of ECL solution, mixed according to the directions supplied with the kit. Wrap the blot in plastic and develop several exposures on X-ray film to ensure the best exposure time for your blot. The suggested exposure times range between 10 sec and 10 min.

References

1. D. G. Payan, J. P. McGills, and E. J. Goetzl, *Adv. Immunol.* **39,** 299 (1986).
2. M. S. O'Dorisio and A. Paneria (eds.), "Neuropeptides and Immunopeptides: Messengers in a Neuroimmune Axis." New York Academy of Sciences, New York, 1990.
3. B. B. Mishell and S. M. Shiigi (eds.), "Selected Methods in Cellular Immunology." Freeman, San Francisco, 1980.
4. D. M. Weir, L. A. Herzenberg, C. Blackwell, and L. A. Herzenberg (eds.), "Handbook of Experimental Immunology," Vols. 1–4. Blackwell Scientific Publications, Oxford, 1986.
5. J. E. Colligan, A. M. Kruisbeck, D. H. Margulis, E. M. Shevach, and W. Strober, "Current Protocols in Immunology," Vols. 1 and 2. Green Publishing Associates, Wiley Interscience, New York, 1991.
6. J. Westermann and R. Pabst, *Immunol. Today* **11,** 406 (1990).
7. L. J. Wysocki and V. L. Sato, *Proc. Natl. Acad. Sci. U.S.A.* **75,** 2844 (1978).
8. D. W. Mason, W. J. Penhale, and J. D. Sedgewick, *in* "Lymphocytes: A Practical Approach" (G. G. B. Klaus, ed.), p. 48. IRL Press, Oxford, 1987.
9. C. D. Severson, D. L. Burg, D. E. Lafrenz, and T. L. Feldbush, *Immunol. Lett.* **15,** 291 (1990).
10. J. P. McGillis, S. Humphreys, and S. Reid, *J. Immunol.* **147,** 3482 (1991).
11. J. P. McGillis, S. Humphreys, V. Rangnekar, and J. Ciallella, *Cell. Immunol.* **150,** 405 (1993).
12. J. Meuller, B. Brun del Re, H. Buerki, H.-U. Keller, M. W. Hess, and H. Cottier, *Eur. J. Immunol.* **5,** 270 (1975).
13. L. T. Yam, C. Y. Li, and W. H. Crosby *Am. J. Clin. Pathol.* **55,** 283 (1971).
14. D. G. Payan, J. P. McGillis, and J. L. Organist, *J. Biol. Chem.* **261,** 14321 (1986).
15. J. P. McGillis, M. L. Organist, and D. G. Payan, *Anal. Biochem.* **164,** 502 (1987).

16. J. P. McGillis, M. L. Organist, K. H. Scriven, and D. G. Payan, *J. Neurosci. Res.* **18,** 190 (1987).
17. M. L. Organist, J. P. Harvey, J. P. McGillis, and D. G. Payan, *Biochem. Biophys. Res. Commun.* **151,** 535 (1988).
18. M. L. Organist, J. Harvey, J. P. McGillis, M. Mitsuhashi, P. Melera, and D. G. Payan, *J. Immunol.* **139,** 3050 (1987).
19. A. Altman, K. M. Coggeshall, and T. Mustelin, *Adv. Immunol.* **48,** 227 (1990).
20. R. H. Schwartz, *Science* **248,** 1349 (1990).
21. M. Lotz, J. H. Vaughn, and D. A. Carson, *Science* **241,** 1218 (1988).
22. K. A. Smith, *Annu. Rev. Immunol.* **2,** 319 (1984).
23. T. D. Geppert, L. S. Davis, H. Gur, M. C. Wacholtz, and P. E. Lipsky, *Immunol. Rev.* **117,** 5 (1990).
24. G. R. Crabtree, *Science* **243,** 355 (1989).
25. K. Ullman, J. P. Northrop, C. L. Vereiji, and G. R. Crabtree, *Annu. Rev. Immunol.* **8,** 421 (1990).
26. G. Shaw and R. Kamen, *Cell (Cambridge, Mass.)* **46,** 659 (1986).
27. D. Caput, B. Beutler, K. Hartog, R. Thayer, S. Brown-Shimer, and A. Cerami, *Proc. Natl. Acad. Sci. U.S.A.* **83,** 1670 (1986).
28. T. Lindsten, C. H. June, J. A. Ledbetter, G. Stella, and C. B. Thompson, *Science* **244,** 339 (1989).
29. S. Gillis, M. M. Ferm, W. Ou, and K. A. Smith, *J. Immunol.* **120,** 2027 (1978).
30. S. Gillis and K. A. Smith, *Nature (London)* **268,** 154 (1977).
31. S. Gillis and K. A. Smith, *J. Exp. Med.* **146,** 468 (1977).
32. D. A. Melton, P. A. Krieg, M. R. Rebagliati, T. Maniatis, K. Zinn, and M. R. Green, *Nucleic Acids Res.* **12,** 7035 (1984).
33. J. M. Chirgwin, A. E. Przybyla, R. J. MacDonald, and W. J. Rutter, *Biochemistry* **18,** 5294 (1979).
34. P. Chomczynski and N. Sacchi, *Anal. Bioc.* **162,** 156 (1987).
35. L. H. Elliott, W. H. Brooks, and T. L. Roszman, *Clin. Invest.* **86,** 80 (1990).
36. J. Sambrook, E. F. Fritsch, and T. Maniatis (eds.), "Molecular Cloning: A Laboratory Manual," Cold Spring Harbor Laboratory Press, Cold Spring Harbor, NY, 1990.
37. J. F. Harper and G. Brooker, *J. Cyclic Nucleotide Res.* **1,** 207 (1975).
38. G. Grynkiewicz, M. Poenie, and R. Y. Tsien, *J. Biol. Chem.* **260,** 3440 (1985).

[9] Methods in Immunotoxicology

Rob J. Vandebriel, Johan Garssen, and Henk Van Loveren

Introduction

Immunotoxicology is the discipline that is concerned with the study of adverse effects of toxic compounds on the immune system. Assessment of potential immunotoxicity is often carried out in the context of general toxicity testing.

An array of rodent assays to assess effects of compounds on the immune system have been or are being developed. They can be divided into nonfunctional and functional assays. Nonfunctional assays provide parameters that may change on effects on the immune system. They, however, do not provide information on the immune system as a functional entity. Functional assays more closely reflect the *in vivo* situation. A wide range of both nonfunctional and functional rodent assays, their characteristics, and some notes on how to perform them are addressed here.

Although, to our knowledge, the assays described here are not validated in neuroimmunological testing, this overview provides a basis to start testing for immune competence.

Rodent Assays for Immunotoxicity

Nonfunctional Assays

Organ Weights

The immunological organs that are suited to weigh in immunotoxicity studies are (a) the thymus, which plays a decisive role in the development of the immune system and is affected by many immunotoxic compounds, (b) the spleen, which is involved in the induction of immune responses and which is also the repository for many recirculating lymphocytes, and (c) the lymph nodes, which are important for the induction of immune responses. It is important to weigh the draining lymph nodes. Thus, for oral exposure the mesenteric nodes and for inhalatory exposure the bronchial nodes should be weighed. In view of systemic effects, distant lymph nodes such as popliteal nodes can also be weighed. Especially for mesenteric nodes there is a string of such nodes within nonlymphoid fatty tissue. This nonlymphoid tissue must be removed for accurate determination of weight. In addition to the weight, the cellularity of these organs is an indicative parameter for effects on the immune system.

Pathology

In addition to histopathology of the thymus, spleen, and draining and distant lymph nodes, histopathology of the mucosal immune system (Peyer's patches in the gut and bronchus- and nose-associated lymphoid tissue in the respiratory tract) and the skin immune system can be performed, depending on the route of exposure. Next to hematoxylin–eosin-stained paraffin-embedded sections, immunoperoxidase staining is a valuable means of evaluation. For mice and rats many monoclonal antibodies (mAbs)* are commercially available to detect differentiation antigens, cell adhesion molecules, and activation markers on hematolymphoid and stromal cells involved in immune responses. Several markers are listed below.

T lymphocytes	CD2, CD3, CD4, CD8, CD44, T-cell receptor
B lymphocytes	CD19, CD20, surface Immunoglobulin
Macrophages	OX41, OX42, ED1 through 9 (rat); Mac-1, Mac-2, MOMA-1 (mouse)
Myeloid cells	HIS54 (rat)
Granulocytes	HIS48 (rat), Gr-1 (mouse)
NK cells	L322 (rat), 3A4 (mouse)
Dendritic cells	IF119 (rat), NLDC145 (mouse)
Thymic epithelium	HIS37, 38, 39, MTS-1, ER-TR-4, 5 (rat)
Adhesion molecules	CD54 (ICAM-1); CD 11/18 (LFA-1/MAC-1)
Activation markers	CD25 (IL-2R)

Staining these markers is mostly performed on acetone-fixed frozen tissue sections of 6–8 μm, usually by a three-step immunoperoxidase procedure.

*mAb, monoclonal antibody; Ig, immunoglobulin; Ab, antibody; ELISA, enzyme-linked immunosorbent assay; ip, intraperitoneal(ly); FACS, fluorescence-activated cell sorter; TH, helper T cell; CTL, cytotoxic T cell; TH1, T-helper 1 cell; TH2, T-helper 2 cell; mRNA, messenger RNA; RT, reverse transcription; PCR, polymerase chain reaction; cDNA, copy DNA; ds, double-stranded; MPS, mononuclear phagocyte system; iv, intravenous(ly); NK, natural killer; LGL, large granular lymphocyte; LPS, lipopolysaccharide; DTH, delayed-type hypersenstivity; FCA, Freund's complete adjuvant; PPD, purified protein derivative (from *Mycobacterium tuberculosis*); SRBC, sheep red blood cell; pfc, plaque-forming cell; [^{3}H]Thy, [^{3}H]thymidine; STM, *Salmonella typhimurium* cell wall extract; Con A, concanavalin A; PHA, phytohemagglutinin; MLR, mixed lymphocyte reaction; MHC, major histocompatibility complex; sc, subcutaneous; C, complement; PMN, polymorphonuclear leukocyte; CMV, cytomegalovirus; REC, rat embryo cell; EAE, experimental allergic encephalomyelitis; HCB, hexachlorobenzene.

The first step comprises the mouse anti-rat or mouse anti-mouse mAb specific for the marker under study; the second step, rabbit anti-mouse immunoglobulin (Ig); and the third step, swine anti-rabbit Ig. The latter two antibodies (Abs) are conjugated to horseradish peroxidase. The peroxidase activity can be developed by 3,3-diaminobenzidine tetrahydrochloride and H_2O_2 as substrate (resulting in a brown color), while the sections can be counterstained with Mayer's hematoxylin to facilitate evaluation. Negative controls are prepared by omitting the Ab in the first step, or replacement by an irrelevant one, preferably of the same isotype. Under these conditions only endogenous peroxidase activity of polymorphonuclear cells (when present) should be found, and immunolabeling should be absent.

In general, histopathological evaluation provides a semiquantitative estimation of effects. For subtle effects morphometrical analysis can be of help to determine the values of parameters such as cell size, cell surface, intensity of staining, and specific T-cell and B-cell areas within spleen and lymph nodes and cortical and medullary areas within the thymus.

Basal Immunoglobulin Level

As exposure to many immunotoxic compounds results in changes of the total Ab levels in serum (1), this assay is very valuable. Antibody levels are a function of (the humoral aspects of) the immune system which react to antigens that are for the larger part unknown. This parameter will not give much information on the possible mechanisms of immunotoxicity, but should be regarded as a screening parameter. Although most experience is on IgM and IgG, both other classes of Ig are also very important, IgA in mucosal immunity and IgE in allergic manifestations, and should therefore also be measured.

Total IgM and IgG can be analyzed by means of a sandwich enzyme-linked immunosorbent assay (ELISA). Total IgA and IgE can be analyzed similarly, except that for coating the microtiter plates monoclonal anti-rat IgA or monclonal anti-rat IgE are used, respectively. For detection of Ig in serum samples peroxidase-conjugated sheep anti-rat IgA or monoclonal anti-rat κ chains are used, respectively.

Bone Marrow

Bone marrow is an important hemopoietic organ and source of precursors for lymphocytes as well as other leukocytes. Changes in the bone marrow are therefore likely to result in alterations of immunocompetent cell populations and thus are an indicator for potential immunotoxicity. In order to count the number of bone marrow cells, they are collected by flushing 4 ml Impuls cytometer fluid through the femur using a 21-gauge needle. Before flushing, both ends of the femur are removed using a scalpel. The concentration of nucleated cells is determined using a Coulter counter. Additionally, a visual differential count of the cells can be done in May–Grünwald Giemsa-stained cytospin preparations.

Enumeration of Leukocytes in Bronchoalveolar Lavage, Peritoneal Cavity, and Skin

Mononuclear phagocytes that reside in the alveoli of the lung play an important role in clearing inhaled particles including microorganisms from the lung. Numbers of cells as well as alterations in their function can be an end point of toxicity on (inhalatory) exposure. In order to harvest these cells from the lungs an excised lung is placed in a pressure chamber, connected to a cannula through which lavage fluid can be introduced into the lung, and transferred from the lung into a test tube. This procedure is then repeated several times to obtain an optimal yield (2).

Enumeration of mononuclear cells in the peritoneal cavity is performed by harvesting these cells by three or four cycles of intraperitoneal (ip) injection of lavage fluid, followed by gentle massaging of the abdomen, and aspiration of the fluid with the syringe that was also used for injection.

Enumeration of cells of Langerhans and other immunocompetent cells in the skin is done using histopathological techniques, as described above.

Fluorescence-Activated Cell Sorter (FACS) Analysis

Evaluation of phenotypic markers is one of the most sensitive indicators for predicting immunotoxic compounds. A 91% concordance for correctly identifying immunotoxic compounds in the mouse based on FACS analysis alone was observed (3). Of the markers routinely used in immunotoxicology, i.e., surface Ig (pan B-cell), Thy 1.2 or CD3 (pan T cell), $CD4^{+}CD8^{-}$ [helper T cell (TH)], $CD4^{-}CD8^{+}$ [cytotoxic T cell (CTL)], and $CD4^{+}CD8^{+}$ (immature T cell), the CD4/CD8 ratio showed the highest concordance for identifying immunotoxic compounds (3).

When enumerating the cell populations, both absolute cell numbers and percentages should be reported, but the absolute cell numbers are by far the most meaningful.

In addition to enumerating the cell populations, FACS analysis is used to determine the activation state of various cell types based on changes in detectable activation markers, such as F4/80, Mac-2, transferrin receptor, and interleukin 2 (IL-2) receptor. The usefulness of activation markers as predictors of immunotoxic compounds has yet to be established.

Cytokine Determination

Cytokines are soluble proteins that perform communication between cells of the immune system. Their crucial roles have been established in a wide array of immune responses. As ongoing immune responses can be monitored by cytokine determinations, these determinations have the potential to be early indicators of immunotoxicity. Also, these determinations should provide a more detailed understanding of the immune deviation caused by immunotoxic compounds than other end points. Finally, in autoimmunity and allergic manifestations, some of which are caused by immunotoxic compounds, the ratios between T-helper 1 (TH1) and T-helper (TH2) cells can change. TH1 and TH2 cells can only be distinguished by determining their cytokine production patterns (4). In conclusion, measuring levels of (production of) cytokines is a promising new tool for immuntoxicity testing.

Cytokines can be measured by (a) bioassay, (b) ELISA, and (c) messenger RNA (mRNA) expression. Since proteins (or protein moieties) recognized by mAbs in ELISA can exist that, for one reason or another, do not contain their biological activity, *in principle* the measurement of biological activity (a) is superior to that of cytokine proteins (b). In the same line of thought, mRNAs encoding cytokine proteins can exist that do not actually lead to the respective protein. Hence, *in principle* the measurement of cytokine proteins (b) is superior to that of cytokine mRNA (c).

Measurement of cytokines in biological assays has, however, significant drawbacks compared to the other two methods: (a) for measuring an array of cytokines many different bioassays have to be set up and the cell lines they require maintained, which makes this technique cumbersome, (b) bioassays depend on the availability of recombinant cytokines to use as a calibration standard and anticytokine mAbs to show that the biological effect is caused by the cytokine under study and not (partially) by other one(s), and (c) cytokines can only be measured in body fluids (blood, urine, peritoneal fluid, nasal lavage, bronchoalveolar lavage) or cell supernatants but not in (intact) tissue, which further restricts the applicability of this type of testing.

Measurement of cytokines using ELISA also depends on the availability of recombinant cytokines to use as a calibration standard and anticytokine mAbs, and these assays too can only be measured in body fluids or cell supernatants. Cytokines may, in some cases, exert their effects only within a certain organ or tissue. Thus, cytokine measurements in body fluids or cell supernatants do not always provide the proper or complete picture. They can, however, still be powerful tools in immunotoxicity testing.

Although anticytokine mAbs can be used to detect cytokine proteins *in situ* (in tissue), such immunohistochemical techniques are semiquantitative. Yet, the localization of cytokines may yield significant information on the functioning of the immune system.

In order to determine cytokines tools have to be available. For all mouse cytokines ELISAs are commercially available. For rat, to our knowledge only tumor necrosis factor α (TNF-α) and γ-interferon (IFN-γ) ELISAs are commercially available. The difference in availability between mouse and rat is much smaller for probes than for ELISAs: for rat IL-1 to -6, IL-10, TNF-α, transforming growth factor α (TGF-α), TGF-β, and IFN-γ have been cloned (and sequenced). ELISAs are available for most mouse cytokine receptors, but none for rat. Whereas all cytokine receptors have been cloned for mouse, only a few rat cytokine receptors (IL-2R, IL-4R, IL-6R, TNF-R, and several TGF-R's) have been cloned.

As ELISAs for cytokine measurements are generally obtained commercially as complete kits, they are not discussed here in detail. As ELISA kits for cytokine measurement differ considerably in price, sensitivity (area), and sensitivity to interfering compounds, such as soluble receptors, it is worthwhile to compare kits from different firms for each specific application.

Two methods exist to quantify mRNA: (a) blotting and subsequent hybridization and (b) reverse transcription and subsequent polymerase chain reaction (RT/PCR).

In the first method, mRNA (or total RNA) is blotted onto a filter. Labeled DNA (probe) is then bound (hybridized) to a specific mRNA on the basis of their nucleotide sequence homology (5). The amount of label hybridized to the filter directly relates to the amount of the specific mRNA. Two blotting techniques exist, namely Northern blotting and dot blotting. In Northern blotting RNA is first electrophoretically separated before blotting whereas in dot blotting RNA is directly blotted onto the filter.

In the second method, mRNA is first reverse-transcribed into copy DNA (cDNA) by means of the enzyme reverse transcriptase (5). This reaction has to be primed with a short stretch of synthetic DNA.

By means of PCR (6, 7), the fraction of the cDNA that is derived from the gene under study is rendered double-stranded (ds). Then, the number of these dsDNA molecules is amplified enormously. A set of two primers, each set specific for the gene under study, is used. A primer is a short stretch of synthetic single-stranded DNA of a specific sequence. The two primers of a set must bind to the different strands of dsDNA at different sites. The primer sequences are usually chosen from within the coding region of the gene. Polymerase chain reaction consists of a number of cycles (usually 25–35). One cycle consists of the following steps: the primer is hybridized to the nucleic acid at 60°C, the primer is elongated by means of the enzyme *Thermophilus aquaticus* (Taq) DNA polymerase at 72°C, and the parent and the newly synthesized nucleic acid strands are separated at 94°C. In the following cycle the newly synthesized strand can be used as a template in combination with the other primer. The net result of a PCR is that in each cycle the number of molecules originating from the gene under study is (theoretically) doubled. All molecules synthesized during PCR are of one size, ranging between (and including) the two primer binding sites.

Not surprisingly, the advantage of RT/PCR over blotting techniques is its enormous sensitivity. However, a lot of work has to be put into setting up the PCR in order to make this technique truly semiquantitative (8).

Finally, if mAbs specific for a certain cytokine are not available, but the gene encoding the cytokine has been cloned, the localization of the cytokine can be evaluated using *in situ* hybridization. As discussed above, this is especially relevant for studies in the rat.

Importantly, mRNA detection *in situ* shows the cell actually producing the cytokine mRNA, whereas immunohistochemical localization may show cells that do not produce the cytokine but have internalized it.

In situ hybridization techniques are semiquantitative, but the localization of cytokine mRNAs may yield significant information on the functioning of the immune system.

Functional Assays

Phagocytic Activity

A nonspecific first line of defense to many pathogens is executed by phagocytic activity. Macrophages in particular are able to phagocytose many particles, including bacteria, and are able to lyse and inactivate them. Alterations in phagocytic activity are therefore an important parameter for immunotoxicity. Not only can the capacity to ingest particles *in vitro* be measured, but *in vivo* activity can also be measured by determining the clearance of bacteria such as *Listeria monocytogenes* (see below).

The phagocytic assay that is most predictive for altered macrophage function is based on the phagocytic ability of fixed macrophages of the mononuclear phagocyte system (MPS). In the MPS, macrophages provide the first line of defense for blood-borne particles including pathogens and nonpathogens. The macrophages of the MPS line the liver endothelium (Kupffer cells), the spleen, the lymph nodes (reticular cells), the lung (interstitial macrophages), and other organs such as the thymus and bone marrow. Mice are injected intravenously (iv) with ^{51}Cr-labeled sheep erythrocytes. Over 15 min 5-μl blood samples are taken from the clipped tail every 2 or 3 min, and a final blood sample is taken after 30 min. One hour after injection the animals are sacrificed and the liver, spleen, lungs, thymus, and kidneys are removed, weighed, and counted in a gamma counter (9). Blood clearance of the radiolabeled cells is expressed as vascular half-life and as phagocytic index which is determined by the slope of the clearance curve. Organ distribution is expressed as percentage organ uptake and cpm/mg tissue (specific activity). The assay is capable of detecting both stimulation and inhibition of the MPS.

Natural Killer Activity

The major role *in vivo* of cells with natural killer (NK) activity probably is to provide surveillance against virus-infected and neoplastic cells (10). Most of the cells showing NK activity are morphologically associated with large granular lymphocytes (LGLs). In spleen and peripheral blood many cells with high NK activity are found. Lymph nodes show less NK activity, whereas thymus and bone marrow show only marginal activity. Natural killer activity can also be demonstrated in the bronchus-associated lymhoid tissue. Large granular lymphocytes can migrate from the circulation into the extravascular tissue of the lung and can even be in contact with the lumen of the alveoli. As the lungs constitute a major site for neoplastic disease (metastatic spread) and viral infections, this presence probably is of great importance. In experimental animals suppression of NK cell activity has been shown to lead to an increase in the number of metastases of transplanted tumors. However, the clinical significance of altered NK cell activity in humans has not been clearly established. Asymptomatic individuals with low NK cell responses may be at some risk for developing upper respiratory infections and increased morbidity. Hence, testing NK activity is an important tool for assessing potential immunotoxicity.

To determine NK activity, cell populations are cultured together with NK-sensitive target cells such as the YAC lymphoma cell line. The YAC cells are radiolabeled with ^{51}Cr, and lysis of Cr from the target cells is measured within 4 hr.

Antigen-Specific Antibody Responses

A minority of antigens is capable of inducing humoral immune responses without involvement of T cells [e.g., lipopolysaccharide (LPS)]. Sensitization of animals to LPS will yield Ig responses that can be measured by ELISA.

Most Ab responses require not only B cells but also the help of T cells. An excellent antigen in this respect is tetanus toxoid. Rats are immunized at Day 0, followed by a booster at Day 10. Primary as well as secondary IgG and IgM responses can be measured in serum at Day 10 (just prior to the booster) and Day 21, respectively. Primary IgM responses are least under control of T cells. As tetanus toxoid is an antigen that is also used for immunization of man, responses to this antigen may be helpful in studies aimed at extrapolation of animal data to man (recall antigen). Determination of such responses can be done using an ELISA. Another widely used T-cell-dependent antigen is ovalbumin. This antigen is used for induction of Ab responses of all classes (IgM, IgG, IgA, and IgE), which can be measured using an ELISA.

Besides humoral responses, ovalbumin also induces delayed-type hypersensitivity (DTH). Sensitization to ovalbumin in Freund's complete adjuvant

(FCA) results in enhanced responses and offers the possibility to assay in one animal not only humoral responses, but also DTH (11). The DTH is directed not only to ovalbumin, but also to PPD (purified protein derivative, a product from *Mycobacterium tuberculosis*). The response to PPD is induced by FCA. At least in mice, immunization in FCA skews responses in the direction of TH1 (i.e., DTH) and hence suppresses responses in the direction of TH2 (i.e., IgE- and IgA-dependent immune responses).

Antibody Responses to Sheep Red Blood Cells (SRBC)

Spleen Immunoglobulin M and Immunoglobulin G Plaque Forming Cell (PFC) Assay to the T-Cell-Dependent Antigen Sheep Red Blood Cell

Mice or rats are injected iv with SRBC (approximately 2×10^8). The Abs induced can then be measured by the PFC assay. Sheep RBC from a sheep that repeatedly gives a high response ($\geq$ 1500 PFC/10^6 spleen cells) should be used. Animals are sacrificed on Day 4 after injection. Spleen cells are prepared and added to sheep erythrocytes and guinea pig complement and placed in a microscope slide chamber (Cunningham assay, Ref. 12). Alternatively, the spleen cells are added to a test tube containing guinea pig C, sheep erythrocytes, and warm agar. After thorough mixing the mixture is plated on a petri dish and covered with a microscope coverslip (Jerne method, Ref. 13). In either case the preparations are incubated at 37°C for 3 hr and counted using a Bellco plaque viewer. Each plaque is generated from a single IgM Ab-producing B cell. Results are expressed as specific activity (IgM PFC/10^6 spleen cells) and IgM PFC per spleen. By adding rabbit anti-mouse IgG Ab or anti-rat IgG Ab to the mixture, the number of IgG Ab-forming cells can also be determined. This number is calculated by subtracting the number of IgM PFCs from the total number of PFCs. The optimum IgG primary response is observed 5 days after sensitization.

The concordance for the PFC assay is the highest of all functional assays (78%) in correctly predicting immunotoxicity (3). In combination with the NK cell activity assay or FACS analysis the PFC assay results in pairwise concordances of greater than 90% for predictability.

Enzyme-Linked Immunosorbant Assay for Anti-SRBC IgM, IgG, and IgA Antibodies

Antigen preparations, prepared from ghosts of sheep erythrocytes by extraction with KCl, are used to coat the bottom of wells of ELISA plates. Serum samples from rats that are immunized with sheep erythrocytes are titrated on these plates. Rat IgM and IgG are detected by peroxidase-conjugated polyclonal Abs. Immunoglobulin A is detected using mouse anti-rat IgA mAb and peroxidase-conjugated polyclonal rat anti-mouse IgG (14).

The anti-SRBC ELISA measures titers of specific antibodies, whereas the PFC assay determines the number of cells that is responsible for production. The cells that are used for the PFC assay are derived from specialized parts of the body (e.g., spleen), and alterations in the number of Ab-producing cells in such an organ due to exposure do not give information on other inaccessible pools of Ab-producing cells. In contrast, ELISAs yield data on the total production of Ab, and alterations in titers due to exposure indicate changes in immune potential of the exposed animals. Thus, ELISAs are preferable to screen for immunotoxicity. However, the PFC assay yields information that is complementary to rather than overlapping with data provided by ELISA.

Mitogen Responsiveness to B-Cell Mitogens

The proliferative response of B cells to mitogenic stimulation can be measured by uptake of [^{3}H]thymidine ([^{3}H]Thy). Like Ab responses, responsiveness to LPS is another estimate of humoral immune responses, as only B cells respond to this mitogen. *Salmonella typhimurium* cell wall extract (STM) is a more potent mitogen than LPS, at least for rat (15). One of the reasons for the insensitivity of mitogen assays is the fact that the cells must remain in culture for several days to obtain a peak response. Hence, cells have the capability to recover from the immunomodulatory effects of the test compounds during this period. This problem is common to many *ex vivo/in vitro* assays, including the MLR and CTL assays (see below). As in the NK assay the culture period is only 4 hr, this is less of a concern in that assay.

Mitogen Responsiveness to T-Cell Mitogens

The proliferative response of T cells to mitogenic stimulation can be measured by uptake of [^{3}H]Thy (16). In both rats and mice, concanavalin A (Con A) and phytohemagglutinin (PHA) are T-cell mitogens. Pokeweed mitogen stimulates the proliferation of both T and B cells and thus lacks specificity. Although both Con A and PHA stimulate T cells, the Con A-responsive T cells are relatively immature compared to the PHA-responsive T cells. Multiple concentrations of the mitogen should be used to ensure the peak response is obtained as both Con A and PHA produce a bell-shaped dose–response curve. Thus, if the concentration of mitogen is too high, the response may be suboptimal.

As mitogen responses of lymphocytes are extremely robust, the assay lacks sensitivity. Other assays based on cellular proliferation, such as PFC assays and mixed lymhocyte reactions (see below), are more sensitive.

Mixed Lymphocyte Reaction

In the mixed lymphocyte reaction (MLR), responder T cells are cocultured with allogeneic stimulator cells. The foreign histocompatibility antigens expressed on the allogeneic stimulator cells serve as the activating stimuli. These antigens usually are major histocompatibility complex (MHC) class I or class II molecules. They are present on all nucleated cells and on antigen-presenting cells, respectively. As a sufficiently high number of T cells will respond to the stimulator cells, priming these responder cells is unnecessary. If the allogeneic stimulator cells contain T cells, their uptake of [^{3}H]Thy has to be prevented by gamma-irradiation or mitomycin C treatment.

Spleen cells or peripheral blood cells from, e.g., Wistar rats are used as responder cells and cocultured with splenocytes from, e.g., PVG rats. The stimulator cells (of PVG origin) are gamma-irradiated (2000 rad, 15 min). Four days after the start of the coculture [^{3}H]Thy is added. One day later, the cells are harvested and the radioactivity is counted. As a control, responder cells are also cocultured with their own syngeneic gamma-irradiated lymphocytes. The net MLR response is the difference in cell proliferation between lymphocytes cocultured with allogeneic cells and those cocultured with syngeneic cells.

Cytotoxic T-Lymphocyte Assay

The CTL assay is a continuation of the MLR response in which the T cells further differentiate into cytotoxic effector cells. Usually, in mice the P815 mastocytoma cell line is used as the sensitizing and target cell (17). Spleen cells are cocultured with the P815 cells. After 5 days the spleen cells are harvested and added to fresh ^{51}Cr-radiolabeled P815 cells. After the cells are incubated for 4 hr, the percentage cytotoxicity is determined by measuring the release of ^{51}Cr into the supernatant. A culture period of 5 days is necessary for the T cells to differentiate into cytotoxic effector cells. This prolonged period of culture enables the spleen cells to recover from any immunomodulatory effects of the compound (see above), making this assay less useful in immunotoxicity testing. This assay again only uses a specialized part of the body, i.e., the spleen. Thus, a holistic assay is preferable, and further research into developing such an assay is certainly warranted.

Delayed-Type Hypersensitivity Responses

Delayed-type hypersensitivity responsiveness reflects the cellular immune system, especially those aspects pertaining to interleukin 2 and γ-interferon-dependent responses (TH1 responses). They include attraction and activation of nonspecific mononuclear leukocytes (macrophages and monocytes). Two antigens that are often used in DTH assays, namely PPD and ovalbumin, have been described above. Another antigen is *L. monocytogenes,* which is particularly interesting since the DTH assay can be carried out in the context of host resistance experiments using this pathogen. The DTH responses can be measured upon sensitization to *L. monocytogenes* after subcutaneous (sc) injection of the antigen in the ears. Prior to and 24 or 48 hr after challenge, the increment in ear thickness can be measured with a micrometer. Background ear swelling responses of similar, nonimmunized control animals are subtracted from the swelling responses found in immunized animals.

The protein antigen keyhole limpet hemocyanin (KLH) produces the classical DTH response both with and without the use of adjuvant. The use of adjuvant in DTH studies should be avoided.

Delayed-type hypersensitivity response assays represent holistic assays for evaluating cell-mediated immunity. Since sensitization and challenge occur in the intact animal, all components of the immune system are present to respond in a physiologically relevant manner. This type of holistic assay is preferable for evaluating effects on cell-mediated immunity as compared to *in vitro* assays such as the MLR or CTL assay since these assays require several days of culture before evaluation enabling the cultured cells to recover from immunomodulatory effects (see above). The DTH response assay is extremely predictive (100% concordance) for identifying immunotoxic compounds when used in combination with the NK assay and the PFC assay (3).

Host Resistance Models

Listeria monocytogenes

Relevant mechanisms of defense against *L. monocytogenes* are phagocytosis by macrophages, and T-cell-dependent lymphokine production that enhances phagocytosis. In contrast to T-cell-dependent immunity, humoral immunity is not relevant in terms of protection against infection in this model. Animals are infected via the iv or the intratracheal route. Clearance of *Listeria* can be assessed by determining the numbers of viable bacteria in the spleen or lungs, respectively. Serial dilutions of homogenates of the organs, prepared in mortars using sterile purified sea sand, are plated onto sheep blood agar plates. After incubating them for 24 hr at 37°C, colonies are counted to determine the number of viable bacteria. Differences in the numbers of bacteria indicate clearance of the bacteria.

Besides clearance of bacteria, histopathology due to a *Listeria* infection can also be a valuable parameter (18). Pulmonary infection with *Listeria* induces histopathological lesions that are characterized by foci of inflammatory cells such as lymphoid and histiocytic cells, accompanied by local cell degeneration and influx of granulocytes. Ozone exposure of rats for 1 week prior to infection results in lesions that are much more severe than in nonexposed animals and that are still present at time points at which both ozone-associated and infection-associated effects alone would have been resolved. Besides the severity and duration of the histopathology, also the quality of the lesions is influenced by prior exposure to ozone. Mature granulomas are found in *Listeria*-infected rats that are exposed to ozone.

When the mouse is used as an experimental animal in host resistance studies using *Listeria*, morbidity is the usual end point. Bacterial clearance can, however, also be conducted. In the mouse, resistance to *Listeria* is genetically regulated. *Listeria* can be stored at −70°C at a stock concentration of 10^8 colony-forming units (cfu) per ml. Usually three challenge levels are selected to produce 20, 50, and 80% mortality in the control animals. Morbidity is monitored daily for 14 days. Using iv administration of *Listeria*, this assay is extremely reproducible. Because *Listeria* is a human pathogen, appropriate precautions are needed when using this organism.

Streptococcus pneumoniae

This bacterial model is among the most sensitive to detect changes in host resistance. This may be due to the fact that several immune defense mechanisms participate, in varying degrees, in the protection from this organism. The first line of defense is the complement (C) system. Activation of the C system can result in direct lysis of certain strains. However, some strains are resistant to lysis by C. Complement can still participate directly in the removal of these bacteria as a result of C component C3 being deposited on their cell surface which facilitates phagocytosis by polymorphonuclear leukocytes (PMNs) and macrophages. In the later stages of the infection Ab plays a major role in controlling the infection. Thus, compounds affecting C, PMNs, B-cell maturation and proliferation, or the production of Ab can be evaluated with this model system.

Stock preparations are maintained at −70°C in defibrinated rabbit blood. Aliquots can be grown in culture at various dilutions to obtain the desired challenge concentration. Alternatively, the bacterial concentrations can be monitored by measuring the culture turbidity. The inoculum can be administered ip or iv. Three inocula are prepared to give a 20, 50, and 80% mortality. The number of colony-forming units administered to the animals is determined by assaying serial dilutions of the inoculi on blood agar plates. Due to the rapid onset of the infection, mortality observations are recorded twice daily for 7 days (19). Since some strains of *Streptococcus* are pathogenic in humans, appropriate precautions are needed when using this organism.

Cytomegalovirus

Cytomegalovirus (CMV) infections are widely distributed throughout the human population. Approximately 60–90% of the population is infected. The vast majority of the naturally occurring primary CMV infections are clinically asymptomatic. Especially in immunocompromised hosts such as transplantation patients more severe diseases may occur. As immunosuppression may be an important factor for development of CMV-associated diseases, a CMV model may be of interest especially for immunotoxicity testing.

Several aspects of the immune system play a role in the resistance of mice against CMV. Antibodies play a role in the neutralization of CMV and in antibody dependent cell-mediated cytotoxicity. CMV-specific CTL can be detected in CMV-infected mice. Natural killer activity appears to be most effective especially during the initial stages of CMV infections. A role for macrophages in resistance against CMV is doubtful. In the rat cellular immunity plays a role in the resistance against CMV.

Rodents can be inoculated ip with CMV of either rat or mouse origin. At several time points after infection, CMV concentrations in tissue are determined using a plaque-forming unit assay. Rat embryo cell (REC) monolayers are prepared in 24-well plates. Different organs (salivary gland, lungs, kidney, liver, and spleen) are homogenized using a tissue grinder and stored at 10% w/v suspensions at −135°C until use. The confluent REC monolayers are infected with 10-fold serial dilutions of the 10% (w/v) organ suspensions. After centrifugation the organ suspension is removed and 0.6 or 1% agarose is added. After incubation for 7 days at 37°C, the cells are fixed in 3.7% formaldehyde solution, the agarose layer is removed, and the monolayer is stained with 1% aqueous methylene blue. Plaques are counted with the aid of a stereoscopic microscope (20).

Influenza Virus

Influenza virus is a host resistance model used in mice (21) and rats. Morbidity is the end point routinely used to evaluate decreased host resistance.

Since the virus is administered by intranasal instillation, it may involve local immune mechanisms of the lung and not adequately reflect systemic immunocompetence.

As influenza virus is a human pathogen, appropriate precautions need to be followed when using the virus.

Trichinella spiralis

The life cycle of the helminth *T. spiralis* is as follows. After ingestion of infected meat, the encysted larvae are excysted in the stomach and passed down to the jejunum, where they mature within 3 to 4 days. After copulation the adult females penetrate the intestinal mucosa. This is associated with an inflammatory response, comprising mast cells and eosinophils. The penetrated worms produce viviparous larvae, that emigrate through the lymph and blood flow toward striated muscle tissue within 1 to 3 weeks after infection, where they get encapsulated. In these capsules, which are surrounded by inflammatory cells of the host, larvae can stay alive for a long time. The adult worms that reside in the gut are expelled from the gut within approximately 2 to 3 weeks. In this expulsion T-cell-dependent immunity plays a crucial role (22). Antibody responses to *T. spiralis* also play a role in the resistance to this parasite. During infection, IgM, IgG, IgA, and IgE are all induced.

Immunosuppression results in a significant increase in the number of muscle larvae compared to those in immunocompetent animals. This may be due not only to decreased resistance, but also to increased numbers of adults worms and to the longer periods that the worms reside in the gut. Inflammatory responses in the gut and around encysted muscle larvae are very scarce as compared to immunocompetent animals, and Ab responses are diminished. Thus, end points in this model are numbers of worms in the gut and numbers of muscle larvae. Determination of the inflammatory infiltrate around encysted muscle larvae and of IgM, IgG, IgA, and IgE titers are other end points.

Animals are infected with muscle larvae by gastric intubation. As animals can only be infected by consumption of infected tissue, there is no danger of spreading the infection in the colony. For animal care personnel, standard hygienic procedures are sufficient to preclude risk of being accidently infected.

Because the *T. spiralis* model can demonstrate differences in immunocompetence and is applicable in both rats and mice, and since humans also can be a target for infection, the model is well suited to assess immunotoxicity.

Plasmodium yoelii

Plasmodium yoelii is a nonlethal strain which produces a self-limiting parasitemia in mice. The host resistance to this organism includes specific Ab, macrophage involvement, and T-cell-mediated functions. Animals are injected with 10^6 parasitized erythrocytes. Parasitemia is monitored by taking blood samples from the animals. In control animals peak responses usually occur between 10 and 14 days after injection. Determination of the degree of parasitemia can be done manually by evaluating blood smears or, based on a different size of infected cells, flow cytometry can be used to enumerate the number of these cells. Incorporation of acridine orange into infected cells containing the *Plasmodium* is an easy and accurate method to determine the degree of parasitemia (23).

Plasmodium yoelii is not infectious in humans and infection of other mice can only occur through contact with contaminated blood.

Tumor Models

B16F10 Melanoma

This tumor cell line is a malignant melanoma that is syngeneic to the C57BL/6 mouse. It was selected for its tendency to metastasize to the lung (24). Natural killer cells and macrophages as well as T cells have been shown to play a role in host protection. This assay is referred to as an artificial metastasis model since the tumor cells are injected iv, usually in the tail vein, and reside in the lung which is the first capillary bed they encounter. The B16F10 tumor cells can be grown in culture prior to their use in the assay. Between 1×10^5 and 5×10^5 cells are used as challenge. Untreated mice that receive the highest number of tumor cells can be used to monitor the tumor burden in order to select the optimum day of assay.

Two parameters are routinely used to assess tumor burden. One is the measurement of DNA synthesis in the lungs of tumor-bearing mice. Since background DNA synthesis of mice without tumors is extremely low, the DNA synthesis measured results from the tumor present. To measure DNA synthesis, mice are pulsed ip with 10^{-6} *M* 5-fluorodeoxyuridine 1 day prior to sacrifice, followed 30 min later with an iv injection of 2 μCi of [^{125}I]iododeoxyuridine. Upon sacrifice the lungs are removed, placed in Bouin's fixative solution, and counted.

A second assessment of tumor burden is the visual enumeration of the tumor nodules following fixation in Bouin's solution. The visibility of the black nodules of the melanin-producing B16F10 tumor cells allows for enumeration of up to 200–250 nodules on the surface of the lungs. A good correlation has been shown between enumerated tumor nodules and radioactivity present in the lungs.

PYB6 Fibrosarcoma

This fibrosarcoma is syngeneic to the C57BL/6 mouse. Host resistance includes NK activity and T-cell-mediated killing (25). PYB6 can be grown in culture, but should be passed in an animal prior to being used as challenge. Animals are injected in the thigh with 1–5 $\times$ 10^3 tumor cells, and mice are palpated weekly to detect the development of tumors. End points evaluated include incidence of tumors, time to tumor appearance, and tumor size.

MADB106 Adenocarcinoma

This tumor cell line is a mammary adenocarcinoma which is syngeneic to the Fischer 344 rat. Natural killer cells appear to play the major role in host defense. Survival time is the usual end point. Following an iv injection of 2×10^6 tumor cells, control rats begin to die 2 to 3 weeks later. Compounds that decrease host resistance to the tumor can decrease both the percentage survival and the survival time of treated animals (26).

Autoimmune Models

Immunization of Lewis rats with H37RA adjuvant induces autoreactive T cells that react with components of cartilage tissue. This leads to inflammatory responses in the joints, known as adjuvant arthritis (27). Sensitization of the same strain with guinea pig myelin induces autoreactive T cells that react with cartilage. This in turn leads to signs of paralysis, known as experimental allergic encephalomyelitis (EAE) (28). Exposure to immunotoxic compounds may lead to alterations in the courses of these induced autoimmune diseases. Whereas hexachlorobenzene (HCB) strongly enhances the severity of EAE, arthritic lesions are strongly suppressed in HCB-exposed rats. Although the quite opposite effects in both models are not yet understood, and clear dose–effect relationships have to be established, this type of information should be evaluated in risk assessment.

Allergy Models Based on Smooth Muscle Hyperresponsiveness

Adverse effects due to allergy are mediated by different immune mechanisms. They are classified as types I–IV hypersensitivity according to the mechanism that is responsible for the adverse immune response (29). Type I hypersensitivity is diagnosed using the skin prick test or Prausnitz-Kustner test (passive cutaneous anaphylaxis) and can be confirmed by a radioallergosorbent test on serum of the patient. Diagnosis of type II hypersensitivity is performed by detection of autoantibodies in serum and, in case of skin-associated type II hypersensitivity, within the epidermis. Type III hypersensitivity can be diagnosed using the hemagglutination and precipitin tests *in vitro*. *In vivo* the arthus reaction (skin) or bronchoprovocation tests (lungs) can be performed. Type IV hypersensitivity (DTH) is discussed above.

The autonomic nervous system innervates smooth muscle and thus regulates smooth muscle function. In this way the functions of the airways and the gastrointestinal tract are controlled. One aspect of allergy (especially types I, III, and IV hypersensitivity) is the occurrence of hyperresponsiveness of smooth muscle to constricting agents, resulting in bronchonarrowing (airways) and possibly diarrhea (gastrointestinal tract). Asthma patients generally suffer from an increased bronchial responsiveness which may be caused, among others, by an imbalance in the regulation of airway smooth muscle tone by the autonomic nervous system. Certain aspects of the immune system can influence the function of the autonomic nervous system and thus smooth muscle functions. The immune system probably plays an important role in the modulation of bronchial reactivity.

Because the immune system can influence smooth muscle functions, these functions are measured in rodents *in vitro* (30). Animals are sensitized and challenged in order to induce local or systemic immune responses. Smooth muscle tissue is dissected from the animals and tested for reactivity *in vitro*. Because of the close anatomical and physiological association between tracheal and bronchial musculature, tracheal muscle is used.

Conclusions

A wide array of rodent assays have been described here that in general are used for immunotoxicity testing. Hopefully this overview provides the reader insight into which test(s) can be useful in specific fields of neuroimmunological research.

References

1. J. G. Vos, E. I. Krajnc, and P. Beekhof, *Environ. Health Perspect.* **43,** 115 (1982).
2. D. Van Soolingen, *Lab. Anim.* **24,** 197 (1990).
3. M. I. Luster, C. Portier, D. G. Pait, K. L. White, C. Gennings, A. E. Munson, and G. J. Rosenthal, *Fundam. Appl. Toxicol.* **18,** 200 (1992).
4. P. Scott, *Curr. Opinion Immunol.* **5,** 391 (1993).
5. J. Sambrook, E. F. Fritsch, and T. Maniatis, "Molecular Cloning: A Laboratory Manual," 2nd Ed. Cold Spring Harbor Laboratory Press, Cold Spring Harbor, NY, 1989.
6. H. A. Erlich, (ed.), "PCR Technology: Principles and Applications for DNA Amplification." Stockton Press, New York, 1989.
7. H. A. Erlich, D. Gelfand, and J. J. Sninsky, *Science* **252,** 1643 (1991).
8. A. O'Garra and P. Vieira, *Curr. Opinion Immunol.* **4,** 211 (1992).
9. K. L. White, V. M. Sander, D. W. Barnes, G. M. Shopp, and A. E. Munson, *Drug Chem. Toxicol.* **8,** 299 (1985).
10. R. B. Herberman and J. R. Ortaldo, *Science* **214,** 24 (1981).
11. J. G. Vos, *Arch. Toxicol.* **(Suppl. 4)**, 95 (1980).
12. A. J. Cunningham and A. Szenberg, *Immunology* **14,** 559 (1968).
13. N. K. Jerne, C. Henry, A. A. Nordin, H. Fun, M. C. Koros, and I. Lefkovits, *Transpl. Rev.* **18,** 130 (1974).
14. H. Van Loveren and J. G. Vos, *in* "Advances in Applied Toxicology" (A. D. Dayan and A. J. Paine, eds.), p. 143. Taylor & Francis, Philadelphia, 1989.

15. S. A. Minchin, D. Leitenberg, L. L. Stunz, and T. L. Feldbush, *J. Immunol.* **145,** 2427 (1990).
16. J. Anderson, G. Moller, and O. Sjorberg, *Cell. Immunol.* **4,** 381 (1972).
17. M. J. Murray, L. D. Lauer, M. I. Luster, R. W. Luebke, D. O. Adams, and J. H. Dean, *Int. J. Immunopharmacol.* **7,** 491 (1985).
18. H. Van Loveren, P. J. A. Rombout, Sj. Sc. Wagenaar, H. C. Walvoort, and J. G. Vos, *Toxicol. Appl. Pharmacol.* **94,** 374 (1988).
19. K. L. White, H. H. Lysy, J. A. McCay, and A. C. Anderson, *Toxicol. Appl. Pharmacol.* **84,** 209 (1986).
20. C. A. Bruggeman, W. M. H. Debie, G. Grauls, G. Majoor, and C. P. A. Boven, *Arch. Virol.* **76,** 189 (1983).
21. P. Thomas, R. Fugmann, C. Aranyi, P. Barbera, R. Gibbons, and J. Fenters, *Toxicol. Appl. Pharmacol.* **77,** 219 (1985).
22. J. G. Vos, E. J. Ruitenberg, N. Van Basten, J. Buys, A. Elgersma, and W. Kruizinga, *Parasite Immunol.* **5,** 195 (1983).
23. R. W. Luebke, D. L. Andrews, C. B. Copeland, M. M. Riddle, R. R. Rogers, and R. J. Smialowicz, *Int. J. Immunopharmacol.* **13,** 987 (1991).
24. I. J. Fidler, D. M. Gersten, and I. R. Hart, *Adv. Cancer Res.* **28,** 149 (1978).
25. J. L. Urban, R. C. Burton, J. M. Holland, M. L. Kripke, and H. Schreiber, *J. Exp. Med.* **155,** 557 (1982).
26. R. J. Smialowicz, R. R. Rogers, D. G. Rowe, M. M. Riddle, and R. W. Luebke, *Toxicology* **44,** 271 (1987).
27. J. Holoshitz, Y. Naparstek, A. Ben-Nun, and I. R. Cohen, *Science* **219,** 56 (1983).
28. A. Ben-Nun, H. Wekerle, and I. R. Cohen, *Eur. J. Immunol.* **11,** 195 (1981).
29. R. R. A. Coombs and P. G. H. Gell, *in* "Clinical Aspects of Immunology" (P. G. H. Gell and R. R. A. Coombs, eds.), p. 317. Davis, Philadelphia, 1963.
30. J. Garssen,F. P. Nijkamp, H. Van Der Vliet, and H. Van Loveren, *Am. Rev. Respir. Dis.* **144,** 931 (1991).

[10] Effects of Tachykinins on Chondrocyte and Synoviocyte Function

Dale A. Halliday, Julian D. McNeil, William H. Betts, and Raffaele Scicchitano

Introduction

Tachykinins have been shown to activate and to modulate the activities of proinflammatory cells such as lymphocytes (1), neutrophils (2, 3), mast cells (4), and macrophages (5). In addition, tachykinins, particularly substance P (SP), may affect connective tissue cells including synovial fibroblasts (6) and smooth muscle cells (7). The possibility that tachykinins may be involved in the pathogenesis of inflammatory diseases such as asthma (8) and arthritis (9–12) has also been investigated in detail. We have therefore examined the effects of tachykinins particularly SP on chondrocyte function.

Although the chondrocyte was once considered to be a relatively inert cell, it is now appreciated that in order to maintain cartilage health, the opposite is the case. Chondrocytes must not only synthesize cartilage matrix components (i.e., collagen and proteoglycans), but must also have the capacity to dismantle their extracellular milieu which they can do by secreting the matrix metalloproteinases, mammalian collagenase, and stromelysin (proteoglycanase). In examining the effects of neuropeptides on chondrocytes we have selected collagenase synthesis as a catabolic function and proteoglycan synthesis as an anabolic function. In addition we have used calcium mobilization as one of many indices of second-messenger activation. Prostaglandin production has been measured in both chondrocytes and synoviocytes as, particularly in the latter cells, it represents an important response to a variety of cytokines released during inflammatory processes.

Using these assays, we have shown that intact tachykinins or SP fragments [SP(1–4) and SP(1–6)] do not affect chondrocyte proteoglycan or protein synthesis (13). Nor does SP stimulate prostaglandin E_2 (PGE_2) production (13). However, the C-terminal fragment of SP, SP(7–11), increased PGE_2 and collagenase production in bovine chondrocytes (14). In addition SP(7–11), but not intact SP, SP(1–4), SP(1–6), SP(9–11), or SP(8–11), nor the tachykinins neurokinin A (NKA) and neurokinin B (NKB), caused an increase in the intracellular calcium concentration ($[Ca^{2+}]_i$) (14). On the basis of these data, we hypothesized that, in the joint, cleavage of SP by neutral endopeptidases, which are present in the synovial fluid and which yield

Methods in Neurosciences, Volume 24

SP(7–11), may be of biological importance in chondrocyte-mediated cartilage pathology (15). In this chapter, we describe the methodologies which we have used to investigate the effects of tachykinins on chondrocyte function.

Materials and Methods

Neuropeptides

The neuropeptides used in these experiments are all purchased from AUSPEP, Melbourne, Australia. Neuropeptides are obtained lyophilized and stored as a powder at −20°C. Stock solutions (10^{-3} *M*) are prepared in phosphate-buffered saline (PBS) which contains 0.01 *M* acetic acid to prevent oxidation of the neuropeptide. Stock solutions are stored for up to 1 month in 100-μl aliquots in Eppendorf tubes in which the air has been replaced by N_2. Tubes are stored at −70°C until use, each aliquot being used once only. Peptides should be used immediately after resuspension in most instances or kept at 4°C on ice while awaiting use.

Cell Cultures

Chondrocytes

Bovine chondrocytes are isolated as described by Kuettner *et al.* (16). The hide from bovine hocks is removed and the resulting surface cleaned and sterilized with 70% ethanol. An incision is made to expose the joint. Cartilage is shaved aseptically from the articular surfaces of the exposed metacarpophalangeal joint using a fresh scalpel blade. Care must be taken not to incorporate underlying bone or adjacent soft tissue. The cartilage slices are placed immediately into a petri dish containing sterile PBS. The cartilage slices are washed with PBS before being digested for 18 hr at 37°C in Dulbecco's modified Eagle's medium (DMEM) containing the following enzymes and supplements: 10% heat-inactivated fetal bovine serum (FBS; Cytosystems, Castle Hill, NSW, Australia), 2 mg/ml bacterial collagenase isolated from *Clostridium histolyticum* (EC 3.4.24.3, Sigma, St. Louis, MO), 1 mg/ml hyaluronidase isolated from bovine testicle (Sigma), 20 m*M* HEPES, 3% penicillin/streptomycin, and 1% L-glutamine. Prior to its use, the enzyme solution is passed through a 0.22-μm Millipore Millex-GS filter (Millipore Products Division, Bedford MA).

Articular shavings are added to this mixture and stirred continuously with a sterilized magnetic stirrer at slow speed, throughout the incubation. Following digestion of the extracellular matrix, dispersed chondrocytes are washed with PBS and counted with a hemocytometer and percentage viability is determined by trypan blue exclusion. The chondrocytes in suspension are pelleted by centrifugation at 500*g* for 5 min at room temperature, recovered, and seeded at high density (5×10^5 cells/ml) directly into 24-well tissue culture plates (Flow Laboratories, McLean, VA) in DMEM containing 10% (v/v) FBS, 1% penicillin/streptomycin, and 1% L-glutamine. The chondrocytes are then cultured at 37°C in an atmosphere of 5% CO_2. It is important to culture the chondrocytes at high density under these conditions to maintain their differentiated phenotype. Chondrocytes seeded at high density produce type II collagen (as assessed by SDS-polyacrylamide gel electrophoresis) and continue to produce keratan sulfate as measured by ELISA assay, as has been demonstrated in our own and other laboratories (16). Chondrocytes grown in this manner do not begin to divide until 4 to 5 days after the initial seeding, after which they rapidly proliferate to form a monolayer *in vitro*. Experiments with neuropeptides are routinely performed when the chondrocytes have just formed complete monolayers.

Synoviocytes

Both human and bovine synoviocytes are grown from explants obtained from the synovial joints of patients undergoing joint replacements or fresh bovine hocks within 3 hr of slaughter. Synovium is dissected free of subsynovial fat and/or joint capsule, diced into 1-mm^2 pieces, and maintained in a small volume of tissue culture medium in 25 cm^3 tissue culture flasks (Falcon tissue culture ware from Cytosystems, Australia). The tissue culture medium consists of DMEM which contains 20 m*M* HEPES buffer, 10% heat-inactivated FBS, 1% penicillin/streptomycin, 1% L-glutamine, and 1% Fungizone (Bristol-Meyers Squibb, Victoria, Australia). Confluent synoviocytes are established more rapidly from bovine than from human synovium. Synoviocytes are passaged into larger (50 cm^3) tissue culture flasks following removal of FBS by washing with PBS and recovery of cells from the plastic surface with trypsin. This is achieved by incubating the monolayer for 10 min with just enough 2.5% (w/v) trypsin (EC 3.4.21.4, Cytosystems, NWS, Australia) in PBS, pH 7.8, prewarmed to 37°C, to cover it (i.e., 300–400 μl for a 25-cm^2 tissue culture flask). After the second subculture, synoviocytes form a uniform population of type II or fibroblast-type cells and are routinely used from the second to the sixth subculture. For experiments, synoviocytes are seeded into 24-well tissue culture plates at a density of 10^5 cells/well. Cells treated in this fashion usually become confluent within 48 hr. Experimental cultures are exposed to neuropeptides for 24 hr in 250 μl of serum-free medium.

Chondrocyte Proteoglycan Production

Labeling of Proteoglycans in Chondrocyte Culture

Isolated chondrocytes in 24-well tissue culture plates in DMEM supplemented with FBS achieve confluence in about 5–7 days. The FBS-containing medium is removed and the cell layers are washed twice with PBS to remove residual FBS prior to use. Chondrocytes are then exposed to 5 μCi/ml of $Na_2{}^{35}SO_4$ [65 MBq/ml in aqueous solution (Amersham Int., Amersham, UK)] for 18 hr in serum-free DMEM, in the presence of neuropeptide, or control medium to which has been added only the neuropeptide diluent containing the highest possible concentration of acetic acid, viz, 10^{-5} *M*. The [^{35}S]sulfate is incorporated into sulfated proteoglycans produced by the cells during the incubation. Unincorporated [^{35}S]sulfate is separated from that incorporated by precipitation of the labeled proteoglycans with cetylpyridinium chloride (CPC, see below). In this assay 10% FBS yields optimal stimulation of chondrocyte proteoglycan production and is therefore used as a positive control. At the end of the experiment, culture supernatants are collected, rendered cell-free, and stored at −20°C until assayed.

Cetylpyridinium Chloride (CPC) Assay of Glycosaminoglycan in Cell Supernatants and Cell Layers

Glycosaminoglycan production (which includes release into the culture supernatant and incorporation into cell layers) is measured using a modification of the method of Marsh *et al.* (17). After incubation with medium or SP, culture supernatants are recovered. The cell layer is washed three times with 1 ml PBS. Hyaluronan [20 μl of 1 mg/ml solution of human umbilical cord hyaluronan (Sigma)] is added to the supernatants and the PBS washings of the cell layer as a carrier. The washings and supernatants are pooled. An equivalent volume of 1% (w/v) CPC containing 100 m*M* NaCl is added and allowed to precipitate for 3 hr at 37°C. The resultant precipitate is spun for 10 min at 1300*g* at room temperature. Following centrifugation, the pellet is washed twice with 1% CPC. Samples are then suspended in scintillation fluid (Readysafe, Beckman Instruments) and counted on a Beckman LS6000LL scintillation counter. The cell layer is solubilized with 1 ml 0.2 *M* NaOH for 2 hr prior to CPC assay.

Determination of Proteoglycan Monomer Size by Sepharose CL-4B Chromatography

Confluent cultures of bovine chondrocytes are radiolabeled for 18 hr with 20 μCi/ml $Na_2{}^{35}SO_4$ in the presence or absence of neuropeptides. After radiolabeling, supernatants are pooled and kept at −20°C until analysis.

Samples (1 ml) are eluted under dissociative conditions with 4 *M* guanidinium hydrochloride (GuHCl) in 0.5 *M* sodium acetate, pH 5.8, on a Sepharose CL-4B column (volume, 60 cm^3), and 1.5-ml fractions are collected.

Cell layer-associated proteoglycans are extracted for 24 hr at 4°C by adding 1 ml 4 *M* GuHCl in the presence of 0.05 *M* Na_2EDTA to each well.This is done in the presence of a mixture of protease inhibitors consisting of 5 m*M* benzamidine hydrochloride, 0.5 m*M* phenylmethylsulfonyl fluoride, 0.1 *M* 6-aminohexanoic acid, and soybean trypsin inhibitor (0.001% w/v) to inhibit endogenous proteases. The resultant extract is pooled and fractionated in the same manner as for the culture supernatants.

Proteoglycans in media or cell layers can be easily quantified using the CPC assay; however, considerable variation between samples may occur if care is not taken to remove all unincorporated radiolabel in the washing steps.

Total Protein Production

Total protein production is measured by incubation of cells with 2 μCi/ml L-[4,5-^{3}H]leucine [9.25 MBq in aqueous solution (Amersham)] for 24 hr in the presence or absence of SP. Protein present in the cell supernatants and cell layers is determined by trichloroacetic acid (TCA) precipitation. The cell layer is recovered by trypsinization as described previously and cells are disrupted by sonication in the presence of 0.2% (v/v) Triton X-100. A total of 0.2 volumes of 50% TCA are added to the supernatants or cell sonicates and incubated for 30 min at 4°C. Following centrifugation at 1300*g* for 5 min at room temperature the resultant pellet is washed twice in 10% TCA before resuspension in a small volume of 0.1 *M* NaOH for scintillation counting.

Prostaglandin E_2 Assay

Prostaglandin E_2 present in chondrocyte supernatants is assayed using a radioimmunoassay (RIA) as described by Jaffe and Behrman (18).

1. Rabbit anti-PGE_2 polyclonal antibody is purchased from Sigma and [5, 6, 8, 11, 12, 14, 15(*n*)-^{3}H]-PGE_2 from Amersham. Standard curves are established for each assay at PGE_2 concentrations between 10 pg and 10 ng. Standard PGE_2 (synthesized; Cayman Chemicals, Ann Arbor, Michigan) is diluted in 1 m*M* Na_2CO_3.
2. Aliquots (100 μl) of chondrocyte conditioned medium are added, in 4-ml polycarbonate tubes, to 100 μl RIA assay buffer which consists of 0.1% (w/v) gelatin, 0.9% (w/v) NaCl, 0.01 *M* Tris base, and 0.05% (w/v) NaN_3,

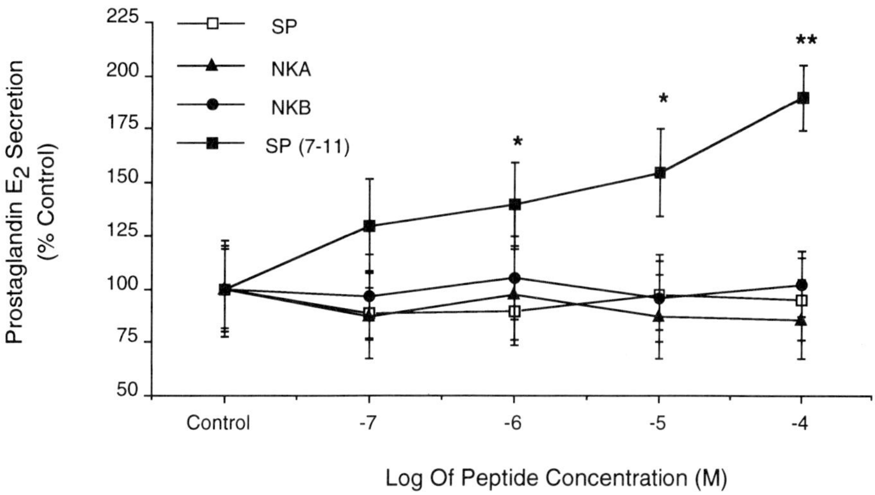

FIG. 1 The effect of SP (□), NKA (▲), NKB (●), and the SP fragment, SP(7–11) (■) on bovine chondrocyte PGE_2 secretion. Confluent chondrocytes were incubated with neuropeptide (0.1–100 μM) for 18 hr. Prostaglandin E_2 secreted into the medium was determined by radioimmunoassay. Values represent means ± SEM for four separate experiments each performed in quadruplicate. Data are expressed as a percentage of the control value which was 16.9 ± 2 ng/ml. The effect of SP(7–11) was inhibited by the presence of 15 μM indomethacin. $^{*}p < 0.05$; $^{**}p < 0.001$ compared with control. Reproduced with permission from D. A. Halliday, J. D. McNeil, W. H. Betts, and R. Scicchitano. *Biochem. J.* **292,** 57 (1993).

pH 7.3. A total of 100 μl of $[^3H]PGE_2$ (Amersham) in 1 mM Na_2CO_3 is added to this mixture. The stock solution of PGE_2 is prepared by adding 20 μl $[^3H]PGE_2$ (7.07 TBq/mmol) to 10 ml of 1 mM Na_2CO_3.

3. Anti-PGE_2 antibody (100 μl) is added (stock solution containing 1 vial anti-PGE_2 reconstituted with 10 ml RIA buffer). This mixture is then incubated at 37°C for 2 hr. Afterward, incubation samples are cooled to 4°C by refrigeration for 1 hr. To separate bound from unbound PGE_2, 500 μl of a solution of assay buffer containing 1% activated charcoal, 1% dextran T70, and 0.05% NaN_3 is added to each sample and mixed. Samples are then centrifuged at 4°C in a precooled centrifuge for 20 min at 2000g. Aliquots (500 μl) of supernatants are carefully removed and radioactivity is determined with a Beckman LS-6000 LL scintillation counter. Standard PGE_2 is assayed under the same conditions. Standard curves are plotted on a logarithmic scale and quantities of PGE_2 in samples are determined from the standard curve. The effect of SP, NKA, NKB, and SP(7–11) on bovine chondrocyte PGE_2 secretion is shown in Fig. 1.

The prostaglandin assay is a standard one which is commercially available and a large number of samples can be processed at any one time. However there are significant differences between the amounts of PGE_2 produced by different preparations of chondrocytes. In some cultures, for example, there was no detectable PGE_2 production. In general, resting synoviocytes produce less PGE_2 than chondrocytes cultured under similar conditions and again some cultures fail to produce detectable levels of PGE_2 for reasons which we could not identify.

Collagenase Production

Preparation of Acid-Soluble Type I Collagen

Acid-soluble type I collagen is prepared from rat tails using the method of Bazin and Delaunay (19). Twelve rat tails are harvested and stored at −20°C until the tendons can be removed. This is achieved by cutting the skin near the tip of the tail, then grasping the tip through the cut with a pair of side-cutting pliers and freeing the tendons by pulling the tail and the tendons apart. The tendons are dissected free of any adherent soft tissue and placed into ice-cold 0.2 *M* NaCl and rinsed three times in this solution before being damped dry. They are then freeze-fractured in a stainless steel mortar and pestle that has been chilled overnight in a −70°C freezer. The tendons are snap frozen with liquid N_2 in the mortar before the pestle is inserted and the tendons shattered with the use of a sledge hammer. More liquid N_2 is added and the process repeated until the tendons are reduced to a powder.

This powder is then stirred in 0.5 *M* acetic acid at 4°C for 48 hr and this solution is then ultracentrifuged at 20,000*g* for 2 hr at 4°C. The supernatant is recovered and dialyzed overnight against 0.02 *M* phosphate buffer, pH 7.8. After dialysis the material is again dissolved in 0.5 *M* acetic acid for 18 hr at 4°C. This solution is then lyophilized in a vacuum freeze-drier for 48 hr. The dry weight of this material is determined and dissolved in 0.5 *M* acetic acid to give a concentration of 2 mg/ml.

Salt Fractionation of Collagen

To prepare native monomeric collagen with intact nonhelical ends (i.e., completely undenatured) from acid-soluble collagen the salt fractionation method described by Chandrakasan *et al.* (20) is used. To do this the salt concentration is adjusted to a final concentration of 3% by adding a stock solution of 25% NaCl dropwise to the collagen preparation. This solution is stirred for a further 18 hr at 4°C. The precipitate from the 3% NaCl "cut" is removed by centrifugation for 2 hr at 10,000*g*. The supernatant is collected and reprecipitated with a 4% NaCl "cut" and the pellet collected after centrifugation at 10,000*g* for 45 min. This native type I collagen is dissolved in 0.5 *M* acetic acid (volume approximately 250 ml) and dialyzed against three changes of volume of 0.2% acetic acid for 24 hr using dialysis tubing with a 10,000 molecular weight cutoff. The concentration of the purified collagen is obtained by adding 0.5 ml of sample to 0.5 ml of 2 *M* $CaCl_2$ in 0.2% acetic acid. The absorbance at 230 nm is measured using 1 *M* $CaCl_2$ in 0.2% (v/v) acetic acid as the blank and the collagen concentration is calculated using the following equation:

$$[\text{Collagen}]\ \text{mg/ml} = A_{230} \times 0.5.$$

Collagenase Assay

A total of 20 μg of collagen is plated into microwell modules (Nunc) on ice in the following buffers. Collagen [stock concentration, 2 mg/ml in 0.2% (v/v) acetic acid] in neutralizing buffer (100 m*M* Tris/HCl containing 200 m*M* NaCl and 0.04% NaN_3, pH 7.8) is gelled to the microwells by incubation for 16 hr at 30°C under humidified conditions, followed by a further 24-hr incubation under dry conditions. The wells are washed in distilled water and allowed to dry at room temperature. Collagenase activity, i.e., matrix metalloproteinase 1 (MMP-1), in the culture medium is assayed using the spectrophotometric method of Nethery *et al.* (21). Samples are mixed with a 1/10th volume of 1.0 *M* Tris and 0.2% NaN_3, pH 7.5. Latent collagenase is activated by incubation at 35°C for 10 min with either 25 μg/ml trypsin in 50 m*M* Tris containing 100 m*M* NaCl, 10 m*M* $CaCl_2$, and 0.2% NaN_3, pH 7.5 (assay buffer), or in this buffer in the presence of 1 m*M* 4-aminophenylmercuryacetate (APMA). Trypsin activity is inhibited with a fivefold molar excess of soybean trypsin inhibitor.

Assays are incubated for 18 hr at 35°C, after which the wells are washed with deionized water and allowed to dry. The wells are stained with 100 μl (per well) of Coomassie brilliant blue R-250 (0.25 mg/ml in 50% methanol, 10% acetic acid, 40% water) for 25 min at room temperature. Wells are rinsed and allowed to dry and the absorbance is read at 590 nm on a spectrophotometer (Titertek Multiscan). Each assay contains the following controls: 25 μg/ml trypsin (measure of native collagen) in assay buffer, assay buffer alone (zero digestion), and conditioned medium from BC-1 cells, a rat mammary carcinoma cell line with high spontaneous tissue collagenase (MMP-1) activity, to act as a positive control for collagenolytic activity. The collagenolytic activity of each sample is expressed as units/ml, one unit of activity being defined as that amount of enzyme required to degrade 1 mg of collagen per min per μl of sample at 35°C.

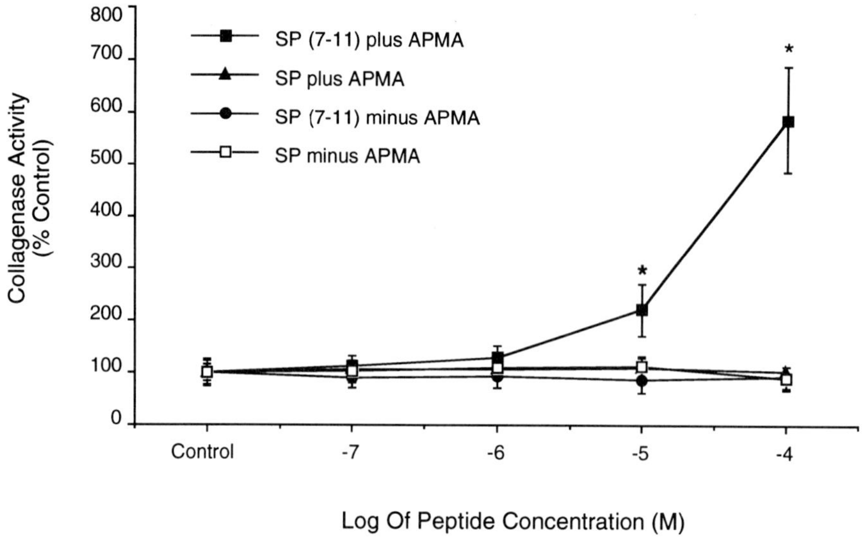

FIG. 2 Effect of SP and SP(7–11) on collagenase secretion by bovine chondrocytes. Confluent chondrocytes were incubated for 24 hr with SP or SP(7–11). TIMP activity was inactivated following reduction and inactivation with 2 m*M* dithiothreitol and 5 m*M* iodoacetamide for 30 min at 37°C. Samples were subsequently dialyzed as outlined in the text. Latent collagenase was activated with 1 m*M* APMA or 25 μg/ml trypsin followed by inactivation with soybean trypsin inhibitor. Collagenase activity was then measured. Values represent means ± SEM for four experiments and are expressed as a percentage of the control which was 13.8 ± 4.1 mU/ml. $^*p < 0.05$; $^{**}p < 0.01$ compared with controls. Reproduced with permission from D. A. Halliday, J. D. McNeil, W. H. Betts, and R. Scicchitano. *Biochem. J.* **292,** 57 (1993).

The effect of SP and SP(7–11) on collagenase secretion by bovine chondrocytes is shown in Fig. 2.

Comments

In order to interpret the measurement of collagenolytic activity, a number of factors must be appreciated. First, mammalian collagenases are generally present in both latent (i.e., procollagenase) and active forms. Therefore activation of procollagenase with an organomercurial compound or enzymatic activation, e.g., with trypsin is advisable as a routine procedure in order to measure both latent and activated activities. Second, the presence of inhibitors of collagenase may mask the real amount of the enzyme present.

In order to overcome this, the assay may be performed in the presence of inhibitors of tissue inhibitors of metalloproteinases (TIMPs) according to the method of Dean and Woesner (23). This can be achieved by incubating cell supernatants with 2 m*M* dithiothreitol at 37°C for 30 min followed by a further incubation with 5 m*M* iodoacetamide for 30 min at 37°C. Samples are then dialyzed against collagenase assay buffer prior to analysis. Using this method we have shown that the increase in collagenolytic activity seen in response to exposure to SP(7–11) is not due to reduced TIMP production but is a true increase in enzyme secretion (14). Third, it is important to conduct the assay at 35°C. At this temperature other proteinases present in the medium and which may degrade the collagen gel are not active whereas mammalian collagenase is active. Fourth, the amount of collagenase present in a sample may completely digest the collagen plug and so dilutions of each sample should be assayed to quantify collagenolytic activity accurately.

Measurement of $[Ca^{2+}]_i$ *Using Fura-2AM*

Fura-2AM may be purchased from Calbiochem, (La Jolla, CA). Hanks' balanced salt solution (HBSS) may be purchased from GIBCO (Victoria, Australia). The peptide, *N*-formyl-methionylleucylphenylalanine (fMLP) and the calcium ionophore A23187 may be purchased from Sigma Chemical Co. We used a Perkin-Elmer LS-50 spectrophotometer as a fluorimeter.

Bovine chondrocytes, isolated by collagenase digestion, are washed and incubated in 7 m*M* HBSS containing 1.3 m*M* $CaCl_2$, 0.3 m*M* KH_2PO_4, 0.5 m*M* $MgCl_2$, 0.4 m*M* $MgSO_4$, 138 m*M* NaCl, 4.0 m*M* $NaHCO_3$, and 0.3 m*M* Na_2HPO_4, pH 7.3. Chondrocytes are loaded with 1 μM Fura-2AM for 30 min at 37°C. After incubation, excess and nonhydrolyzed Fura-2AM is removed by washing the cells twice with HBSS. Chondrocytes are resuspended in HBSS at a concentration of 1×10^6 cells/ml and kept in a water bath at 37°C. Chondrocytes in HBSS are added to glass cuvettes and placed in a Perkin-Elmer LS-50 fluorospectrophotometer using excitation and emission wavelengths of 340 and 510 nm, respectively; slit widths are both 10 mm (22). Maximal fluorescence (F_{max}) is determined by the addition of 0.1% Triton X-100. Minimum fluorescence (F_{min}) is determined by the simultaneous addition of 2 m*M* EGTA and 25 m*M* Tris–HCl. The change in $[Ca^{2+}]_i$ is calculated by the formula described by Grynkiewicz *et al.* (22) using the dissociation constant (K_d) for Fura-2AM of 220 n*M*.

The following calculations are used to determine the change in $[Ca^{2+}]_i$ concentration following exposure to tachykinins or other stimuli

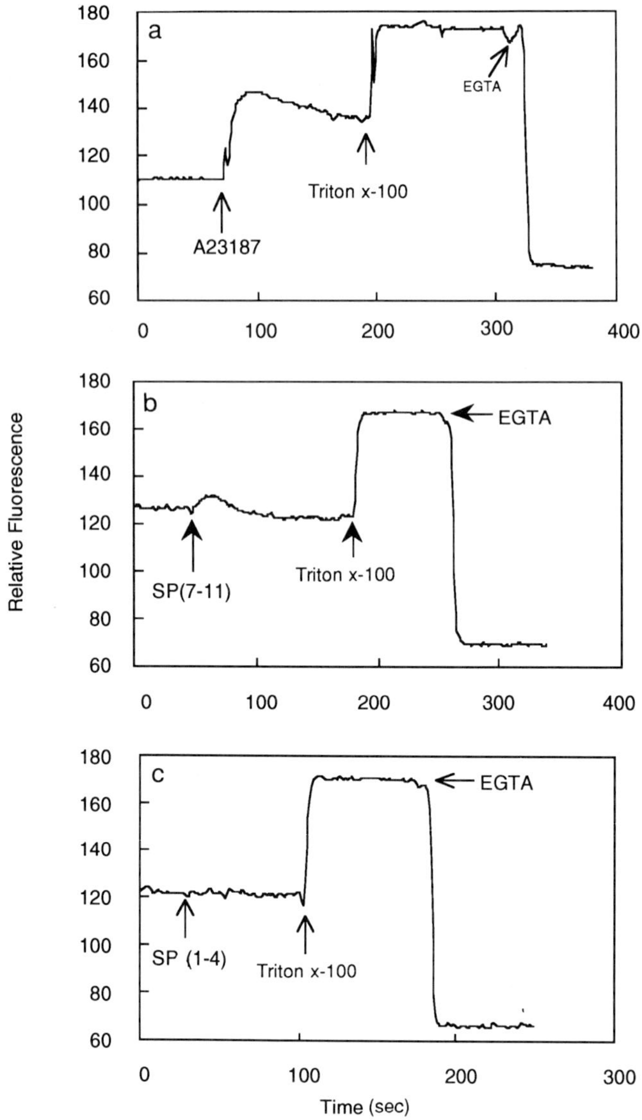

FIG. 3 Changes in $[Ca^{2+}]_i$ in bovine articular chondrocytes. (a) Sustained increase in $[Ca^{2+}]_i$ in response to Ca^{2+} ionophore A23187. Fura-2-loaded chondrocytes were stimulated with 1 μM A23187. F_{max} was obtained by the addition of 0.1% Triton X-100; F_{min} was obtained by chelation of extracellular Ca^{2+} with 2 mM EGTA. (b and c) Transient increases in $[Ca^{2+}]_i$ in response to SP(7–11) (b) and lack of response to the N-terminal fragment SP(1–4) (c). These are representative experiments. Reproduced with permission from D. A. Halliday, J. D. McNeil, W. H. Betts, and R. Scicchitano. *Biochem. J.* **292,** 57 (1993).

$$\text{Resting } [\text{Ca}^{2+}]_i = \frac{F_1 - F_0 \times 220 \text{ n}M}{F_{\max} - F_1}$$

$$\text{Stimulated } [\text{Ca}^{2+}]_i = \frac{F_2 - F_0 \times 220 \text{ n}M}{F_{\max} - F_2}$$

Change in $[Ca^{2+}]_i$ (n*M*) = stimulated $[Ca^{2+}]_i$ − resting $[Ca^{2+}]_i$ where F_1 is the basal or resting fluorescence; F_2, maximal stimulated fluorescence; $F_0 = [Ca^{2+}]_i$ following addition of 2 m*M* EGTA; and F_{max}, maximum fluorescence following addition of 0.1% Triton X-100. Changes in $[Ca^{2+}]_i$ in bovine chondrocytes are shown in Fig. 3. The Fura-2AM assay has the advantage of determining the effects of tachykinins and their metabolites on chondrocyte or synoviocyte calcium movement quickly and can therefore be used as an indicator of biological activity in a particular cell type. The preparation of cells for determination of intracellular calcium measurements is simple and rapid. However, when using heavy metals such as Zn^{2+} or Co^{2+} (as calcium channel blockers), F_{max} values cannot be determined due to interference with the addition of Triton X-100. For these reasons alternate reagents should be used to block calcium channel activity.

Acknowledgments

The authors thank Dr. Michael James for help with the PGE_2 assay and the Research Review Committee and the Special Purposes Fund of the Royal Adelaide Hospital, grants from whom have supported this work.

References

1. R. Scicchitano, J. Bienenstock, and A. Stanisz, *Brain Behav. Immun.* **1,** 231 (1987).
2. A. Wozniak, W. H. Betts, G. McLennan, and R. Scicchitano, *Immunology* **78,** 629 (1993).
3. A. Wozniak, G. McLennan, G. Murphy, W. H. Betts, and R. Scicchitano, *Immunology* **68,** 359 (1989).
4. J-L. Bueb, M. Mousli, Y. Landry, and C. Bronner, *Agents Actions* **30,** 98 (1990).
5. H. P. Hartung, K. Wolters, and K. V. Toyka, *J. Immunol.* **136,** 3856 (1986).
6. M. Lotz, D. A. Carson, and J. H. Vaughan, *Science* **235,** 893 (1987).
7. P. D'Orleans-Just, S. Dion, J. Mizrahi, and D. Regoli, *Eur. J. Pharmacol.* **114,** 9 (1985).
8. T. B. Casale, *J. Allergy Clin. Immunol.* **88,** 1 (1991).

9. J. D. Levine, D. H. Collier, A. I. Basbaum, M. A. Moskowitz, and C. A. Helms, *J. Rheumatol.* **12,** 406 (1985).
10. E. S. Kimball, *Ann. N. Y. Acad. Sci.* **594,** 293 (1990).
11. M. Fitzgerald, *Trends Neurosci.* **12,** 86 (1989).
12. M. Matucci-Cerinic and G. Partsch, *Clin. Exp. Rheumatol.* **10,** 211 (1992).
13. D. A. Halliday, J. D. McNeil, and R. Scicchitano, *Biochim. Biophys. Acta* **1137,** 29 (1992).
14. D. A. Halliday, J. D. McNeil, W. H. Betts, and R. Scicchitano, *Biochem. J.* **292,** 57 (1993).
15. D. A. Halliday, J. D. McNeil, and R. Scicchitano, *Med. Hypotheses* **40,** 227 (1993).
16. K. E. Kuettner, B. U. Pauli, G. Gall, V. A. Memoli and R. K. Shenk, *J. Cell. Biol.* **93,** 743 (1981).
17. J. M. Marsh, O. W. Wiebkin, S. Gale, H. Muir, and R. N. Maini, *Ann. Rheum. Dis.* **38,** 166 (1979).
18. B. M. Jaffe and H. R. Behrman, *in* "Methods of Hormone Radioimmunoassay" (B. M. Jaffe and Behrman, eds.), p. 19. Academic Press, New York, 1974.
19. S. Bazin and A. Delaunay, *in* "Methodology of Connective Tissue Research" (D. A. Hall, ed.), pp. 13–17. Joynson-Bruvvers, Oxford, 1974.
20. G. Chandrakasan, D. A. Torchia, and K. A. Piez, *J. Biol. Chem.* **251,** 6062 (1976).
21. A. Nethery, G. Lyons, and R. L. O'Grady, *Anal. Biochem.* **159,** 390 (1986).
22. G. Grynkiewicz, M. Poenie, and R. Y. Tsien, *J. Biol. Chem.* **260,** 3440 (1985).
23. D. Dean and J. F. Woesner, *Biochem. J.* **218,** 277 (1984).

Section II

The Brain Immune System

[11] Identification of Stressor-Activated Areas in the Central Nervous System

Bruce S. Rabin, Michael A. Pezzone, Alexander Kusnecov, and Gloria E. Hoffman

Activation Markers in the Immune System

Numerous tools have been available to immunologists to assess activation of the various components of the immune system. For example, following injection of antigen, antibody production can be quantitated in the plasma. The presence of T lymphocytes which become sensitized to the antigen can be determined by inducing lymphocytes into mitosis when incubated with the sensitizing antigen. The number of B lymphocytes which are producing antibody to the antigen can be determined by counting individual antibody-producing B lymphocytes. Finally, the role of macrophages in presenting antigen to the T-helper population of lymphocytes can be determined.

Two different populations of helper T lymphocytes, termed the TH1 and TH2 lymphocyte populations, have been identified. Their functional activity can be determined by evaluating the cytokine pattern produced in response to antigenic stimulation. Thus, techniques utilizing the measurement of secreted products of the immune system or their DNA precursors are capable not only of indicating activation of the immune system but also of providing information regarding the mechanism of interaction between various components of the immune system.

Interaction between the Brain and the Immune System

It is now well established that the immune system does not function in a manner that is independent of influences originating within the central nervous system (CNS). There is no longer any question regarding whether stress can influence the function of the immune system (1). Both increases and decreases of immune function may be induced by stress. Just as the immune system is activated by an antigen, so too must the central nervous system be activated by a stressor. An antigen activates the immune system and a stressor activates the central nervous system. The immune system must be able to perceive the presence of an antigen, while the central nervous system must be able to perceive the presence of a stressor. Perception of a stressor by the central nervous system induces biochemical changes within the central nervous system, and measurement of these changes and their location within the central nervous system may help in understanding the mechanism of stressor-induced immune alteration.

Early studies which indicated that the central nervous system could modulate immune function utilized the placement of lesions in specific areas of the brain and determined the effect of such lesions on immune function. If the posterior or anterior parts of the hypothalamus of rodents are lesioned, there is a decreased ability of the animals to produce a normal immune response (2, 3). Interestingly, electrical stimulation of the hypothalamus results in an increase of antibody production in immunized animals (4, 5). Thus, these studies suggest that the hypothalamus plays a critical role in regulating the activity of the immune system. When animals are immunized with an antigen, and the electrical activity of the hypothalamus is monitored, there is an increase in electrical activity at the time of the peak of the immune response (6). In humans, who have brain tumors, a tumor affecting the left side of the brain is associated with an impairment of *in vitro* responsiveness of peripheral blood lymphocytes to phytohemagglutinin (PHA). However, right-sided cerebral tumors do not alter PHA responsiveness (7). Thus, there can be no doubt that there are anatomically discrete areas within the brain which have the capability of regulating immune function. It is possible that the architecture of the brain determines the amount of regulatory input to brain areas which are involved with the release of catecholamines in the spleen or activation of the Hypothalamic–Pituitary–Adrenal (HPA) axis. It will require careful dissection of those areas of the brain which are activated by a stressor and determination of their connections and biochemical content in order to firmly characterize the mechanistic aspects of stressor-induced immune alteration.

Activation Markers in the Central Nervous System

Studies have identified the presence of a marker which appears in the nucleus of cells which are functionally activated. This marker, termed the c-*fos* protooncogene, produces a protein product to which an antibody can be produced. The protein product has a size of approximately 62 Da. There are epitopes on the c-Fos protein which are shared by other molecules, but there are also epitopes which appear to be specific for c-Fos. Thus, production of antibody to the Fos-specific epitopes can be used to identify cells which have been activated. We have found this technique extremely useful and have identified those areas of the rat forebrain and brain stem which become c-*fos* reactive following either an unconditioned aversive stimulus or a conditioned aversive stimulus (10).

Use of c-*fos* Protooncogene as Activation Marker

It is important that antisera used to detect the c-Fos protein product be specific for c-*fos*. Sera should be carefully screened against brain tissue that is derived from animals that are in a resting state, in a quiet room, and in the dark. This would produce the lowest amount of activation of the c-*fos* marker. The antisera should produce no, or only minimal, staining in the visual or auditory areas of the brain. Animals maintained in a room with the lights on or that undergo an injection of hypertonic saline can be used as positive controls. Procedures for this are described elsewhere (10).

Interpretation of the significance of an area of the brain which becomes c-*fos* positive must be done with caution. It is possible that a c-*fos*-positive neuron is sending a signal to an area of the brain which will then become activated to do something which will alter immune function. It is also possible that the signal that is being sent will inhibit the activity of another brain area. Thus, finding the presence of c-Fos, although indicating activation of those particular neurons, may or may not be associated with activation of other brain areas. In addition, it is possible that activated neurons may not synthesize the c-Fos protein product. Thus, finding c-Fos in various areas of the brain should only indicate the minimum number of brain areas that are activated.

c-Fos Procedure

We have used the following procedures to identify c-Fos-containing neurons within the central nervous system:

Handling of Animals

The protein product of the c-*fos* oncogene is synthesized approximately 30–45 min after the neuron is activated. This allows us to expose our experimental animals to the stressor, in our animal quarters, and then transport them to the laboratory for perfusion. If less than 30 min elapse following transport of the animals to the laboratory and sacrifice of the animals, those areas of the brain which are activated by transporting the animals will not yet have synthesized the c-Fos product. Thus, the only activated areas which we identify are those which have been activated by the stressor (provided at least 30–45 min has elapsed between exposure of the animal to the stressor and sacrifice), areas in the visual cortex which are activated by light, and the auditory areas.

Fixation of the Brain

Animals are given an intraperitoneal injection of 0.5 ml of sodium pentobarbital (50 mg/ml). They are then placed into a fume hood as the fixative with which the animals are perfused contains acrolein and paraformaldehyde, which are volatile irritants. The thorax is opened and a small incision is made in the left atrium and a catheter which is connected to tubing that is in the perfusion fluid is placed into the ventricle and positioned at the aortic bulb. The perfusion fluid is allowed to flow by gravity or by a peristaltic pump. A second incision is then made immediately in the right atrium. This allows the perfusion fluid to flow through the tissues of the animal and drain through the atrium.

Two different perfusion fluids are used. The first is isotonic saline which contains 2% sodium nitrite. This produces vasodilatation which later facilitates movement of the fixative throughout the tissues. After approximately 3 min of perfusion with the sodium nitrite solution, the fixative solution is used. We use 4% paraformaldehyde which contains 2.0% acrolein (approximately pH 7.2). Perfusion then continues for approximately 15 min after which, the musculature of the animal has hardened. The fluid which has passed through the animal drips into a pan containing 10% (w/v) sodium bisulfite. The perfusion fluids drain into the animal by gravity or by the use of a peristaltic pump. The animal is usually placed onto a piece of rigid plastic mesh which rests on top of a large pan. After fixation the animals are flushed with saline for 10 min to remove any residual acrolein from the vasculature.

After fixation, the brain and/or spinal cord is removed and placed into a 25% solution of sucrose in the cold. The sucrose solution is changed two to three times, after which the tissue can be blocked and sectioned at 25 μm on a freezing-sliding microtome.

Staining Procedure

If the tissues are to be stained immediately after sectioning, they are placed into physiologic phosphate-buffered saline. If they are going to be stained at a later time, they are placed into a cryoprotectant solution. After the sections are removed from the cryoprotectant, they are rinsed in phosphate-buffered saline (PBS) and then treated with 1% (w/v) $NaBH_4$ (sodium borohydride to neutralize the acrolein) solution for 15–20 min and rinsed in PBS until all bubbling subsides. The tissue is then incubated with the anti-c-*fos* antiserum which is diluted in 0.4% Triton X-100 solution made in PBS at 4°C for 48 hr. A variety of antisera to c-Fos are available from commercial sources. Antisera directed to the N-terminal portion of the c-Fos molecule have the highest degree of specificity. Depending on the antiserum, dilutions ranging from 1 : 2,000 up to 1 : 50,000 may be used. Each antiserum will have to be titrated in the individual laboratory performing the assay.

Following incubation with the primary antibody, the tissue is rinsed and then incubated with the secondary labeled antibody. We typically used a biotinylated goat antiserum to the appropriate primary antibody species. Incubation proceeds for 1 hr at room temperature after which the tissue is rinsed three times in PBS. The tissue is then incubated with an avidin–biotin complex reagent at room temperature for 1 hr. The tissue is then rinsed in 0.175 *M* sodium acetate and the c-*fos* antibody–peroxidase complex stained with a solution of $NiSO_4$ (25 mg/ml), 3,3′-diaminobenzidine (0.2 mg/ml) and H_2O_2 (0.83 μl of a 3% dilution/ml of reaction solution) in 0.175 *M* sodium acetate. After 30–40 min the tissue is transferred into acetate solution to stop the reaction, rinsed in PBS, and then mounted on gelatin/chrom alum-coated glass slides. The tissue is then dehydrated through graded ethanol solution, cleared in Histoclear, and coverslipped with Histomount. C-Fos is evident as a blue-black reaction product in cell nuclei.

As an example of studies which can be performed subsequent to identification of stressor-induced activation of c-Fos in the brain, we have evaluated the effect of lesioning of the paraventricular nucleus (PVN) on immune alteration in the spleen of stressed rats (11). The PVN becomes intensely positive for c-Fos following exposure of an experimental rat to a conditioned or unconditioned stressor (8). When the PVN was lesioned, there was significantly more suppression of the ability of spleen lymphocytes to respond to nonspecific mitogens than was present in sham-operated animals. This suggests that the PVN functions to ameliorate the effect of stress on spleen lymphocyte mitogenic activity.

It is possible to use double immunohistochemical staining procedures to identify the hormone content of the Fos-positive neurons. This allows, for example, the identification of activated neurons which contain such peptides as Corticotropin-Releasing Hormone (CRH), oxytocin, or vasopressin. The double-staining procedures are described elsewhere (10).

Examples of the use of the c-*fos* protooncogene to identify activated neurons in experimental animals that have been stressed are shown in Figs. 1–5. Male Lewis rats received a 1.6 mA electric footshock every 4 min over 64

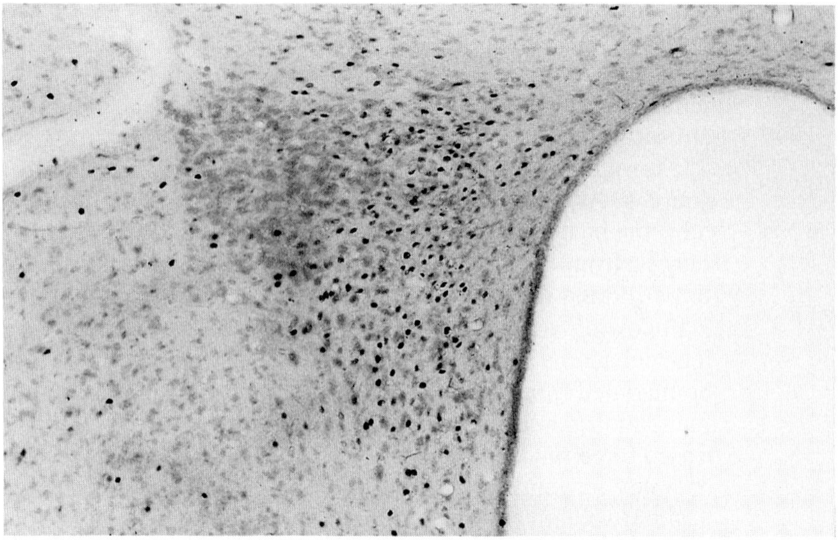

FIG. 1 Identification of c-Fos-positive neurons in the medial parvocellular division of the paraventricular nucleus following footshock.

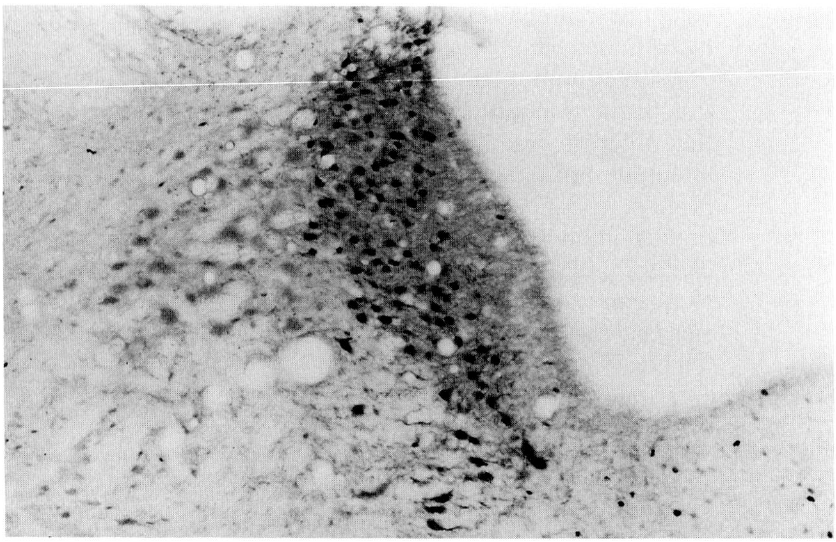

FIG. 2 Identification of c-Fos-positive neurons in the locus coeruleus following footshock.

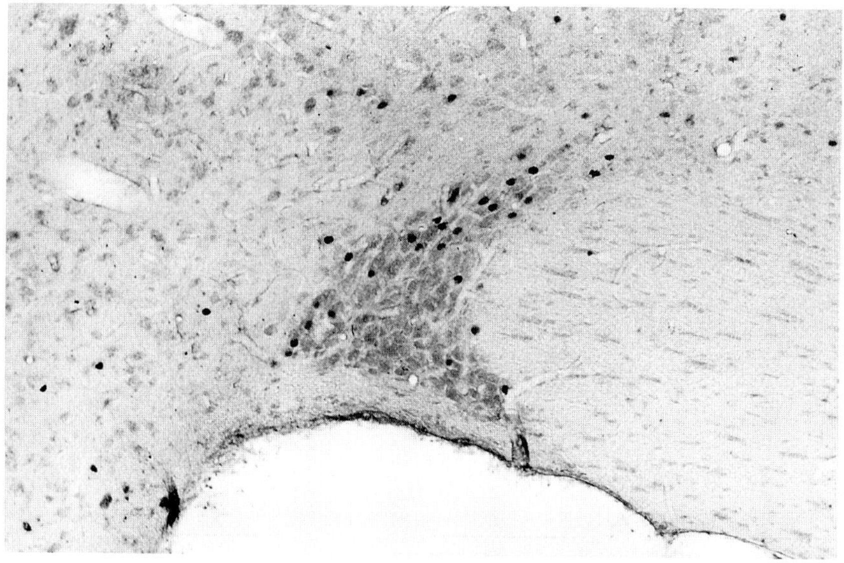

FIG. 3 Identification of c-Fos reactivity in neurons of the dorsal border of the supraoptic nucleus following footshock.

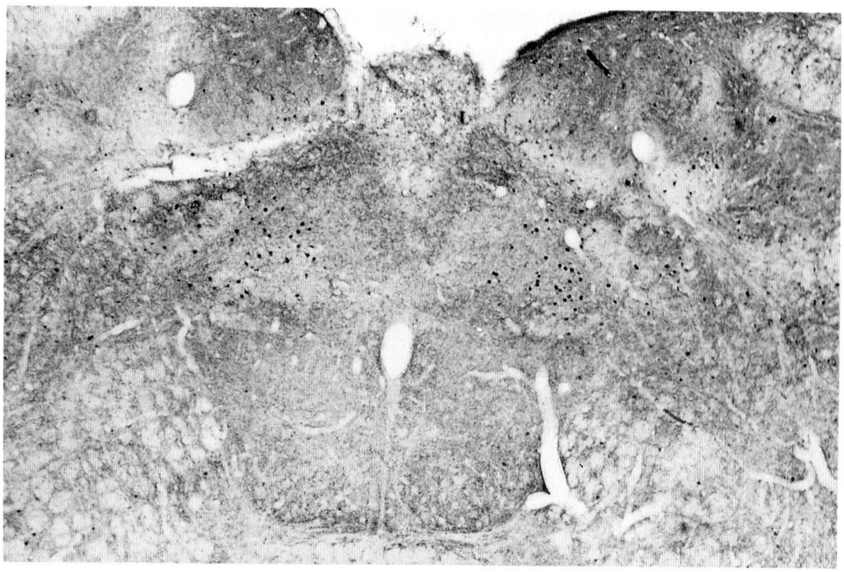

FIG. 4 Identification of c-Fos reactivity in neurons of the nucleus tractus solitarius following footshock.

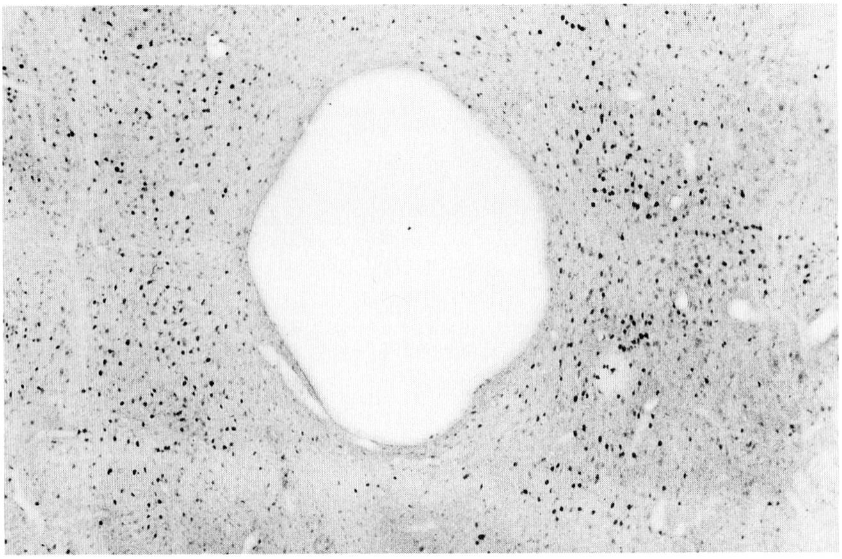

FIG. 5 Identification of c-Fos reactivity in neurons of the periaqueductal gray following footshock. Ventral is to the right and dorsal to the left.

min. A total of 16 footshocks were given. The animals and tissue were then processed as described.

The technique of c-Fos immunohistochemistry, used to study activated neurons of the brain, has contributed significantly to our knowledge of behaviorally activated brain areas. This information can now be used to gain a better understanding of the mechanism of stressor-induced brain activation and immune function alteration.

References

1. B. Rabin, S. Cohen, R. Ganguli, D. T. Lysle, and J. E. Cunnick, *CRC Crit. Rev. Immunol.* **9(4),** 279 (1989).
2. R. J. Cross, M. R. Markesbery, W. H. Brooks, *et al., Brain Res.* **196,** 79 (1980).
3. R. J. Weber and C. B. Pert, *in* "Central and Peripheral Endorphins: Basic and Clinical Aspects" (E. E. Muller and A. R. Genazzani, eds.), p. 35. Raven Press, New York, 1984.
4. E. A. Kroneva, *Fiziol. Chel.* **2,** 469 (1976).
5. A. B. Tsypin and V. H. Malstev, *Pathol. Fixiol. Exkp. Ter.* **11,** 83 (1972).
6. H. O. Besedovsky, E. Sorkin, D. Felix, *et al., Eur. J. Immunol.* **7,** 323 (1977).

7. H. M. Blomgren, V. Blom, and H. Ullen, *Cancer Immunol. Immunother.* **21,** 31 (1986).
8. M. A. Pezzone, W-S. Lee, G. E. Hoffman, and B. S. Rabin, *Brain Res.* **597,** 41 (1992).
9. M. A. Pezzone, W-S. Lee, G. E. Hoffman, K. M. Pezzone, and B. S. Rabin, *Brain Res.* **608,** 310 (1993).
10. G. E. Hoffman, M. S. Smith, and J. G. Verbalis, *Front. Neuroendocrinol.* **14(3),** 173 (1993).
11. M. A. Pezzone, H. Dohanics, J. G. Verbalis, and B. S. Rabin, *Soc. Neurosci.* **18,** 678 (1992).

[12] Methodological Approaches for Studying Neuroimmune Connection of Identical Functional Blocks

G. A. Belokrylov and E. I. Sorochinskaya

Introduction

Systematic approaches to the analysis of experimental results are necessary in any field of science. However, it is extremely difficult to systematize information concerning neuroendocrine immune connections because of the great discrepancies in the results. One of the reasons for these discrepancies is the use of approaches which are not sufficiently valid for solving such a complicated and difficult problem as neuroendocrine immunomodulation. The approach we use to study this problem is based on the following principles: (i) similar functional blocks are used as the basis of our methodology; (ii) only chemically individual compounds are used; (iii) preparations and solvents must not be pyrogenic; and (iv) definite methodical parameters must be maintained during the entire experiment.

Similar Functional Blocks as Basis of Methodology

A functional block is a structure which is related to a particular function. The evolution and the specialization of functions which have been determined mainly by recombination and transposition of identical blocks have resulted in the creation of unique highly specialized systems (1). For this reason functionally different and sometimes contrary systems may constitute polypotent or polyfunctional blocks due to the structure–function connections between these systems. Neuroendocrine immunoactive compounds such as thymosin α_1 (2) and β_4 (3), prothymosin α_1 (4), the endogenous regulator of prothymosin α_1, parathymosin (5), oxytocin (6), γ-aminobutyric acid (GABA) (7), Thy-1 antigen (8), and vasoactive intestinal peptide (VIP) (9) have all been found in mammalian thymus and brain. Hormones which are not thymic hormones, for example, oxytocin and vasopressin, have been synthesized simultaneously *de novo* (6).

In brain and in the gastrointestinal tract (GIT), the so-called brain–gut peptides that display neuroendocrine immune activity (11, 12) are present

Methods in Neurosciences, Volume 24

simultaneously: bombesin, gastrin, cholecystokinin (CCK), VIP, substance P, and neurotensin (11). Most of these peptides penetrate the blood–brain barrier.

The neuroendocrine immunoactive substances of different mammalian species are distributed not only in the brain, thymus, and GIT; but also, in the case of neuroimmunoregulatory peptides, in other organs. Different forms of gastrin have been found in the CNS and GIT, as well as in the peripheral nervous system (12, 13), and CCK and VIP have been found in the cerebromedullary liquor (13, 14). Vasoactive intestinal peptide has also been found in the placenta (14), and CCK and neurotensin in white splenic pulp (9). Vasopressin and oxytocin are present in the ovaries, testes, and adrenal glands as well as in the CNS. Peripheral synthesis of oxytocin has been confirmed in bovine corpus luteum. The gene for the hypothalamic peptide hormone oxytocin is highly expressed in the bovine corpus luteum and granulosa cells (6). Prothymosin α_1 has been found in liver, kidney, lungs, and spleen; parathymosin has been found in liver and kidney in higher concentrations than thymosin α_1 (5). The neuroendocrine immunoactive peptide thymosin β_4 is present in practically every cell, not just in erythrocytes (3). Thy-1 antigen is the main marker of the murine T cells and along with the peptides noted has displayed neuroimmunomodulatory properties (8). It has been found on T cells and neurons as well as on the membranes of many other lymphoid and nonlymphoid cells, such as astrocytes, macrophages, neutrophils, derma cells, myoblasts, and mammary epithelium (8).

Neuroendocrine immunoactive compounds may be synthesized *de novo* and secreted by separate lymphoid and even nonlymphoid mammalian cells. For example, adrenocorticotropic hormone (ACTH) and β-endorphin have been synthesized by lymphocytes and macrophages; the ACTH synthesis has been possible in the absence of hypophysis. The number of lymphocytes containing immunoreactive ACTH increases in the presence of vasopressin and corticotropin-releasing factor (CRF) (6). Rodent and human lymphocytes synthesize CRF-like factor, immunoreactive thyreotropin (TSH), growth hormone, chorionic gonadotropin, follicle-stimulating hormone, and luteinizing hormone (LH) (16). Mucous and polynucleated cells synthesize VIP; basocytes synthesize substance P (17); and macrophages synthesize prostaglandin (18), bombesin, and thymosin β_4 (17).

The majority of substances with neuroendocrine immunomodulating properties possess specific receptors on lymphoid cells. Thus, the receptors for metenkephalin, somatostatin, VIP, and substance P (16) have been noted on T lymphocytes. The receptors for VIP and substance P have also been found on B lymphocytes (16). The receptors for endorphin have been found on T lymphocytes, and these receptors are tightly connected with the receptors for interleukin (IL-2) on cell membranes (11). The specific receptors for growth hormone and prolactin (19) have been discovered on thymocytes and directly on the thymus epithelium. On the T-cell membranes the receptors for glucocorticoids, whose density is higher on the less-mature cells, have been found (2). The presence of the specific receptors for estrogens and thyroid hormones has been shown in T-lymphocyte nuclei and in the thymus epithelium (20). The receptors for T4 antigen, the main marker of human T helpers, are found in neurons (11).

Compounds of neuroendocrine origin that have the receptors on the thymus epithelium are able to enhance the synthesis and production of thymic hormones when added to thymus epithelial cell culture. Under the influence of physiological concentrations of prolactin, β-endorphin (but not α- and γ-endorphins), estradiol, progesterone, triiodotyronine, and hydrocortisone, the thymulin concentrations in this cell culture have been increased (19). In turn, thymic peptides, thymosin fraction 5, and its constituent thymosin α_1 and β_4, in particular, are able to enhance hormone production of neuroendocrine origin. Thymosin fraction 5 and thymosin β_4 have been found to stimulate LH release *in vivo,* following infusion into lateral ventricle, as well as after infusion into isolated median eminence pituitary cultures (18, 21). Thymosin fraction 5 stimulates the ACTH and β-endorphin production in normal or tumor pituitary cell (AtT-20 line) cultures *in vitro* (21) and enhances the growth hormone and prolactin concentration in the tumor pituitary cell culture of the GH3 line (21). In adrenal fasciculata cell culture both thymosin fraction 5 and its constituent thymosins α_1, α_7, and β_4 are inactive. When injected directly into the third ventricle of the cerebrum, fraction 5 (but not the analogous preparation made from kidney tissue) enhances the production of corticosterone. The increase in the serum corticosteroid concentration is accompanied by an increase in the weight of the adrenal glands, but not of the gonads or thymus. Thymosin α_1, but not thymosin β_4, displays the same property.

An increase in corticosterone levels in the rodent blood has been found as well after an intraperitoneal injection of thymosin fraction 5 (21, 22), lymphokine-containing (LAF, MIF, IL-2) supernatants (23), and corpuscular and soluble antigens (23). Thymosin fraction 5 elevates the serum corticotropin, β-endorphin, and cortisol when administered intravenously to prepubertal monkeys (21). The rise in steroid may be secondary to the release of thymosins and/or lymphokines and the stimulation of glucocorticoid release during an immune response may constitute a mechanism by which the immune system can limit the extent of its activation.

The thymus is directly connected with the central nervous system structures by parasympathetic fiber originating from vagal nuclei in the brain stem, and by orthosympathetic fibers from the stellate and other ganglia of the thoracic chain. Acetylcholinesterase-positive fibers are mainly found in the subcapsular cortex and the corticomedullary junction. Noradrenergic fibers enter with arterial and subcapsular plexuses and are projected throughout the thymic cortical parenchyme including the corticomedullary boundary (11). Catecholamine, discovered not only in brain but in thymus as well, may play the mediatory role in neuroimmunomodulation. In mice, the injection of 100 μg 6-oxydopamine (in a volume of 10 μl) into cisterna magna, but not intraperioneally, has led to a decrease in epinephrine in the hypothalamus, midbrain, and pons medulla, and to a suppression of the primary immune response and the immunological memory (24).

The data reported above have allowed the formulation (25) of two levels of neuroendocrine–immune system interrelationships. The first level is based on the interactions between the neuroendocrine system and the thymus as the organ which induces proliferation and differentiation of stem cells into mature T lymphocytes. The second level is at the periphery and connects neuroendocrine signals with the humoral products which have been secreted by immune cells during specific reactions to various antigens (25). Substances which influence not only the neuroendocrine system, but also the immune system have been synthesized in the thymus; thymic peripheral cells are then able to synthesize *de novo* substances of neuroendocrine origin. For this reason thymus should be considered as a immunoneuroendocrine organ which is part of a united defense system: identical blocks can provide homeostasis during their functioning in target cells. This approach is the basis of our methodology for studying neuroendocrine–immune system connections.

Individuality of Biologically Active Compounds

The next point to be taken into consideration in our investigations is the composition of preparations to be studied. As a basis of our methodological approach we use only chemically individual compounds in our investigations. Traditionally in studying the role of an organ and its function on the molecular level purified tissue extracts are used. These extracts are complex mixtures of substances of different origins. Many of the data reported deal with experiments and clinic trials of thymosin fraction 5 (26), thymostimulin (27), thymomodulin (128), and thymalin (8); the exact total composition of these substances is unknown. Sometimes the whole activity of the complete polymeric molecule or of the extract could be modeled fully by a molecular fragment or a component of the extract. For example, leukokinin stimulation of the phagocytic activity of polymorphonuclear leukocytes can be attributed to a small daughter peptide, tuftsin (29), and the inhibition of various macrophage functions with hydrolyzed immunoglobulin G (IgG) has been reproduced with the tripeptide, threonyllysylarginine, which is a component of this hydrolysate (30). However, more often individual components of extracts and hydrolysates display properties which are distinct from the activity of the whole mixture. Thus, thymosin fraction 5 has been effective in partially or fully inducing and maintaining immune function (26), but thymosin fraction 5 components reveal quite different effects (2): thymosin α_1 is inactive in those assays where thymosin fraction 5 displays activity, thymosin α_5 converts T cells to T-helper cells, and thymosin α_7 changes immature T cells to cells with suppression function. Thymosins β_3 and β_4 appear to act at very early stages of the maturation sequence, and thymosin β_1 is inactive. Thymosin α_1 enhances, whereas thymosin β_4 suppresses, the human autologous and allogeneic mixed lymphocyte reaction (31). When the modes of action are alike, the effective doses of the separate components can be 100 to 1000 times less than that of the whole mixture (32).

Moreover, some trace amounts of impurities, often very minor, drastically affect activity and may lead to a marked decrease, abolishment, or even inhibition of action: the tripeptide lysylprolylarginine can block the stimulation of phagocytosis induced by the tetrapeptide threonyllysylprolylarginine on phagocytic cells (29). This should be taken into account when comparing the results of assays using different preparations. The extracts of the whole thymus tissue (thymosin fraction 5, thymostimulin, thymalin, etc.) contain mainly polypeptide mixtures. Hydrolysates such as thymomodulin include polypeptides and mixtures of amino acids which themselves have marked immunomodulating activity (33, 34) and are an independent part of immunogenesis regulation. Both extracts and hydrolysates may include lymphokines of thymocytic origin and other immunoactive substances (GABA, oxytocin, vasopressin, VIP) whose presence or even synthesis in the thymus have been shown. Simultaneously in preparations of lymphocytic origin (for example, lymphocytic chalone) the thymic peptide FTS, which masks inhibitory chalone activity, may be present (35).

Negative results which have been obtained (36) in an attempt to prepare an immunologically active preparation from calf brain may be explained not by the absence of the immunostimulator in the brain but by the use of the preparation from the whole brain opposite the cortex where the immunomodulator has been predominantly localized. The absence of the immunostimulator in white matter (8), whose quantity has been significantly higher than that in gray matter (cortex) has made it impossible to prepare the immunostimulator from the whole cerebrum.

The use of mixtures of biologically active compounds extracted from organs has not proved advantageous because of the presence of substances from other specialized systems. Thymosin fraction 5 which consists of no less than 50 peptides (37) has been able to induce *in vivo,* but not *in vitro* (2), steroidogenesis, whereas a component of fraction 5, thymosin α_1, which penetrates the brain–blood barrier, has not revealed this property after intraperitoneal administration to rodents or after the direct injection of not only thymosin α_1, but also thymosin β_4 into the bloodstream of monkeys (21). These facts testify to the connection between the endocrine and immune systems as a whole, but do not prove that the functional connection is directly provided by peptides from the thymosin fraction 5. After the thymus epithelium has synthesized vasopressin which enhances steroidogenesis in pituitary cells (6) and in lymphocytes, it might be possible to determine that the increase in steroidogenesis under the influence of the thymosin fraction 5 has been the result of the vasopressin action due to its presence in the thymosin fraction 5.

The peptide used in the assays should be strictly individual, because its function has to be determined by its structure. For example, a single amino acid substitution can abolish the excessive grooming trait elicited by bombesin or CCK-8 (10). Thymopentin and splenopentin whose structures differ from each other by a single amino acid residue have fully distinct functionality (38). Thymopentin has marked immunomodulating activity, whereas splenopentin is practically immunoinert (38). The substitution of valine in position 37 by leucine within the tetradecapeptide represented by fragment 32–45 of thymopoietin III enhances the T-cell immune response of immunodeficient patients to PHA to a level which is higher than the activity of the fragment itself. The substitution of this valine residue by glycine results in a decrease in activity and substitution by proline or β-alanine and in the full disappearance of activity (39). The peptides leucylglycylisoleucylproline and prolyltyrosylisoleucyllysine (fragments 49–53 and 66–69 of murine Thy-1 antigen) which contain both immunologically inert amino acids (leucine, glycine, isoleucine, proline, tyrosine, lysine) and phagocytosis-stimulating amino acids (leucine, tyrosine, proline, lysine) influence neither the immune response nor phagocytic activity of neutrophils. The elongation of the peptide leucylglycylisoleucylproline at the C terminus with immunologically active glutamic acid results in the emergence of a peptide leucylglycylisoleucylprolylglutamic acid which stimulates both the immune response and phagocytosis. The addition of valine, which stimulates both processes, to the C terminus of peptide prolyltyrosylisoleucyllysine results in the ability of the peptide prolyltyrosylisoleucyllysylvaline to enhance phagocytosis without affecting the immune response (34).

In every case the homogeneity of each compound should be confirmed by elemental and amino acid analyses, high-voltage electrophoresis, thin-layer chromatography in several systems, and high-performance liquid chromatography. Homogeneity of the preparations is achieved by the use of defined synthetic methods for obtaining the compounds to be studied. Classical peptide synthesis (40) in solution with minimal protection of side groups avoids the additional stages of preparation of fully protected amino acids and the additional complexities connected with extra deprotection steps. The combination of consecutive and fragmental schemes of synthesis guarantees the shortest inexpensive route to a desired structure and makes it possible to verify the homogeneity of the peptides obtained and their amino acid sequences at every stage of synthesis. This approach makes it possible to obtain functional blocks which can act in different systems of organisms inside large polypeptide molecules.

Necessity of Pyrogen-Free Preparations and Solvents

The essential condition for correct experiments is the use of pyrogen-free saline for dissolving preparations. Most investigators studying the problem of neuroendocrine immune connections have used sterile but not pyrogen-free solutions. Distilled water which is used for solution preparation may be contaminated with bacterial pyrogens because many pyrogenic heterotrophic bacterial products accumulate in water. The ability of bacteria to breed in the cold is also significant (41).

The use of sterile, but not pyrogen-free, solutions has led to serious misinterpretations of results. Preparations which have not been pyrogen-free or have been dissolved in sterile but not pyrogen-free saline increase steroidogenesis. Irrespective of dose (2.0 or 20.0 mg/kg) thymosine fraction 5 enhances (22) the serum corticosterone concentration in 20 min after an intraperitoneal injection into rats as compared with the basal level (55.3 ± 15 ng/ml for noninjected animals) to levels which are equal to the results for intraperitoneal injections of sterile but not pyrogen-free saline. The corticosterone concentration increases to 161.6 ± 38.8 ng/ml for a dose of 2 mg/kg and 209.3 ± 44.6 ng/ml for a dose of 20 mg/kg, as compared with 146.5 ± 45.6 ng/ml after saline application. Saline enhances the serum corticosterone concentration 2.6 times compared to the basal level, whereas thymosin fraction 5 which has been dissolved in saline increases the level 2.9 and 3.8 times, depending on the dose (2.0 or 20.0 mg/kg). The administration of sterile but not pyrogen-free saline to cisterna magna of mice increases the plasma corticosterone concentration during the first hour from 23 ± 8.4 for noninjected mice to 220 ± 1.3 ng/ml (24). Increase in body temperature and in concentration of the neuroendocrine axis hormones have been observed as well after subcutaneous injection of sterile, but not pyrogen-free, saline (10). Subcutaneous injection of such saline (2 ml/kg) reduces the grooming behavior of rats induced with i.c.v. ACTH (3 μg in 4 μl saline) and attenuates their rise in body temperature (10). Increases in body temperature and enhancement of steroidogenesis have not been observed after the use of pyrogen-free saline even after direct administration into the bloodstream (42). In addition, those substances which cause pyrogeneity may induce either B-cell activity at low concentations in the case of endotoxins or T-cell activity when exotoxin has been the source of pyrogeneity. In both cases the immune response increases and sometimes masks the real influence of the preparation to be studied. The use of pyrogen-free solutions is one of the indispensable conditions for obtaining the adequate results in the study of neuroendocrine immune connections.

Methodical Parameters of Experimental Organization

The assays of biologically active preparations for the estimation of neuroendocrine immune connections should be carried out in animals of the same species, sex, and age because specific age and sexual differences are well known. For example, in assays for VIP used in equal doses in cultures of human lymphocytes, lymphocytes from guinea pig lymph nodes, and rat splenocytes, opposite results have been obtained: the suppression of spontaneous proliferation of human thymocytes and the stimulation of guinea pig lymph node cells and rat splenocytes (43). Oxytocin, which modulates the effect of CRF on antehypophyseal ACTH secretion, influences this process differently in different species: it enhances the influence of CRF on ACTH production in rats and suppresses this effect in humans (6). The ACTH-induced behavioral syndrome differs qualitatively from one species to another (44, 45). In each of three species studied different symptoms have prevailed: excessive grooming in rats, penile erection and anorexia in rabbits, stretching and yawning in mice. Neuroendocrine mechanisms of peptide-induced grooming may also differ among species (10). Moreover, the dependence of functional characteristics of thymic hormones on the genetic status of an experimental recipient has been shown (46): thymosin fraction 7 treatment of murine spleen cell cultures has enhanced the plaque-forming cell response of BALB/c spleen cells while it has suppressed this response in CBA mice.

The choice of preparation doses and administration modes is important for the evaluation of the preparation role in neuroimmunomodulating processes. For example, glucocorticoids, which are considered immunodepressive hormones, do not always have a suppressive effect. The inhibitory effect of corticosteroids *in vitro* and *in vivo* has been found only when using pharmacological doses. Unlike T-helper cells, T-suppressor cells are less sensitive, and natural killer cells are resistant to pharmacological concentrations of steroids. At low ($0.01–0.11^{-6}$ *M*) physiological concentrations, steroids reveal a so-called "permissive effect" and stimulate *in vitro* and *in vivo* T, but not B, lymphocyte proliferation (18, 21). The effect of estrogens on the mitotic activity of lymphocytes and on cell-mediated immunity is like the corticosteroid effect: low concentrations stimulate and high concentrations inhibit immunocompetent cell mitosis (18, 20). In assays of biologically active preparations, stimulating properties are usually revealed at lower doses: diminishing a thymosin fraction 5 dose 200 times (from 1000 μg/kg to 5 μg/kg) results (47) in a threefold increase in PFC values (from 31.2 $\pm$ 1.0 to 95 $\pm$ 4.7 as compared with 13.2 $\pm$ 0.9 in the control). Decreasing the dose of the aminio acid preparation levamine 10^7 times (from 1 mg/kg to 0.0001 μg/kg) increases PFC values from 18.4 $\pm$ 2.7 to 25.1 $\pm$ 1.7 as compared with 11.0 $\pm$ 1.6 in the control (48). The promotion of cell differentiation is influenced by using low concentrations of different individual peptides and their mixtures. Thymopentin-induced Thy-1 antigen expression on bone marrow T precursor membranes takes place at concentrations of 10^{-5}–10^{-6} μg/ml but not at a concentration of 10^2 μg/ml (49), and with thymosin fraction 5 at concentrations of 10^{-2}–10^{-4} μg/ml, but not at 10^2–10^3 μg/ml (50).

It is important to use the same type of administration method throughout the experiment because the values for effective doses depend on the way a preparation is applied. Equal values for a biological response have been achieved after intravenous injections of thymopentin at a dose that is 10 times less than the level for subcutaneous or intraperitoneal administration (51). The effect is also markedly changed depending on the mode and the duration of application: to eliminate noradrenaline from cerebrum demands a single injection whereas no less than 10 intraperitoneal injections are needed to attain peripheral functional sympathectomy (45). It is important to note that the observed variations in expression of different T-cell markers are characteristic mainly for polypeptide and/or amino acid mixtures. The difference between the effects of individual components testifies to the necessity of using individual substances.

When choosing a dose of the preparation to be studied it is important to take into account the initial levels of a substance. The increase in steroidogenesis induced by biologically active preparations has been observed only for a plasma corticosterone basal level not higher than 50 ng/ml (22). At the initially low levels of corticosteroids in murine serum (less normal) the quantity of blood monocytes increases leading to an enhancement of the immune response to sheep red blood cells (SRBC). Moreover, it is possible to overcome dose tolerance: the twofold increase of hemagglutinin titer at a tolerogenic (2×10^9) SRBC dose. The immunomodulating effect of peptides is more significant at the initially decreased indexes of immunity (52).

The choice of a mitogen for the evaluation of cell-mediated immunity and the search for an antigen for the estimation of the humoral immune response must take into consideration that the neuroendocrine immune homeostasis provides a system of common functional blocks that have been localized predominantly in brain and thymus and are connected to one another structurally and functionally. The control of homeostasis has been provided by T cells which are connected with the majority of neuroendocrine immunoactive compounds. Therefore it is more correct to use for the initial evaluation of the functional activities of such compounds those mitogens and antigens whose effect has been directed to T cells, and then to compare their activities with their influence on B-cell functions. Unlike classical adjuvants, the peptide functional blocks are marked by their ability to immunostimulate only using suboptimal, but not optimal, antigen doses (52, 53). Thymosin fraction 3 does not increase the immune response to a large dose (2.5%) of SRBC in mice (54). At the same time, the thymosin fraction 5 reveals the marked immunomodulating activity over a wide range of doses (1000–0.05 μg/kg) for the SRBC immunization of animals at a dose of 2×10^6 (47). Thymopentin activates the precursors of cytotoxic lymphocytes only at suboptimal, but not optimal, allogeneic stimulation (53). Moreover, the use of suboptimal antigen doses is advisable because SRBC are able to induce T suppressors in murine spleens when used in a large (2×10^9–5×10^9) dose (55). A dose of 5×10^9 SRBC enhances the rodent serum corticosterone level and diminishes the thyroxin concentration; whereas after decreasing the SRBC dose 10 times (to 5×10^8), the thyroxine level is unchanged and the corticosterone concentration changes less markedly (23).

When choosing the site for the antigen application it is advisable to use direct administration into the bloodstream. Intraperitoneal antigen injections may lead to the enhancement of steroidogenesis because of the direct contact of antigen with peritoneal macrophages. This contact induces the synthesis and production of IL-1 which, like thymosin fraction 5, may enhance the ACTH production in tumor cell (AtT-20 line) cultures (11).

Taking into account all of the above-mentioned considerations we have used one species (mice), one line (CBA) of one sex (male), of equal age (5 weeks old) and equal weight (14–16 g) for the estimation of immunomodulation and pubertal male rats (2–2.5 months old and 80–90 g body weight) for the evaluation of neuroimmune activity. For antigen doses we have taken into account the previously reported data about the efficacy of using suboptimal, but not optimal, antigen doses for the evaluation of peptide activities (47, 52–55).

Thymectomy has been carried out (56) surgically using a low ether anesthesia and an artificial respiration apparatus. As the control sham-thymectomized animals are used for whom all the operation stages have been carried out except for the thymus extraction. Special attention should be paid to the completeness of the thymus extraction. That is especially important for assays to determine the effects of preparation on the conditioned reflex;

even a minimal part of the nonablated thymus (3–5 mm in the diameter) normalizes fully the decreased ability to form the food-instrumental reflex. The age of the animals when the thymectomy is performed is important because thymectomy of 8-week-old CBA mice has led to the elimination of Thy-1^+ cells from the spleen, but has not changed their functional activity (responses to PHA and SRBC). If the operation is performed at an earlier age (4 to 6 weeks old), the quantity of cells as well as the functional activity is diminished (57). Therefore we use 4- to 5-week-old mice weighing 12–14 g for thymectomy.

The estimation of the behavioral effects due to substances is carried out according to classic methods (58).

Induction Assays of T-Cell Differentiation

Cells of chest, thigh, and leg bone marrow are freed from erythrocytes using a 0.65% solution of ammonium chloride. With this procedure the leukocyte suspension contains no less than 85–90% viable cells, unlike the effect of 0.83% ammonium chloride solution in which the leukocyte viability is no more than 70% (59). Then the cells are washed with a cold Hanks' solution five times, centrifuged at 1200 rev/min for 7 min at 4°C five times, and mixed with the preparations to be studied so that 1 ml of the solution contains 3×10^7 nucleated cells and $1.0–10^{-6}$ μg/ml of a preparation. The mixture of the preparation and the cells is incubated with periodical shaking at 37°C for 1.5 hr, then it is washed with Hanks' solution five times, and the cell susceptibility to the brain tissue antisera is evaluated in a complement-dependent cytotoxicity assay. The antiserum is raised by the immunization of rabbits with the CBA murine cortex tissue in which the Thy-1 antigen identical to the Thy-1 antigen of T cells is mostly localized (8). The immunization is carried out subcutaneously without Freund's adjuvant. The antiserum (60) is heated at 56°C for 30 min and then absorbed twice with the murine liver homogenate and murine and sheep red blood cells (SRBC) (1 ml of the antiserum for 0.1 ml of the dense sediment of each kind of cell) for 1 hr at room temperature. After the absorption the antiserum is diluted with distilled water (1 : 10) and the antigen–antibody complexes are deleted by the reprecipitation with carbon dioxide. The anticortex serum is used at a 1 : 50 dilution; in this case the antiserum causes a depth of thymocytes of 88.0 ± 1.3% in the presence of complement (fresh guinea pig serum, 1 : 3) and does not interact with the bone marrow cells of CBA mice. In the control (cells in Hanks' solution in the presence of complement at a dilution of 1 : 3), the viability of lymphocytes is no less than 85–90%. No less than 200 cells are calculated; the viability is tested by the exclusion trypan blue method (0.2%, Sigma). Each assay is repeated no less than two to three times.

Immunoglobulin M Plaque-Forming Cell (IgM pfc) Assay

Peptides or amino acisd are dissolved in pyrogen-free saline prepared from double-distilled water and pure grade sodium chloride. The peptide or amino acid solutions are prepared just before injection or *in vitro* assay. The peptides are injected subcutaneously in 0.5 ml of sterile pyrogen-free saline for 5 days in doses of 2×10^{-8}–10^{-15} *M* per mouse per day (corresponding to 1.3×10^{-6}–6.5×10^{-14} *M*/kg). Amino acids are injected in equimolar quantities. Control animals are given sterile pyrogen-free saline. The mice are then intravenously (use the tail vein because immunization into this vein produces pfc in the spleen) immunized once with 2×10^6 SRBC or with Viantigen (polysaccharide from *Salmonella typhi abdominalis,* 0.001 μg per animal). On the fourth day after the immunization the mice are decapitated and IgM-pfc is calculated in the spleen by the method of local hemolysis in agarose (Sigma). To determine the number of pfc to Viantigen, SRBC are coated with Viantigen (20 μg/ml) for 1.5 hr at 37°C. The SRBC are washed with the saline at least eight times to eliminate nonbound Viantigen. To determine IgM-pfc to SRBC and Viantigen, each spleen is weighed. The spleen homogenates are prepared in Medium 199 at a concentration of 50 mg/ml. A total of 0.1 ml of SRBC (8–9 $\times 10^8$/ml) or SRBC coated with Viantigen and 0.1 ml of spleen homogenate is added to 2 ml of 0.5% agarose and the mixture is poured into a 90-mm petri dish. The petri dishes are incubated for 1 hr at 37°C, then 2 ml of fresh guinea pig complement (1 : 10) is added; 40 min later the number of hemolysis zones is calculated. The IgM pfc values are calculated per 10^6 nucleated cells.

In Vivo and *in Vitro* Assay of Phagocytosis by Peritoneal Murine Neutrophils

The exudates for the phagocytosis assays *in vivo* and *in vitro* are collected 2.5 hr after the intraabdominal injections in mice of 10% sterile peptone solution, when the exudate contains the maximum quantity of neutrophils (97–98%). The exudate cells are used at a final concentration of 12.5 million/ml. The phagocytosis experiments are performed with a 24-hr culture of *Staphylococcus aureus* at a final concentration of 250×10^6/ml. Peptides and amino acids are injected subcutaneously for 5 days, the peritoneal exudate cells are collected and incubated for 15 min at 37°C, then the suspension of *S. aureus* is added, and the mixture of cells is incubated at 37°C for 15 min. For *in vitro* assays the peritoneal exudate cells are coincubated with the preparations to be studied at 37°C for 15 min, followed by the addition of the *S. aureus* suspension with additional incubation at 37°C for 15 min. The cell suspension is centrifuged for 7 min at 1200 cpm and the precipitate is stained with Romanowski Giemsa reagent. The phagocytic index (the percentage of neutrophils taking part in phagocytosis) and the phagocytic number (the average of microbe cells captured by one neutrophil) are estimated. All experiments are run in triplicate. The results are expressed as the average of 900–1000 neutrophils. The lipopolysaccharide (LPS) prodigiosane (0.005%) is used as a reference.

Using the methods reported above we have obtained results that may be summarized by the following theses. In addition to previously known neuromediatory properties of some amino acids (61) we have determined the immunomodulating activity of amino acids included in proteins (33, 34). Alanine, asparagine, aspartic acid, cysteine, glutamic acid, serine, threonine, tryptophan, and valine promote the differentiation of T-cell precursors to mature T lymphocytes and stimulate the thymus-dependent immune response, but not the thymus-independent immune response. Arginine under the same conditions does not influence T-cell differentiation, but inhibits the immune response; aspartic and glutamic acids reveal the most immunomodulating activities. We have found immunomodulating activity not only in amino acids but also in their mixtures: panangine, levamine, and cerebrolysine. Moreover, the neuromediator γ-aminobutyric acid (GABA) which is a fatty acid stimulates the immune response as well. When injected in doses that cause or do not cause the trophic effect, amino acids influence the immune response in different ways: doses that do not elicit the trophic effect lead to the reliable enhancement of immunogenesis. Amino acids in peptides determine the immunomodulating activity of the peptides; those peptides which have not incorporated immunostimulating amino acids do not reveal immunomodulating properties, but, the presence of immunoactive amino acids in these peptides does not determine the activity of the peptides. Neurotensin, containing glutamic acid, asparagine, and arginine, does not influence the immune response, but enhances the functions of neutrophils and macrophages. Amino acids and peptides influence the immune response and phagocytosis in different ways: glutamic acid, aspartic acid, threonine, and valine stimulate the immune response as well as phagocytosis, whereas proline, lysine, tyrosine, and leucine do not influence the immune response, but enhance the phagocytic activity of neutrophils. Arginine inhibits the immune response, but stimulates phagocytosis. Pentagastrin and CCK-8 stimulate the immune response without any effect on phagocytosis (62, 63). The immunomodulating properties of hormonally active and hormonally inactive forms of pentagastrin and CCK-8 have not been distinguished. Pentagastrin analogs demonstrate marked immunostimulating properties. Like that nonsulfated CCK-8 which does not display neuronal activity, significant immunostimulating activity is revealed (64). The common fragment of Thy-1 antigen and thymosins (pro-, para-, α_1, and α_{11}), threonylthreonyllysylaspartic acid, enhances both processes and restores the strongly reduced ability to produce food-instrumental reflex in thymectomized mice. It should be noted that the same property has been characteristic of aspartic acid which has been incorporated in this peptide, during assay in equimolar doses. These facts suggest the possibility of neuroimmune correlations at the level of a single amino acid. Further work is necessary to determine if separate amino acids play a role as common functional blocks by which to realize the neuroendocrine immune connections.

References

1. A. M. Ugolev, "The Digestion Evolution and the Function Evolution Principles." Nauka, Leningrad, 1985.
2. T. L. K. Low and A. L. Goldstein, *in* "Thymic Hormones and Lymphokines" (A. L. Goldstein, ed.), p. 21. Plenum, New York, 1984.
3. E. Hanappel, *in* "Thymusfaktoren Thymuspräparete: Biol. Eigensch. und klin. Aspekte," p. 64. Stuttgart, New York, 1987.
4. A. A. Haritos, G. Goodall, and B. L. Horecker, *Proc. Natl. Acad. Sci. U.S.A.* **81,** 1008 (1984).
5. A. A. Haritos, S. B. Salvin, R. Blacher, S. Stein, and B. L. Horecker, *Proc. Natl. Acad. Sci. U.S.A.* **82,** 1050 (1985).
6. V. Geenen, J.-J. Legros, P. Franchimont, M.-P. Defresne, J. Boniver, R. Ivell, and D. Richter, *Ann. N. Y. Acad. Sci.* **496,** 56 (1987).
7. N. R. Hall and A. L. Goldstein, *in* "Psychoneuroimmunology" (R. Ader, ed.), p. 521. Academic Press, New York, 1981.
8. G. A. Belokrylov, *Usp. Sovrem. Biol.* **102,** 39 (1986).
9. D.L. Felten, S. Y. Felten, S. L. Carlson, J. A. Olschowska, and S. Linot, *J. Immunol.* **135,** 755 (1985).
10. D. L. Colbern and D. A. Twombly, *Ann. N. Y. Acad. Sci.* **525,** 180 (1988).
11. J. E. Morley, N. E. Kay, G. F. Solomon, and N. P. Plotnikoff, *Life Sci.* **41,** 527 (1987).
12. J. F. Rehfeld, N. Gotterman, L. J. Larson, and P. S. Emson, *Fed. Proc.* **38,** 2325 (1979).
13. J. F. Rehfeld, *Nature (London)* **271,** 771 (1978).
14. J. Fahrenkrug and Schaffatitzky de Muckadell, *J. Neurochem.* **31,** 1445 (1978).
15. D. J. J. Carr and J. E. Blalock, *in* "Progress in Immunology VI", (B. Cinader and R. G. Miller, eds.), p. 619. Academic Press, Orlando, FL, 1986.

16. D. G. Payan, J. P. McGillis, and E. J. Goetzl, *Adv. Immunol.* **39,** 299 (1986).
17. J. Biennenstock, M. Perdue, A. Stanisz, and R. Stead, *Gastroenterology* **93,** 1431 (1987).
18. N. R. Hall and A. L. Goldstein, *in* "Immune Modulation Agents and Their Mechanisms" (R. L. Fenichel and M. A. Chirigos, eds.), p. 533. Dekker, New York, 1984.
19. M. Dardenne, W. Savino, and M.-C. Gagnerault, *Endocrinology* **125,** 3 (1989).
20. T. Paavonen, *Med. Biol.* **65,** 229 (1987).
21. N. R. Hall, B. L. Spangelo, J. M. Fark, Jr., T. L. O'Dononue, and A. L. Goldstein, *in* "Neural and Endocrine Peptides and Receptors" (T. W. Moody, ed.), p. 683. Plenum, New York, 1986.
22. J. P. McGillis, N. R. Hall, G. V. Vahouny, and A. L. Goldstein, *J. Immunol.* **134,** 3952 (1985).
23. H. O. Besedovsky and A. del Rey, *in* "Progress in Immunology" (B. Cinader and R. G. Miller, eds.), Vol. VI, p. 578. Academic Press, Orlando, FL, 1986.
24. R. J. Cross, J. C. Jackson, W. H. Brooks, D. L. Sparks, W. D. Markesbery, and T. L. Roszman, *Immunology* **57,** 145 (1986).
25. G. F. Solomon, M. A. Flatarone, D. Benton, J. E. Morley, E. Bloom, and T. Marinodan, *Ann. N. Y. Acad. Sci.* **523,** 43 (1988).
26. T. L. K. Low, G. B. Thurman, C. Chincarini, J. E. McClure, G. D. Marshall, S.-K. Hu, and A. L. Goldstein, *Ann. N. Y. Acad. Sci.* **332,** 33 (1979).
27. A. Pugliese, A. Biglino, M. Mascolo, G. Schippacassi, R. Falchetti, and P. A. Tovo, *Boll. Ist. Sieroter. Milan.* **66,** 5 (1987).
28. P. Cazzola, P. Mazzanti, and N. M. Kouttab, *Immunopharmacol. Immunotoxicol.* **9,** 195 (1987).
29. M. Fridkin and Ph. Gottlieb, *Mol. Cell Biochem.* **41,** 73 (1981).
30. C. Auriault, M. Joseph, A. Tartar, and A. Capron, *FEBS Lett.* **153,** 11 (1983).
31. C. N. Baxevanis, G. J. Reclos, S. Perez, D. Kokkinoroulos, and M. Papamichail, *Immunopharmacology* **13,** 133 (1987).
32. Y. Ohta, K. Sueki, Y. Yoneyama, E. Tezuka, and Y. Yagi, *Cancer Immunol. Immunother.* **15,** 108 (1983).
33. G. A. Belokrylov, I. V. Molchanova, and E. I. Sorochinskaya, *Int. J. Immunopharmacol.* **12,** 841 (1990).
34. G. A. Belokrylov, O. Ya. Popova, I. V. Molchanova, E. I. Sorochinskaya, and V. V. Anokhina, *Int. J. Immunopharmacol.* **14,** 1285 (1992).
35. M. Lenfant and L. Millerioux, *Int. Arch. Allergy Appl. Immunol.* **68,** 387 (1982).
36. M. Dardenne and J.-F. Bach, *Immunology* **25,** 343 (1973).
37. N. R. Hall and A. L. Goldstein, *in* "Immunoregulation" (N. Fabris, E. Garaci, J. Hadden, and N. Mitchison, eds.), p. 141. Plenum, New York, 1983.
38. E. H. Goldberg, G. Goldstein, D. B. Harman, and E. A. Boyse, *Transplantation* **38,** 52 (1984).
39. A. Takashi, S. Hiroshi, and S. Hishosi, *J. Appl. Biochem.* **7,** 408 (1985).
40. M. Bodanszky, "Principles of Peptide Synthesis." Springer Verlag, New York, 1984.
41. A. V. Sorokin, "Pyrogens." Medicina, Leningrad, 1965.

42. V. N. Gurin and A. A. Romanovsky, *in* "Neuropeptides and Thermoregulation," p. 35. Navuka i technika, Minsk, 1990.
43. O. Soder and P. M. Hellstrom, *Int. Arch. Allergy Appl. Immunol.* **84,** 205 (1987).
44. A. Bertolini, R. Poggioli, and A. V. Vergoni, *Ann. N. Y. Acad. Sci.* **525,** 114 (1988).
45. K. Miles, J. Quintans, E. Chelmicka-Schorr, and B. G. W. Arnarson, *J. Neuroimmunol.* **1,** 101 (1981).
46. Cs. Kerekgyarto, J. Erdei, B. Mandi, E. Olveti, and J. Fachet, *Folia Biol. (Prague)* **33,** 237 (1987).
47. G. A. Belokrylov and V. S. Turovsky, *Immunologia (U.S.S.R.),* **34** (1984).
48. G. A. Belokrylov and I. V. Molchanova, *Byull. Eksp. Biol. Med.* **113,** 165 (1992).
49. I. V. Miroshnichenko, A. A. Yarilin, I. D. Ryabinina, V. F. Martynov, L. I. Leontjeva, and E. I. Sorochinskaya, *Immunologia (U.S.S.R.),* **85** (1986).
50. A. A. Yarilin, I. V. Miroshnichenko, M. G. Mikhna, E. B. Polushkina, I. D. Ryabinina, M. D. Lutsik, V. D. Zazhirey, E. A. Sokolova, V. A. Liftshits, O. M. Tepelina, and G. K. Korotaev, *Immunologia (U.S.S.R.),* **23** (1986).
51. T. Audhya and G. Goldstein, *Int. J. Pept. Protein Res.* **22,** 187 (1983).
52. G. H. Werner, F. Floe'h, D. Migliore-Samour and P. Jolles, *Experientia* **42,** 521 (1986).
53. C. Y. Lau and G. Goldstein, *J. Immunol.* **124,** 1861 (1980).
54. A. L. Goldstein, Y. Asanuma, J. R. Battisto, M. A. Hardy, J. Quint, and A. White, *J. Immunol.* **101,** 359 (1970).
55. G. A. Belokrylov and A. P. Surovtseva, *Byull. Eksp. Biol. Med.* **101,** 730 (1986).
56. G. A. Belokrylov, *Zh. Mikrobiol. (U.S.S.R.),* **55** (1978).
57. M. J. Doenhoff, E. Leuchars, R. S. Kerbel, V. Wallis, and A. J. S. Davies, *Immunology* **37,** 397 (1979).
58. I. M. Kisselev and G. A. Belokrylov, *Byull. Eksp. Biol. Med.* **15** (1982).
59. J. E. Niderhuber and E. Moller, *Cell. Immunol.* **3,** 559 (1972).
60. G. A. Belokrylov, *Zh. Mikrobiol.* 2328 (1976).
61. J. C. Watkins, *Neurochem. Int.* **12(Suppl.),** 1 (1988).
62. G. A. Belokrylov, *Byull. Eksp. Biol. Med.* **102,** 213 (1986).
63. G. A. Belokrylov, I. V. Molchanova and O. Ya. Popova, *Byull. Eksp. Biol. Med.* **103,** 584 (1989).
64. I. V. Molchanova, G. A. Belokrylov, O. Ya. Popova and V. N. Kalikhevich, *Byull. Eksp. Biol. Med.* **114,** 631 (1992).

[13] Computer-Assisted Microscopic Image Analysis in Neuroimmunology

George B. Stefano

Introduction

Microscopic computer-assisted image analysis represents a new methodology in studying both living and dead tissues/cells. However, as with any new methodology certain considerations must be noted. In this chapter a rationale is provided for what components of a typical image analysis system are essential and how they relate to each other. Additionally, in the form of a preliminary exercise the potential of this methodology is examined within the context of differentiating drug treatments to invertebrate immunocytes. In this chapter the term image analysis is used in the context of the extraction from image data of a set of numerical descriptors of the objects, in this case cells. The terms image analysis and image processing are sometimes loosely used as though they were synonymous; however, this masks a broad distinction in types of algorithms used with image data.

Image Processing

There are a large number of algorithms which process the pixels in an image and yield a new image improved in some way. Examples include contrast enhancement, pseudo color, edge enhancement by digital spatial filters, and geometric correction (1–3). The distinctive feature of these algorithms is that they produce as an output another image generally with the same amount of information as that of the input. Normally this is done to make the image easier to interpret either by a human observer or by subsipient computer processing step. The term image processing is reserved for this type of task. This follows the usage of authors who make a distinction between modifying an image and extracting data from it (1–3).

Image Analysis

Frequently the user of image data does not actually want a modified or improved picture but rather some sort of tabular data characterizing the objects in the image. This could be as simple as the number of cells in an

Methods in Neurosciences, Volume 24

image or it could be large tablets giving many parameters such as area, location, perimeter, density, and orientation, for each cell. The key point here is that the input to the algorithm is a picture (perhaps preprocessed by another algorithm) but the output is not. This is related to the distinction between raw data and information.

A video frame may contain megabits of data but if the desired information is the centroid of a cell, most of the image data is in a sense either superfluous or redundant. The task of the algorithm is to filter the tremendous volume of data and extract the relevant numbers. The term image analysis is reserved for this type of algorithm.

In neurobiology image analysis algorithms are normally used to categorize cells either to tabulate different types or to evaluate treatment effects. Any meaningfully defined parameter of geometric objects is potentially calculable and usable as a parameter. Examples range from the obvious such as area to esoteric concepts such as fractal or fractional dimension (4). Of particular interest are measures which are invariant under size change or rotation since cells of the same type can have a range of sizes and the absolute orientation of the cell is normally an artifact of the slide orientation (although the orientation of cells relative to each other may be an interesting parameter). A wide variety of methods have been used including Fourier transforms (1, 5) but the most widely used factor for characterizing cell shape is the classical shape factor (*SF*; 6–8).

Immunocyte Conformational Analysis

Shape Factor

The shape factor quantifies the degree to which a cell or other object deviates from circularity. It is by definition the area of an object divided by the area of a circle of the same perimeter. A shape factor of one would represent a perfect circle, objects with either elongated or ruffled outlines will have shape factors less than one. The shape factor can also be defined in terms of perimeters as the square of the perimeter of a circle of the same area as the object divided by the actual perimeters. Thus, $SF = A_c(A_T = (L_T/L_c)^2$, where A_T is the area of a circle with the same perimeter as the given cell and L_T is the perimeter of a circle with the same area as the given cell and A_c and L_c area the actual area and perimeter of the cell.

Shape Factor in Neuroimmunology

The shape factor has been a standard measure for characterizing the response of cells to opioid peptides. Opioid peptides have a high degree of phylogenic conservation (6, 7, 9) and diverse functions (10). For example, they have been shown to play a role in both immunomodulation and autoimmunoregulation in both vertebrates and invertebrates (6, 7, 9, 11, 12). Many of the autoimmunoregulatory functions associated with these peptides were determined by image analysis of cellular conformation based on measurements of cellular area and perimeter and were mathematically expressed by the use of the shape factor. The lower the value, the longer the cellular perimeter and the more ameboid the shape. Changes in cellular shape ranged from rounded (inactive) to ameboid (active).

Furthermore in subsequent reports it was determined that the immunoreactive cells of *Mytilus* resemble the granulocyte/monocyte–macrophage lineage of vertebrates (9, 13). As a result the author and collaborators determined the effects of two monokines, tumor necrosis factor (TNF) and interleukin 1 (IL-1), on *Mytilus* immunocytes. In a dose-dependent fashion these cytokines increased the relative reflectance of the cells and also caused the cells to flatten as indicated by the measured increase in their area and their perimeter. Typically, they display form factor values of 0.40, indicating an activated state. As a rule, control cells during the observation period remain rounded and generally inactive.

Immunocytes also respond to lipopolysaccharide (LPS; 14). However, LPS-stimulated immunocytes exhibit a "round"-spreading conformation (Fig. 1) even though they have a low form factor value (average, 0.39). This introduces a new problem into the interpretation of conformational change as a measure of pharmacology as well as the potential to determine the physiological state of the cell in question. In order to meet this need for greater accuracy and detail in describing conformational changes of responsive cells the following mathematical models were developed (see Ref. 8 for detailed mathematical explanations).

Elliptical Shape Factor

A shortcoming of the shape factor is that it does not distinguish between (i) a cell whose perimeter is increased by ruffling while the overall shape remains circular and (ii) a cell whose edge remains smooth while overall shape elongates. Consider the two shapes in Fig. 2: Fig. 2B an ellipse and Fig. 2C a ruffled circle. Both of these shapes have the same shape factor but clearly the nature of the deviation from circularity is different in the two cases. In order to quantify the different kinds of changes involved more closely two new factors were defined, the elliptical shape factor and the circularity (8).

Both of these are based on the comparison of a cell with an ellipse of the same area and rotational moment of inertia. Because of the constraint of rotational moment at inertia this equivalent ellipse shares the same degree

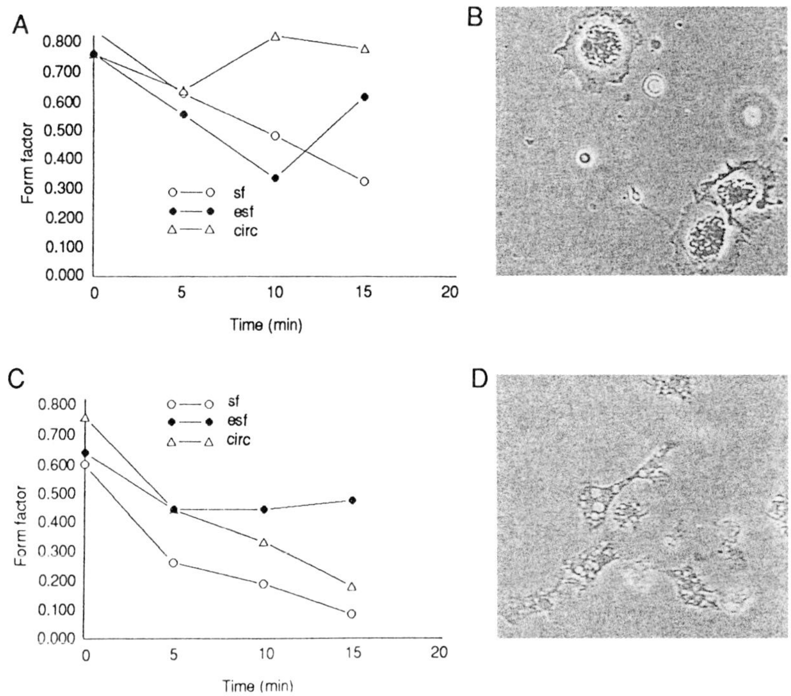

FIG. 1 Effect of lipopolysaccharide (LPS) on immunocyte conformation (A, B). (C, D) More polymorphic inducing properties of D-Ala^2-Met^5-enkephalin on immunocyte conformation. (○) Shape factor; (◆) elliptical shape factor; (△) circularity. Taken with permission from Schoen *et al.* (8). Reprinted from *Cell. Mol. Neurobiol.*, **12,** 357 (1992). Copyright 1992, with kind permission of Pergamon Press, Ltd., Headington Hill Hall, Oxford OX3 OBW, UK.

of elongation as the cell making it a more suitable comparison object than a circle of the same area. Given this equivalent ellipse we can now define the elliptical shape factor as the square of the perimeter of the equivalent ellipse divided by the square of the perimeter of the cell (L_c): $ESF = (L_e/L_c)^2$, where L_e is the perimeter of the equivalent ellipse. The elliptical shape factor will be one for any degree of elongation as long as the elongation results in an elliptical object. ESF values less than one indicate either a ruffled edge or a more complex elongation.

Given an equivalent ellipse we can also derive a measure of the elongation from the major and minor axes. We define the circularity as the ratio of the minor(a) to the major(b) axis: $CIRC = b/a$. The circularity will be one for a roughly circular form even if the edges are ruffled but will decline for elongated forms.

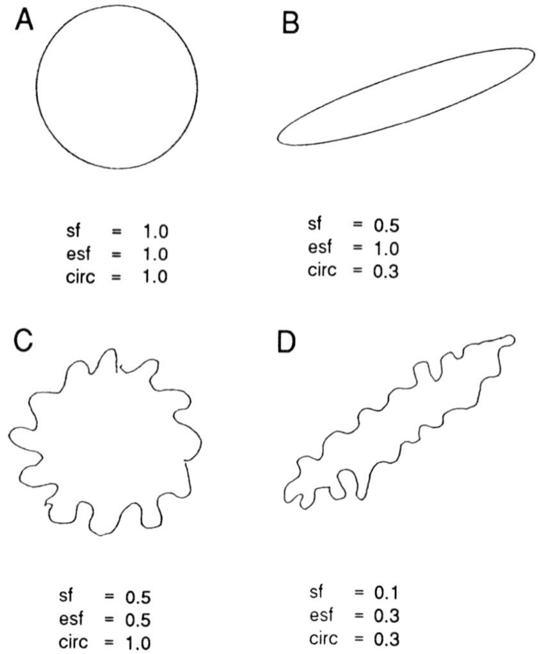

FIG. 2 Shape factors of typical objects. sf, Shape factor; esf, elliptical shape factor; circ, circularity. Taken with permission from Schon *et al.* (8). Reprinted from *Cell. Mol. Neurobiol.*, **12,** 357 (1992). Copyright 1992, with kind permission of Pergamon Press, Ltd., Headington Hill Hall, Oxford OX3 OBW, UK.

These relations also are examined in Fig. 2. The ellipse shown in Fig. 2B has an ESF value of 1.0, but a circularity of 0.3. This indicates that it is smooth (because of the high ESF) but elongated (because of the low circularity). In contrast the ruffled circle in Fig. 2C has a low ESF but a high circularity indicating that it has a ruffled edge but its overall form is circular. Thus the combination of ESF and circularity expresses the difference between these two forms while the traditional shape factor does not. Note that the ruffled ellipse in Fig. 2D has both a low ESF (because of ruffling) and a low circularity) because it is elongated).

Application of ESF to Neuroimmunology

In Fig. 1 we see that the classical shape factor declines under both LPS and DAMA (D-Ala^2-Met^5-enkephalinamide) stimulation. However, studying the ESF and circularity shows that the nature of the response is different under these two stimuli. With LPS treatment the circularity remains high, while ESF declines, indicating that the cells maintained roughly circular overall shape while their edges become more complex. When stimulated by DAMA Figs. 1C and 1D, the circularity of the cells declined more than that in the ESF, indicating that the elongation was a relatively more prominent response than ruffling.

Immunocytochemical Quantification: Analysis by Color and Size

Immunocytochemistry is a valuable technique for localizing highly specific substances. However, until now, the technique did not provide information as to the amount of the immunoreactive material being viewed. Given the state of image analysis technology, it is possible to make quantitative estimations of immunoreactive material increases or decreases relative to a control and blank value (15).

A study has been undertaken to determine where interleukin 1α is found in an invertebrate ganglia since earlier reports demonstrated its presence in ganglionic extracts by enzyme-linked immunosorbent analysis (ELISA) (16). Briefly, the immunocytochemical analysis of *Mytilus* (invertebrate bivalve mussel) ganglionic tissues for interleukin 1α immunoreactivity is performed according to the classical peroxidase technique (17) as described in detail elsewhere (18). Tissues are fixated in perfix (Fisher) in the Hitomatic tissue processor (Model 166MP, Fisher) and embedded by automated vacuum control in paraffin. Sections of 4 μm are reacted with polyclonal (Endogen) anti-human recombinant interleukin 1α antibodies. Tissues also are checked for endogenous peroxidase activity.

The morphology of *Mytilus edulis* glia is based on cell area and perimeter determinations by the use of American Innovision, Inc. (San Diego, CA), described earlier. The observational area for measurement determinations and frame grabbing of the posterior central portion of the pedal ganglion is 400 μm in diameter. The percentage of positive immunostaining for interleukin 1α is determined by assigning the "brown"-immunopositive cells a color via the feature detection function of the American Innovision software whereas nonstained cells are assigned another color, and the ratio obtained serves as the prime indicator of not only the specific presence of the material but a relative measure of its quanity as well. This simple comparison of the respective populations of cells within the time course of the experiment provides either an increase or decrease in the appearance of glial immunostaining for interleukin 1α.

In order to determine if various treatments to the pedal ganglia would cause a rise in interleukin 1α levels detectable in either the cells or fibers, the following experiments have been performed (15). The ganglia are removed and maintained in an artificial sea water (ASW; Instant Ocean, Inc., Boston, MA) -50% cell-free hemolymph incubation medium with constant aeration at 23°C for up to 24 hr. A group of ganglia are also treated with DAMA (10^{-9} *M*) for the entire incubation period. At this time the ganglia are processed for the immunostaining of interleukin 1α. In order to detect and quantify the immunostaining products we assign the system a color that is considered positive immunostaining by feature detection. Additionally, size parameters (area) are set to differentiate objects of different sizes such as "globs" with a 4-μm diameter (in this case, indicative of glia) or greater (indicative of neurons) as opposed to those equal to or less than 1 μm which we define as fiber varicosities. Wherever the proximity of objects causes the system to interpret the objects as one, therefore a greater value, the system automatically subtracts that value. Tissues exposed to the entire technique minus the antibody serve as "controls" whereas sections not treated with anything but exhibiting the color of positive immunoreactive material serve as blanks. The control and blank mean values are subtracted from the mean value obtained from analyzing treated tissues.

The end result of our study was that DAMA increased the number of immunostained fibers, not the number of glial cells emitting this "color" (15). This result was further confirmed in this report by ELISA interleukin 1α determinations.

Specific Fluorescent Product Determinations

The presence of HIV nucleocapsid (p24) antigen has been noted in HIV-infected H9 cells (19). The infected cells are immunofluorescent [via UV with fluorescein isothiocyanate (FITC) filter system] with anti-p24 at 45 days after infection. By using feature detection after creating a binary image we are able to differentiate the color intensity of both the specific fluorescent product as well as that of an unknown but present autofluorescent product emitting the same green fluorescence without antibody treatment. This was accomplished by identifying and determining the amount of similar "color" in the nontreated sample and subtracting the value, as noted above, from that obtained in the anti-p24-treated sample (Fig. 3). The intensity found in the anti-p24 cells is in part due to approximately a 16% contribution from the native autofluorescent material. In order for the infection to be regarded as productive, a baseline reading of specific fluorescence has to be present at the 32–36% fluorescent intensity level. Given this ability to estimate p24 relative levels it should be possible to add various pharmacological agents and attempt to alter the course of this infection.

Clearly, "color" identification and size parameters via feature detection

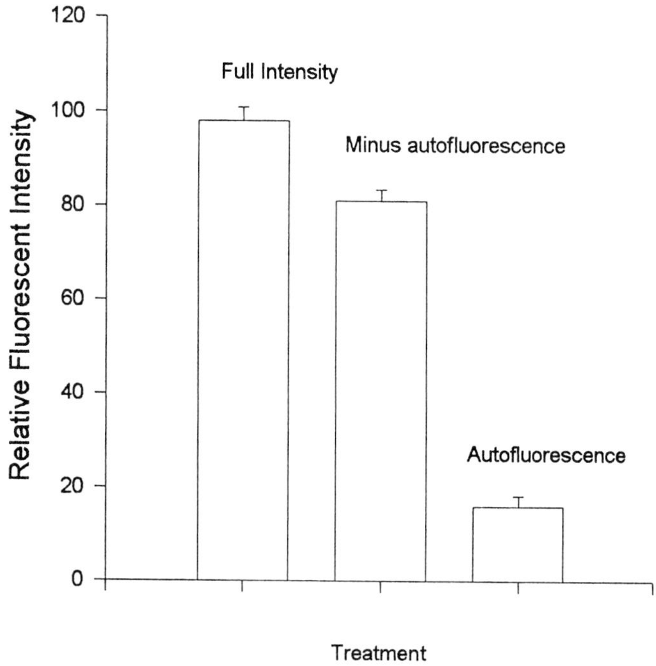

FIG. 3 Relative fluorescent data obtained from image processing which demonstrates that, in H9 cells, a contribution to the total fluorescent value obtained comes from an autofluorescent product. Additionally, the autofluorescent product provides a background "blank" value that must be taken into account if the technique is used to determine relative fluorescent product levels following drug treatments.

can be a valuable tool for the quantification of immunocytochemical materials. Caution, however, must be exercised to ensure that all sections are cut uniformly. Concentration quenching of juxtaposed fluorescent molecules, as well as a high density of immunostaining, may cause erroneous readings. However, this can be tested for by assigning the higher intensity fluorescent product, due to this phenomenon, its own color and then examining all specimens for its appearance. Once found it can be corrected for by subtracting the value of this material with the feature detection determination. An alternate approach is to simply count its occurrence and also use it as a test for the enhanced levels of material you are looking for. Also, the illumination of the specimen must be controlled for uniformity so that bleaching of the immunoreactive material does not occur between samples. This becomes a critical factor when considering fluorescence since the light source (mercury) can degrade and wavelength variability occur with age. Obviously, all aspects of the procedure should be uniformly reproduced between samples.

Of special note, caution should be attached to these procedures especially when dealing with the same chemicals from different venders. Of minor note, values must be recalculated when performing the analysis on different microscopes, since different lenses and objectives may be in place as well as different video cameras.

Overall these computer-assisted microscopic image analysis techniques are quite rapid and cost effective once the initial purchase is made. Indeed, in making the purchase one should consider present and future needs, since one generally uses only a fraction of the entire image analysis program package. In many cases, given the excellent quality of the commercial products, it is better to ensure that the best optics are being employed because it is difficult to work with an image of poor quality.

Conclusion

Image analysis has the potential to differentiate between drug treatments. Furthermore, since many of the compounds that are employed in stimulating immunocytes are endogenous to the organism we may be able to obtain fresh cells and, by observing their conformation and behavior, be able to surmise which molecules are influencing their behavior (12, 20, 21). Thus, the potential to determine the relative physiological state of an organism by noting the "condition" of the immunocytes may be possible. These techniques may also be used to study the growth and development of cells in culture as well as the effects of drug alterations on this process. Clearly, this may even allow for the interpretation of pathological disorders based on cellular appearances/responsiveness in conjunction with other factors (12).

Acknowledgments

This work was in part supported by the following grants: NIMH-NIDA-COR 17138, DA-09010, and the Research Foundation/SUNY.

References

1. R. C. Gonzalaez and P. Wintz, "Digital Image Processing." Addison Wesley, Reading, MA, 1977.
2. E. L. Hall, "Computer Image Processing and Recognition," Academic Press, New York, 1979.

3. M. R. Hord, "Digital Image Processing of Remotely Sensed Data." Academic Press, New York, 1982.
4. B. P. Mandlebrot, *Science* **156,** 636 (1967).
5. A. W. Partin, "The Development of a System for the Quantitative Analysis of Tumor Cell Motility: Application to Prostate Cancer," Thesis, Johns Hopkins Univ., 1988.
6. G. B. Stefano, M. K. Leung, X. Zhao, and B. Scharrer, *Proc. Natl. Acad. Sci. U.S.A.* **86,** 626 (1989).
7. G. B. Stefano, P. Cadet, and B. Scharrer, *Proc. Natl. Acad. Sci. U.S.A.* **86,** 6307 (1989).
8. J. C. Schon, J. Torre-Bueno, and G. B. Stefano, *Adv. Neuroimmunol.* **1,** 252 (1991).
9. G. B. Stefano, *Cell. Mol. Neurobiol.* **12,** 357 (1992).
10. M. K. Leung and G. B. Stefano, *Prog. Neurobiol.* **28,** 131 (1987).
11. J. E. Blalock, *Physiol. Rev.* **69,** 1 (1989).
12. G. B. Stefano, T. V. Bilfinger, and G. L. Fricchione, *Prog. Neurobiol.* **42,** 475 (1994).
13. T. K. Hughes, Jr., E. M. Smith, P. Cadet, J. Sinisterra, M. K. Leung, M. A. Shipp, B. Scharrer, and G. B. Stefano, *Proc. Natl. Acad. Sci. U.S.A.* **87,** 4426 (1990).
14. T. K. Hughes, Jr., E. M. Smith, J. A. Barnett, R. Charles, and G. B. Stefano, *Dev. Comp. Immunol.* **15,** 117 (1991).
15. L. R. Paemen, E. Porchet-Hennere, M. Masson, M. K. Leung, T. K. Hughes, Jr., and G. B. Stefano, *Cell. Mol. Neurobiol.* **12,** 463 (1992).
16. G. B. Stefano, E. M. Smith, and T. K. Hughes, *J. Neuroimmunol.* **32,** 29 (1991).
17. F. Vandesande, "Neuroimmunocytochemistry," pp. 257–272. Wiley, New York, 1983.
18. L. R. Paemen, L. Schoofs, and A. De Loof, *Cell Tissue Res.,* in press.
19. E. M. Smith, T. K. Hughes, Jr., F. Hashemi, and G. B. Stefano, *Proc. Natl. Acad. Sci. U.S.A.* **89,** 782 (1992).
20. G. B. Stefano and T. V. Bilfinger, *J. Neuroimmunol.* **47,** 189 (1993).
21. T. V. Bilfinger and G. B. Stefano, *J. Cardiovasc. Surg.* **34,** 129 (1993).

[14] Cytokines as Mediators of Reactive Astrogliosis

Voon Wee Yong and Vijayabalan Balasingam

Introduction

Astrocytes are stellate-shaped cells that form a major population of glial cells in the central nervous system (CNS). Astrocytes were once thought mostly to function passively as structural support elements for neurons, but many dynamic properties have since been attributed to astrocytes that include the maintenance of ionic homeostasis, metabolism of neurotransmitters, guidance of neuronal migration during development, and production of growth factors. Following many types of injury to the adult CNS, a characteristic reaction of astrocytes occurs in a phenomenon referred to as reactive astrogliosis. Through hypertrophy and hyperplasia, reactive astrocytes become larger, extend thicker, longer processes, and significantly increase their cytoplasmic content of glial fibrillary acidic protein (GFAP), an astrocyte-specific intermediate filament. A convenient marker of astrogliosis in brain sections is GFAP immunoreactivity (GFAP-IR) (reviewed in 1). Astrocytes in the parenchyma of the uninjured cortex do not immunoreact for GFAP, although they contain this protein. Following injury, presumably because GFAP synthesis increases or previously hidden epitopes become exposed as astrocytes swell and intermediate filament disassembly occurs (2, 3), GFAP-positive cells become readily apparent in the cortex (Fig. 1). Other changes of a reactive astrocyte include an increase in the number of mitochondria, glycogen content, and various enzyme levels (reviewed in 4).

For many types of CNS injuries, the process of reactive astrogliosis is dynamic and continues to evolve with time. An end result can be the formation of a densely interwoven glial "scar" which, depending on the type of injury, is composed of many different cell types and myelin debris, collagen dense bundles in the extracellular space, and multiple layers of abnormal basal lamina (reviewed in 5). The formation of glial scars has classically been thought to be undesirable, and included among the many postulated detriments are inhibition of axonal growth or regeneration, the genesis of a site of electrical instability and epilepsy, and interference with remyelination.

More recent evidence, however, suggests that the process of astrocyte reactivity may actually be an attempt by these cells to promote CNS recovery. This concept has evolved from studies indicating that: (i) cultured

Methods in Neurosciences, Volume 24

astrocytes synthesize a number of neurotrophic factors including the neurotropins nerve growth factor and NT-3 (6–8), (ii) astrocytes are conducive substrates for survival and growth of neurons *in vitro* (9, 10), (iii) neurotrophic factors are produced around the locus of a lesion and that the source of these appears to be reactive astrocytes (11–13), and (iv) in previously acallosal mice, a nitrocellulose filter embedded with early postnatal astrocytes could provide a terrain suitable for axons to traverse the cerebral midline to reform the corpus callosum (14).

The possibility that the process of reactive astrogliosis may occur to promote recovery runs contrary to the postulate that gliotic scars serve as impediments to regeneration of axons or myelin. This dichotomy may be better addressed if the molecular mediators of reactive astrogliosis could be identified. The hope would be that the manipulation of levels of such mediators would affect the occurrence, extent, or duration of astrogliosis in order for the resultant neurotrophic consequences to be better defined.

In considering molecular mediators of reactive astrogliosis, it is important to note that, depending on the type of injury (e.g., chronic degenerative diseases versus acute trauma), the mediators may be different. In conditions where the blood–brain barrier has been breached (*anisomorphic* injuries) (15, 16), astrocytes likely encounter a milieu substantially different from the environment seen in *isomorphic* injuries where the blood–brain barrier remains intact (e.g., facial nerve resection models) (16, 17). In this chapter, we consider only molecular mediators of astrogliosis in acute trauma with breach of the blood–brain barrier and where prime candidates as molecular mediators appear to be inflammatory cytokines. It should be noted that we use the term "cytokine" in its traditional sense, for soluble molecules that are synthesized and released predominantly by lymphoid and monocytoid cells (e.g., interferons and interleukins) and which have traditionally been associated with immune functions. Growth factors such as the epidermal growth factor (EGF), although by definition a "cytokine" (cell-secreted product), are referred to here as noncytokine growth factors in order to differentiate them from inflammatory cytokines.

Trauma to the CNS has long been known to involve the recruitment of intrinsic (e.g., microglia) and extrinsic [e.g., monocytes, lymphocytes, and natural killer (NK) cells] inflammatory mononuclear cells (18–21). These inflammatory cells release diffusible cytokine products, and measurements of cytokine levels in the brain following CNS trauma have demonstrated the increase of interleukin (IL 1, IL-6, and tumor necrosis factor-α (TNFα) (20–23). That these cytokines can further propagate inflammation within the CNS has been suggested by reports that a single microinjection of γ-interferon (γ-IFN), TNFα, or IL-2 into the normal CNS resulted in the recruitment of many types of inflammatory cells into the CNS parenchyma (24–26).

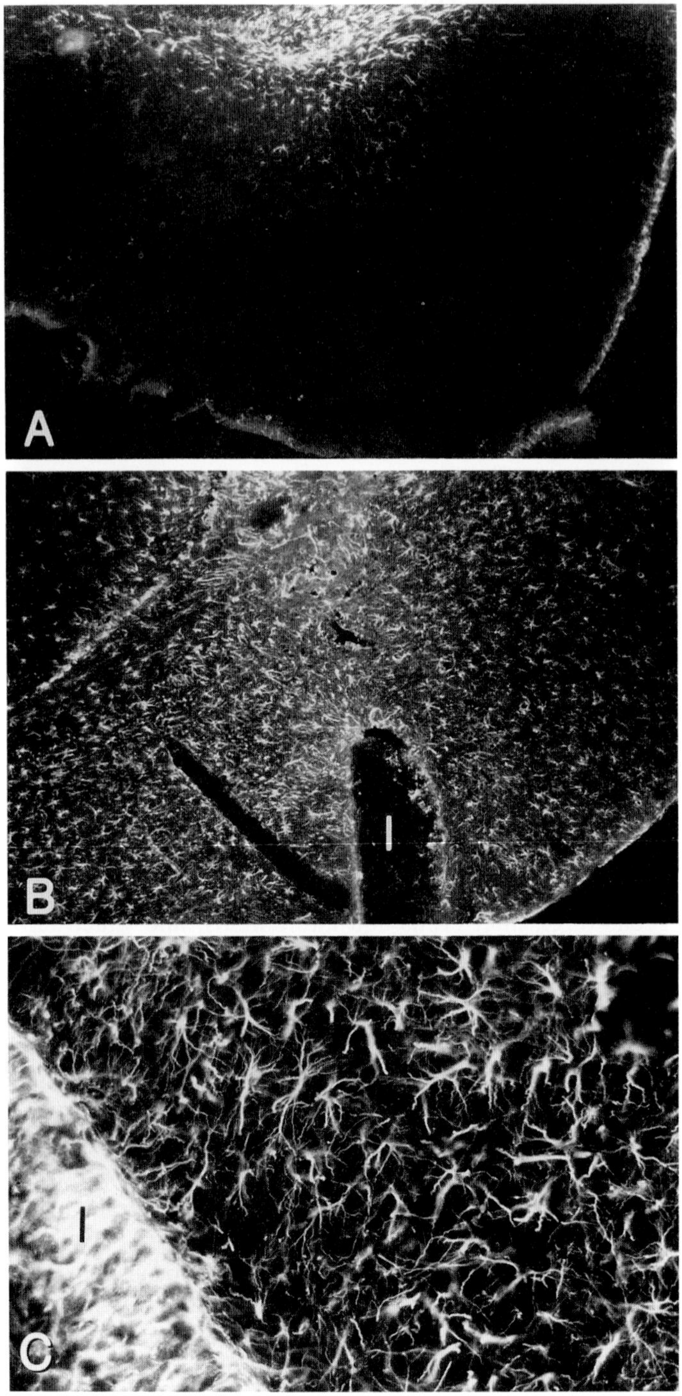
A
B
I
C
I

The presence of increased levels of inflammatory cytokines in the brain raises the question of their effects on neural cells. Of particular interest is the possibility that these cytokines may be the diffusible factors that modulate astrogliosis. This notion is supported by studies where the administration of IL-1 (27, 28) and IL-2 (24) into the adult rodent brain increased the extent of GFAP-IR. Intraocular injections of γ-IFN, TNFα, and IL-1 increased the adherence of inflammatory cells to the vascular endothelium and evoked astrogliosis in rabbits (29). While the list will likely expand, receptors for γ-IFN (30) and IL-1 (31) have been demonstrated on astrocytes. Finally, although the extent to which proliferation of astrocytes contributes to the overall astroglial reactivity remains controversial (17, 32–35), *in vitro* evidence to IL-1, IL-6, and TNFα (28, 36–38) have provided further credence for the role of cytokines as diffusible mediators of astrogliosis.

In this chapter we discuss our efforts, both *in vitro* and *in vivo*, to determine the role that cytokines may play in evoking aspects of the reactive astrogliosis response. *In vitro* experiments in our laboratory have focused mostly on cytokines as regulators of proliferation of *adult* brain-derived astrocytes because astrogliosis is a common consequence following injury to the adult CNS. In contrast, most (39–43), but not all (44, 45), reports indicate that following stab wounds to *embryonic or neonatal* CNS, the presence of astrogliosis is minimal, if at all; neonatal cells *in vitro* may therefore not be informative for adult CNS injuries. As previously mentioned, the extent to which astrocyte hyperplasia contributes to the overall astroglial reactivity remains controversial; nonetheless, proliferation of astrocytes *in vitro* is an easily quantifiable response of increased astroglial metabolic activity whereas the intensity of GFAP-IR (an often used marker *in vivo*) is not.

Methods

Cell Culture

A routine source of adult brain-derived astrocytes for our studies has been the brain biopsy specimens of adult human subjects undergoing surgical

FIG. 1 Detection of the occurrrence of astrogliosis in the cortex by GFAP-IR following the implantation of a foreign object in the brain. (A) Normal brain areas shown are GFAP-IR only in the corpus callosum (top of frame) and in the glia limitans (bottom of frame); significantly, parenchymal cortical astrocytes are not GFAP-IR. Following the insertion of a piece of foreign object (I, a piece of nitrocellulose membrane), GFAP-IR astrocytes are seen in the cortex (B and C). Magnification: (A and B) × 39.5; (C) × 316 (higher magnification of B)

resection to ameliorate intractable epilepsy. The method to obtain cells from these human specimens has been described in detail elsewhere (46). In brief, brain tissues are cut into cubes of 1 mm^3 or less and incubated with 0.25% (v/v) Trypsin (GIBCO Grand Island, NY) and 100 μg/ml DNase (Boehringer-Mannheim, Mannheim, Germany) for 1 hr at 37°C. Following addition of 1% final concentration of fetal bovine serum (FBS, UBI) to inactivate trypsin, the cell suspension is passed through a filter of 132 μm pore size to retain undissociated fragments. The filtrate is centrifuged (15,000 rpm, 30 min, 4°C) in 30% (v/v) Percoll (Pharmacia, Piscataway, NJ) to separate a viable CNS cell layer from myelin, debris, and red blood cells. The viable CNS cell layer is collected, washed twice with phosphate-buffered saline (PBS), and finally suspended in feeding medium of Eagle's minimum essential medium supplemented with 5% FBS, 20 μg/ml gentamicin, and 0.1% dextrose. Cells are placed in 25-cm^2 uncoated flasks at a density of 2×10^6/ml at 37°C. The next day, floating cells (mostly oligodendrocytes) are removed for other studies. Adherent cells (mostly microglia and astrocytes) are allowed to develop morphologically for 1 week; astrocytes tend to stratify themselves above microglia and because the astrocytes also tend to be less adherent, they can be shaken off by rotary shaking (150 rpm, 5 hr) and collected. Because some microglia cells are also shaken off during this process, purity of astrocytes remain, at best, 70% (antibody-dependent complement-mediated lysis of microglia cells is possible, but this also nonspecifically kills adult human astrocytes). The floating cells are collected by centrifugation (900 rpm, 10 min, room temperature) and plated onto 10 μg/ml poly(L-lysine)-coated coverslips at a density of 10^3 to 10^4 cells/coverslip. These cells are used for the experiments described below. Adult human brain-derived astrocytes tend to assume many different morphologies (47) which are quite unlike the flat forms typical of neonatal rodent astrocytes *in vitro*. Another source of adult brain-derived cells has been the adult mouse brain (48). In general, we make the assumption that these adult brain-derived cells are "adult" astrocytes; this assumption is supported by the observations that the basal rates of proliferation of adult human or adult mouse astrocytes tend to be far lower than those of neonatal rodent or fetal human astrocytes (48), much akin to their counterparts *in vivo*.

Assessment of Proliferation of Astrocytes in Vitro

Because the purity of adult human astrocytes is 70% at best, bulk measurement of proliferation of these cells (e.g., by using [^{3}H]thymidine uptake and liquid scintillation counting of a population of cells) can be misleading if the nonastrocytes present in the cultures are undergoing mitosis. For this reason, we have developed a double-immunofluorescence technique (49) that utilizes

GFAP-IR combined with immunofluorescence for bromodeoxyuridine (BrdU); BrdU is a thymidine analog that is taken up by cells in the S phase of the cell cycle. Following incubation of living cells with 10 μM of BrdU (this period varies proportionally to the doubling time of astrocytes; for slow growing adult human astrocytes, a 2-day period of incubation with BrdU is desirable; for fast growing neonatal rodent or fetal human astrocytes, this period is short, e.g., 2 hr) in order that cells in the S phase may incorporate this label into their DNA, cells are fixed in 70% ethanol (v/v) at −20°C for 30 min. A rabbit polyclonal antibody to GFAP (Dako, 1 : 100) (Dako, Carpintesia, CA) is then applied for 45 min at room temperature followed by a goat anti-rabbit immunoglobulin (Ig) conjugated to fluorescein isothiocyanate (FITC) (Cappell, 1 : 100 45 min). Cells are then incubated for 10 min with 2 M HCl to denature DNA; this denaturation allows the BrdU antibody access to BrdU incorporated within the DNA double helix. The HCl is then neutralized by application of 0.1 M sodium borate, pH 9.0, for 10 min. A mouse monoclonal antibody to BrdU (1 : 25, Becton–Dickinson, Mountainview, CA) is applied (45 min), followed by a goat anti-mouse Ig conjugated to rhodamine. All antibodies are diluted in HHG (i.e., 10% goat serum, 2% horse serum, 1 mM HEPES buffer in Hanks' balanced salt solution). Using an immunofluorescence microscope, count the number of GFAP-positive cells (astrocytes); of these, the number and thus the percent with BrdU labeling in their nuclei is documented (Fig. 2).

While the GFAP–BrdU technique allows unambiguous identification of the proliferating astrocyte, a disadvantage is the time required to count the number of astrocytes with labeled nuclei. Nevertheless, for cultures that are not highly enriched, this method is indicated. For cultures that are highly enriched, such as astrocyte cultures derived from fetal human or neonatal rodent brains (over 90% purity) (48), we utilize the quicker method of [^{3}H]thymidine incorporation followed by liquid scintillation counting. We have documented that the results obtained using GFAP–BrdU and [^{3}H]thymidine incorporation are comparable and are reflective of changes in actual cell number (48).

Effects of Cytokines on Proliferation of Astrocytes in Vitro

Using adult human astrocytes as targets, we found that supernatants from activated human T lymphocytes were potent mitogens; in contrast, growth factors that are mitogens for neonatal brain-derived cells (e.g., epidermal growth factor) were not (50). Since lymphocyte supernatants contain a variety of cytokines (and noncytokine growth factors), we incubated the supernatants with neutralizing antibodies to defined cytokines to ascertain whether the mitogenic activity could be further characterized. A neutralizing antibody

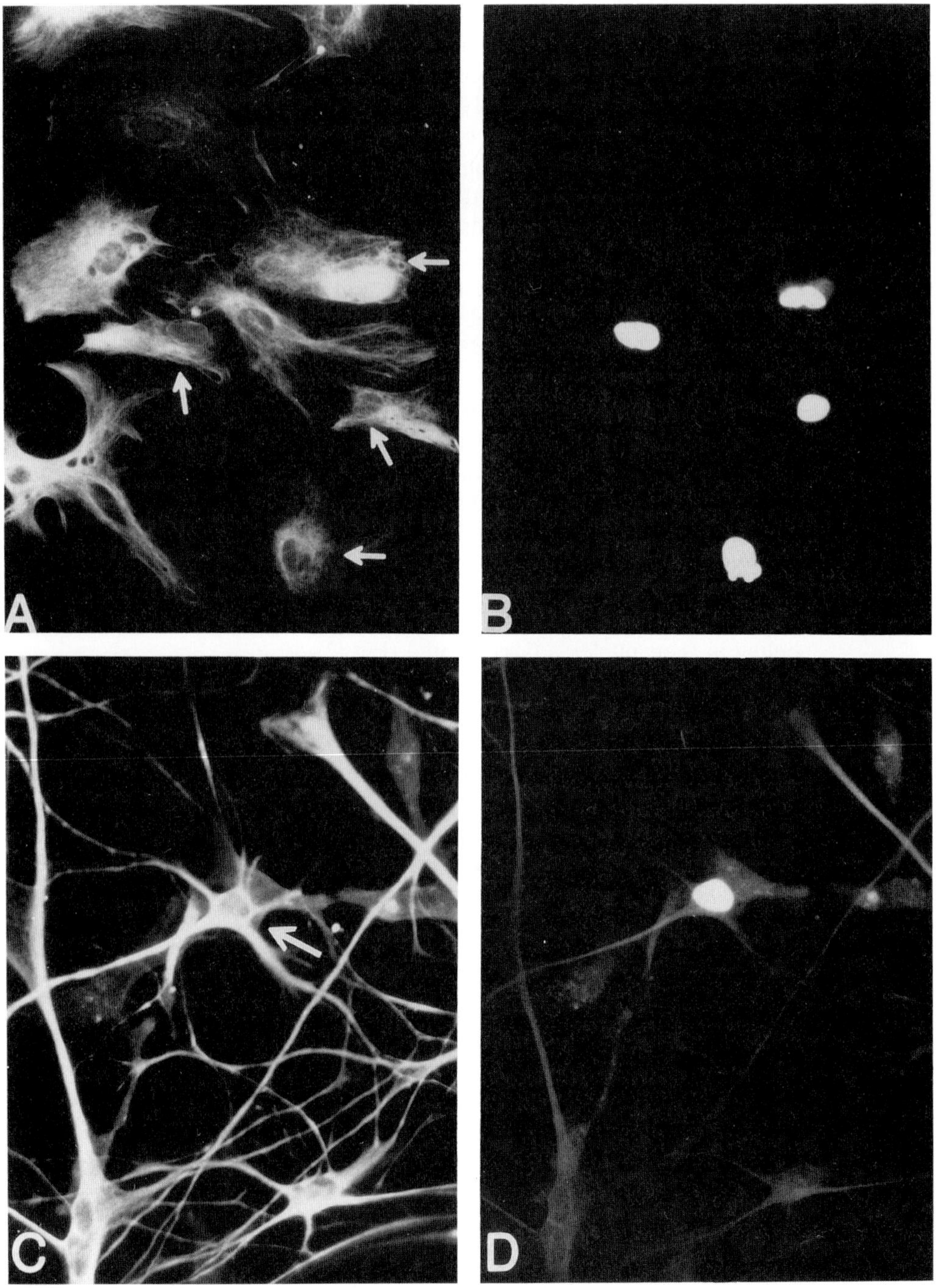
A
B
C
D

to γ-IFN, but not neutralizing antibodies to TNFα or IL-1, dose-dependently abrogated the effects of the lymphocyte supernatants. When recombinant γ-IFN itself was applied to cells, it increased the proliferation of adult human astrocytes (50). This demonstration that γ-IFN, generally thought to be a negative regulator of cell growth, could be a mitogen for some cell type has since been supported by findings by others that γ-IFN promoted proliferation of rat astrocytes (51), rat skeletal muscle cells (52), and human smooth muscle cells (53). When we applied γ-IFN in a piece of Gelfoam (Upjohn, Kalamazoo, MI) over an area of corticectomy (removal of 2 mm^3 of occipital cortex) in the adult rat brain, the extent of resultant astrogliosis was significantly enhanced (50), suggesting that γ-IFN could be a mediator of astrogliosis *in vivo*.

Because the purity of *adult* human astrocytes was 70% at best, it was possible that the remaining 30% of cells (mostly microglia) could have influenced the astrocyte response to an added cytokine mitogen (e.g., γ-IFN could have acted on microglial cells to release the actual mitogen). We considered this unlikely to be the case for γ-IFN since an indirect action via microglial secretory products did not account for the mitogenic effect of γ-IFN (50). Nevertheless, it became necessary to test the effects of γ-IFN on highly purified human astrocyte preparations and this was accomplished by utilizing astrocytes (over 90% purity) derived from *human fetal* brains (48). In this manner we demonstrated that γ-IFN was a mitogen for human fetal astrocytes (48).

When *mouse* astrocytes from adult or neonatal brains were incubated with recombinant murine γ-IFN, a *decrease* in proliferation was found (48). Recombinant human γ-IFN did not alter the proliferation of murine astrocytes, and recombinant murine γ-IFN did not affect the proliferation rate of human astrocytes, corresponding with reports that the interaction of γ-IFN with its receptor occurs in a species-specific manner (54,55). Thus, the effects of γ-IFN were species-specific: for human astrocytes (*fetal* or *adult*), γ-IFN was a mitogen, while for mouse astrocytes (*neonatal* or *adult*), γ-IFN slowed the proliferation rate. Since earlier work has demonstrated that the extent of GFAP-IR in the injured adult rat brain was increased by

FIG. 2 GFAP–BrdU double-immunofluorescence to detect proliferating astrocytes. (A, C) Stained for GFAP, while the corresponding BrdU labeling is (B) and (D), respectively. (A, B) Adult mouse astrocytes. (C, D) Adult human astrocytes. Astrocytes that have incorporated BrdU are indicated by arrows. As previously described (47), many adult human astrocytes bear process-bearing morphology *in vitro*. In contrast, adult mouse astrocytes are mostly flat and fibroblast-like *in vitro* (A), as are neonatal rodent or fetal human astrocytes.

γ-IFN treatment (50), several possibilities exist to explain the discrepancy between the *in vitro* and *in vivo* results: (i) *In vitro* proliferation results are poor indicators of *in vivo* astroglial reactivity, (ii) the different responses of astrogliosis (e.g., proliferation versus GFAP-IR) may be regulated by different factors, or (iii) the response of mouse or rat astrocytes to γ-IFN may well differ, as is the case for human and mouse astrocytes. We consider the first possibility to be most likely because of a recent series of experiments that show that while most cytokines (with the exception of γ-IFN, IL-1, and TNFα) did not affect the proliferation of *mouse* astrocytes *in vitro,* they increased astroglial reactivity when administered into the *mouse* brain *in vivo* (56, see below).

Comments on in Vitro Determinations of Cytokines as Mediators of Astrocyte Reactivity

In general, *in vitro* experiments are useful only in that they provide important guides to cellular processes occurring *in vivo*. Furthermore, for astrocytes in particular, the study of astrocyte reactivity *in vitro* has been limited technically by the number of parameters that can be used reliably to assess astrogliosis in culture. *In vitro,* GFAP-IR is noninstructive since all astrocytes in culture are defined by GFAP-IR, whatever their stages of reactivity may be; measurements of intensity of GFAP-IR (e.g., low in resting and high in reactive cells) are possible only if immunofluorescence signals can be reproducibly compared against a defined background, but this is hampered by variations in background intensity from sample to sample. Proteins such as vimentin, which has a controversial role as a marker of astrocyte reactivity *in vivo* (57, 58), are found on all astrocytes *in vitro* and additionally in other cell types (e.g., oligodendrocytes) which are not known to contain these *in vivo* (59). Measurements of proliferation of astrocytes *in vitro* are often used as a guide to understanding astroglial reactivity *in vivo*; however, our data, as cited above, have shown proliferation *in vitro* to be a poor indicator of astrocyte reactivity *in vivo*. Furthermore, while reports exist on the high proliferation rate of astrocytes in astrogliosis (32, 33), other laboratories have not found significant astroglial mitosis following injury (17, 34–36); this discrepancy requires resolution since the nature of the CNS insult (trauma versus autoimmune disease, or anisomorphic versus isomorphic injuries) may influence the nature of the astroglial reactivity. It has been proposed that changes in GFAP protein content *in vitro* may be representative of astrogliosis in culture (60). It is clear from the above discussions that in order to identify mediators of astrogliosis, *in vivo* experiments are pivotal.

In Vivo Determinations of the Role of Cytokines as Mediators of Reactive Astrogliosis

As stated above, we have determined that the application of γ-IFN to the site of a corticectomy in the adult mouse brain increased the extent of resultant astrogliosis. To address further the hypothesis that immunoregulatory cytokines are mediators of reactive astrogliosis we have taken advantage of neonatal CNS injury where the presentation of astrogliosis is minimal, if present at all, following trauma (39–43). Reasons postulated for this lack of astrogliosis have included the relative immaturity and plasticity of neonatal astrocytes and neurons and the lack of myelin in neonatal animals. Since the immune system in neonatal animals is relatively immature compared to that of adults (61–63), we considered that this, and the consequent lack of cytokine production, might constitute a probable cause of the lack of astrogliosis following neonatal CNS injuries. To test this hypothesis, we created stab wounds (using either a scalpel or a pair of iris scissors) to the cortex of Postnatal Day 3 mouse pups, introduced 20 U of cytokine into the stab wound site at the time of injury, and assessed astroglial reactivity 4 days later. The results showed the conversion of minimal GFAP-IR to significant astrogliosis in neonatal animals treated with various cytokines (56, see below).

Postnatal Day 3 CD1 mouse pups are anesthetized with inhalational methoxyflurane and an incision is made in the skin overlying the skull in the region of the parietal cortex. A 1-mm incision is then made in the skull with a pair of iris scissors followed by the creation of a 1-mm-deep stab wound in the parietal cortex; this cortical stab wound is created with either an 11-gauge scalpel or a pair of iris scissors, both give comparable results. Two microliters of solution containing 20 U of recombinant cytokine dissolved in 0.2% BSA is deposited at a rate of 1 μl/min into the stab cavity using a 22-gauge Hamilton micromanipulator attached to a stereotaxis instrument. The skin incision overlying the skull is closed using Krazy glue and all traces of blood are removed. Pups are kept under a heat lamp for 1 hr before being returned to their mothers; in this manner, the rate of cannabalism by nursing mothers is less than 1%. Four days later, animals are deeply anesthetized with inhalational methoxyflurane to facilitate intracardial perfusion of periodate–paraformaldehyde–lysine (PLP) fixative. The whole brain is removed from the animal and postfixed for 6 hr in PLP, then soaked in 25% sucrose overnight for cryoprotection, and finally frozen and stored at −70°C before being serially sectioned. These sections are either coronal or longitudinal sections, through the injury site, to allow documentation of the occurrence and spatial distribution of astrogliosis.

To document GFAP-IR, 10-μm sections on gelatin-coated slides are

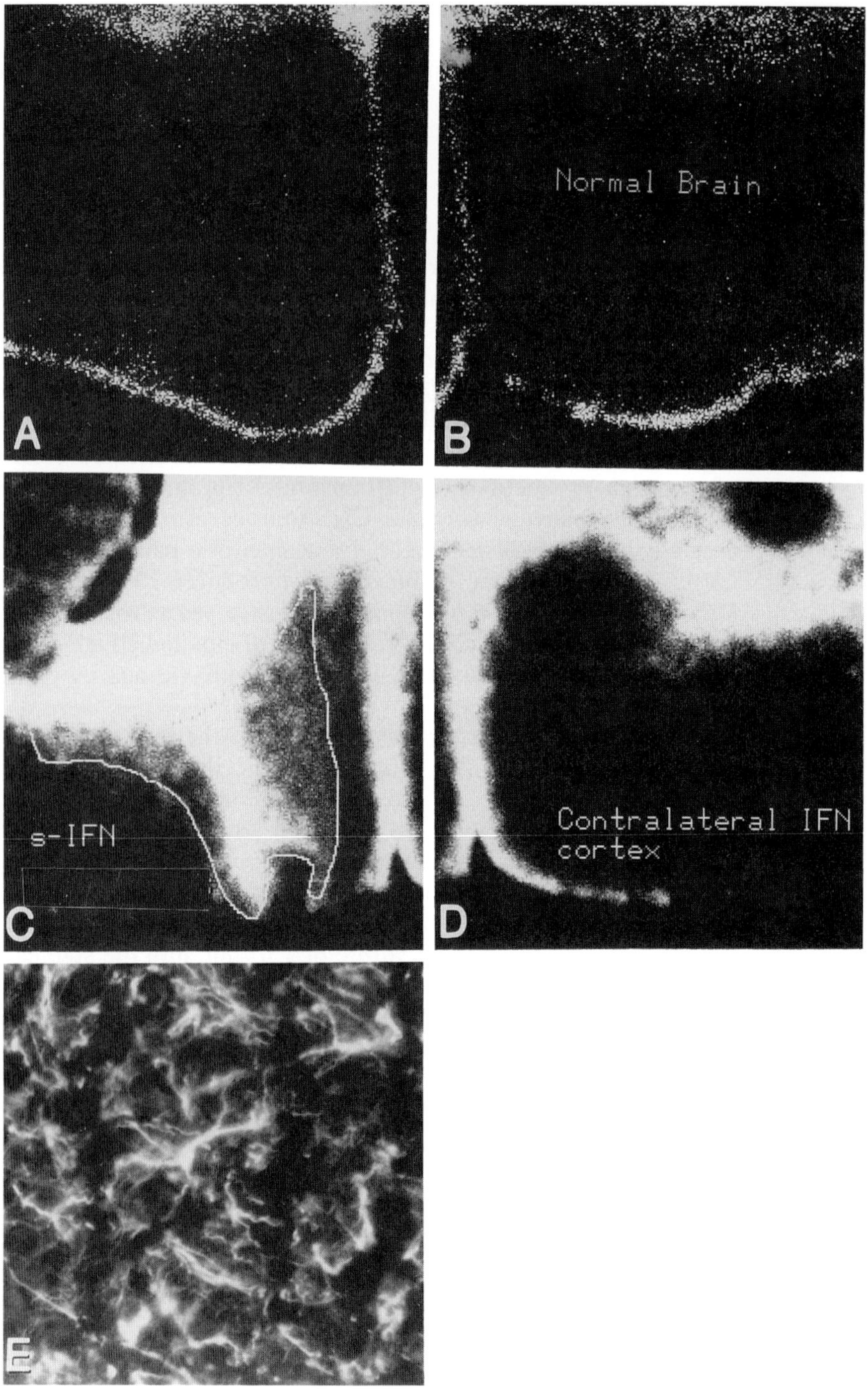
Normal Brain
s-IFN
Contralateral IFN
cortex
A
B
C
D
E

thawed for 1 min in a humidifying chamber, fixed in 70% ethanol for 20 min, and washed with PBS. Each section is treated for 30 min with 3% (v/v) ovalbumin to block nonspecific binding and incubated for 6 hr with a rabbit anti-GFAP polyclonal antibody (Dako, 1 : 100). After being rinsed briefly with PBS, a goat-anti-rabbit Ig conjugated to FITC is introduced for 1 hr. All procedures occur at room temperature. Brain sections are rinsed with PBS, coverglassed with 10% glycerol in PBS (w/v) and coded at this point for subsequent blind analyses. Immunofluorescence analyses are restricted to the cortical regions since astrocytes in these areas become GFAP-positive on becoming reactive. Qualitative determinations utilized a scale of + to ++++ in ascending order of cortical area covered by GFAP-IR astrocytes.

Quantitative assessment of GFAP-IR is performed using a confocal laser scanning microscope (Leica) (56). The dorsal cortex ipsilateral to the lesion site is scanned using a 2.5 × 0.08 NA objective (this low-power objective is used in order to encompass a large cortical area). The image is reconstructed from the averages of 64 passes per raster line (scan-64), in an attempt to obtain a high signal-to-noise ratio. Areas with GFAP-IR are traced out on each section to encompass only regions contributing to a cumulative immunofluorescence intensity with a standard deviation of 30. An example of this measurement is given as Fig. 3.

Qualitatively, all cytokines tested (recombinant murine γ-IFN, IL-1, IL-2, IL-6, TNFα, and M-CSF) (purchased from Genzyme, Cambridge, MA or UBI, Lake Placid, NY), chosen to reflect cytokines released predominantly by T lymphocytes (γ-IFN, IL-2, and M-CSF), NK cells (γ-IFN), or microglia/macrophage (IL-1, IL-6, and TNF-α), result in increased astrogliosis, even though only γ-IFN, IL-1, and TNFα altered proliferation of astrocytes *in vitro* (56). Thus, as inferred earlier, proliferation studies *in vitro* cannot predict the effects of an administered cytokine *in vivo*. Furthermore, there is *no selectivity* to particular cytokines, although *specificity* is demonstrated by the ineffectiveness of *human* γ-IFN in promoting mouse astroglial reactiv-

---

FIG. 3 The application of γ-IFN into a cerebral stab site increases astrogliosis in the neonatal rodent brain. (A, B) Two cortical hemispheres of the normal neonatal brain. Note that GFAP-IR is present only in the glia limitans (bottom of frame) and the corpus callosum (top). When 20 U of recombinant γ-IFN is applied to the cortical stab site of a 3-day-old mouse pup, GFAP-IR in the ipsilateral cortex (C), but not the contralateral hemisphere (D), becomes very significant 4 days after. (A–D) Images acquired by confocal laser scanning microscopy using a 2.5 X objective. Magnification: ×39.5. (E) Higher magnification of the traced area in (C), acquired using a 40X objective, to denote the morphology and reactive nature of the astrocytes.

ity in accordance with reports that the interaction of γ-IFN with its receptor occurs in a species-specific manner (54, 55).

Quantitatively, we compare the effects of recombinant murine γ-IFN with its vehicle (0.2% BSA). Brains from seven animals per group, and two sections per brain, are scanned using confocal microscopy. The results of area of the ipsilateral cortex containing reactive astrocytes show that γ-IFN caused a threefold increase in the extent of GFAP-IR (BSA = $180 \pm 27 \times 10^3\ \mu m^2$; murine γ-IFN = $634 \pm 54 \times 10^3\ \mu m^2$) (56).

Why was there no selectivity among the many cytokines tested? This remains unresolved, although a testable hypothesis is the indirect role of many of these cytokines in causing propagation of an immune response, however immature the immune system may be to begin with, within the CNS. As mentioned, a single application of γ-IFN, TNFα, or IL-2 into the normal adult rodent CNS has resulted in the recruitment of many types of inflammatory cells into the CNS parenchyma (24–26). The demonstration that the single application of cytokine to a cortical stab wound site in neonates converts minimal astroglial reactivity to extensive astrogliosis provides strong evidence for cytokines as molecular mediators of astrogliosis following brain trauma.

Final Comments and Future Directions

If inflammatory cytokines are mediators of astrogliosis, which cytokines are most important and what may their cellular sources be? Both questions remain unresolved. With regards to the cytokine, receptors for γ-IFN (30) and IL-1 (31) have been detected on astrocytes and the list will likely increase. With regards to cellular sources of cytokines, an approach would be to detect immunocompetent cells within the CNS and to determine whether the accumulation of these cells (e.g., macrophages/microglia, NK cells, T lymphocytes, and others) could be temporally and spatially correlated with the evolution of astrogliosis; this approach is being actively pursued in this laboratory. The potential role of *neural cells* as cellular sources of cytokines following trauma needs also to be considered since a multitude of reports now indicate that astrocytes *in vitro* can produce IL-1, IL-3, IL-6, M-CSF, IFN, TNFα, and TGFβ_1 either under basal culture conditions or when stimulated with viruses or other cytokines. Similarly, *in vivo,* astrocytes have been reported to produce γ-IFN, IL-1, IL-3, and TGF (64–67). Reports are emerging that neurons can produce IL-1, IL-2, IL-3, γ-IFN (or a closely related molecule) and TNFα (66–69); these neuronal-derived cytokines may well signal astrocytes to become reactive. Finally, while this chapter has focused on cytokines, the potential role of noncytokine growth factors as possible mediators of astrogliosis cannot be dismissed since levels of acidic fibroblast growth factor, basic fibroblast growth factor, and insulin-like growth factor-1 are upregulated in the injured brain, as are the cytokines described above. Furthermore, Eclancher *et al.* (70) reported that the administration of bFGF to the injured neonatal rodent brain increased the extent of astrogliosis. It is timely to compare and contrast the effects of cytokine and noncytokine growth factors in astrogliosis; the interactions between these (e.g., cytokines cause the release of noncytokine growth factors which then act on astrocytes, and vice versa) also offer intriguing possibilities.

Acknowledgments

We acknowledge those who have contributed to our work on reactive astrogliosis: T. Tejada-Berges, E. Wright, R. Moumdjian, and J. Turley. The skilled technical assistance of F. P. Yong, K. Dickson, and R. Bouckova is also gratefully acknowledged. We thank the Medical Research Council of Canada for support of operating funds. V. W. Yong is a scholar of the Medical Research Council of Canada. V. Balasingam is the recipient of a studentship from the Canadian network for neural regeneration and functional recovery, one of 15 networks of Centres of Excellence supported by the government of Canada.

References

1. W. T. Norton, D. A. Aquino, I. Hozumi, F. C. Chiu, and C. F. Brosnan, *Neurochem. Res.* **17,** 877 (1992).
2. L. F. Eng, F. E. D'Amelio, and M. E. Smith, *Glia* **2,** 308 (1989).
3. D. A. Aquino, F. C. Chiu, C. F. Brosnan, and W. T. Norton, *J. Neurochem.* **51,** 1085 (1988).
4. E. J. H. Nathaniel and D. R. Nathaniel, *in* "The Reactive Astrocyte; Advances in Cellular Neurobiology" (S. Fedoroff and L. Hertz, eds.), p. 249. Academic Press, New York, 1981.
5. P. J. Reier, *in* "Astrocytes" (S. Fedoroff and A. Vernadakis, eds.), Vol. 3, p. 263. Academic Press, New York, 1986.
6. D. M. Araujo and C. W. Cotman, *J. Neurosci.* **12,** 1668 (1992).
7. J. S. Rudge, R. F. Alderson, E. Pasnikowski, J. McClain, N. Y. Ip, and R. M. Lindsay, *Eur. J. Neurosci.* **4,** 459 (1992).
8. K. Frei, U. V. Malipiero, T. P. Leist, R. M. Zinkernagel, M. E. Schwab, and A. Fontana, *Eur. J. Immunol.* **19,** 689 (1989).
9. M. Noble, J. Fok-Seang, and J. Cohen, *J. Neurosci.* **4,** 1892 (1984).
10. R. M. Lindsay, *Nature (London)* **282,** 80 (1979).
11. M. Nieto-Sampedro, E. R. Lewis, C. W. Gotman, M. Manthorpe, S. D. Skaper, G. Barbin, F. M. Longo, and S. Varon, *Science* **217,** 860 (1982).
12. S. David, C. Bouchard, O. Tsatas, and N. Giftochristos, *Neuron* **5,** 463 (1990).

13. N. Y. Ip, S. J. Wiegand, J. Morse, and J. S. Rudge, *Eur. J. Neurosci.* **5,** 25 (1993).
14. J. Silver and M. Y. Ogawa, *Science* **220,** 1067 (1983).
15. H. Mansour, R. Asher, D. Dahl, B. Labkovsky, G. Perides, and A. Bignami, *J. Neurosci. Res.* **25,** 300 (1990).
16. I. Fernaud-Espinosa, M. Nieto-Sampedro, and P. Bovolenta, *Glia* **8,** 277 (1993).
17. M. B. Graeber, W. Tetzlaff, W. J. Streit and G. W. Kreutzberg, *Neurosci. Lett.* **85,** 317 (1988).
18. D. Giulian, *J. Neurosci. Res.* **18,** 155 (1987).
19. V. H. Perry, P. B. Andersson, and S. Gordon, *Trends Neurosci.* **16,** 268 (1993).
20. V. Taupin, S. Toulmond, A. Serrano, J. Benavides, and F. Zavala, *J. Neuroimmunol.* **42,** 177 (1993).
21. M. N. Woodroofe, G. S. Sarna, M. Wadhwa, G. M. Hayes, A. J. Loughlin, A. Tinker, and M. L. Cuzner, *J. Neuroimmunol.* **33,** 277 (1991).
22. M. Nieto-Sampedro and M. A. Berman, *J. Neurosci. Res.* **17,** 214 (1987).
23. M. Nieto-Sampedro and K. G. Chandy, *Neurochem. Res.* **12,** 723 (1987).
24. R. G. Watts, J. L. Wright, L. L. Atkinson, and R. E. Merchant, *Neurosurgery* **25,** 202 (1989).
25. R. D. Simmons and D. O. Willenborg, *J. Neurol. Sci.* **100,** 37 (1990).
26. M. P. Sethna and L. A. Lampson, *J. Neuroimmunol.* **34,** 121 (1991).
27. D. Giulian, J. Woodward, D. G. Young, J. F. Krebs, and L. B. Lachman, *J. Neurosci.* **8,** 2485 (1988).
28. D. Giulian D and L. B. Lachman, *Science* **228,** 497 (1985).
29. C. F. Brosnan, M. S. Litwak, C. E. Schroeder, K. Selmaj, C. S. Raine, and J. C. Arezzo, *J. Neuroimmunol.* **25,** 227 (1989).
30. N. Rubio and C. de Felipe, *J. Neuroimmunol.* **35,** 111 (1991).
31. E. M. Ban, L. L. Sarlieve, and F. G. Haour, *Neuroscience* **52,** 725 (1993).
32. K. Janeczko, *Brain Res.* **456,** 280 (1988).
33. K. S. Topp, B. T. Faddis, and V. K. Vijayan, *Glia* **2,** 201 (1989).
34. Y. Matsumoto, K. Ohmori, and M. Fujiwara, *J. Neuroimmunol.* **37,** 23 (1992).
35. C. M. Morshead and D. van der Kooy, *Brain Res.* **535,** 237 (1990).
36. Y. J. Oh, G. J. Markelonis, and T. H. Oh *Glia* **8,** 77 (1993).
37. K. W. Selmaj, M. Farooq, W. T. Norton, C. S. Raine, and C. F. Brosnan, *J. Immunol.* **144,** 129 (1990).
38. B. P. Barna, M. L. Estes, B. S. Jacobs, S. Hudson, and R. M. Ransohoff, *J. Neuroimmunol.* **30,** 239 (1990).
39. A Bignami and D. Dahl, *Neuropathol. Appl. Neurobiol.* **2,** 99 (1976).
40. W. L. Maxwell, R. Follows, D. E. Ashhurst, and M. Berry, *Phil. Trans. R. Soc. Lond. Biol.* **328,** 501 (1990).
41. M. Berry, W. L. Maxwell, A. Logan, A. Mathewson, P. McConnell, D. E. Ashburst, and G.H. Thomas, *Acta Neurochir [Suppl.]***32,** 31 (1983).
42. J. Gearhart, M. L. Oster-Granite, and L. Guth, *Exp. Neurol.* **66,** 1 (1979).
43. C. P. Barrett, E. J. Donati, and L. Guth, *Exp. Neurol.* **84,** 374 (1984).
44. I. E. Moore, J. M. Bountempo, and R. O. Weller, *Neuropathol. Appl. Neurobiol.* **13,** 219 (1987).
45. P. A. Trimmer and R. E. Wunderlich, *J. Comp. Neurol.* **296,** 359 (1990).

46. V. W. Yong and J. P. Antel, *in* "Protocols for Neural Cell Culture." The Humana Press, New York, 1992.
47. V. W. Yong, F. P. Yong, A. Olivier, Y. Robitaille, and J. P. Antel, *J. Neurosci Res.* **27,** 678 (1990).
48. V. W. Yong, T. Tejada-Berges, C. G. Goodyer, J. P. Antel, and F. P. Yong, *Glia* **6,** 269 (1992).
49. V. W. Yong and S. U. Kim, *J. Neurosci. Methods* **21,** 9 (1987).
50. V. W. Yong, R. Moumdjian, F. P. Yong, T. C. G. Ruijs, M. S. Freedman, N. Cashman, and J. P. Antel, *Proc. Natl. Acad. Sci. U.S.A.* **88,** 7016 (1991).
51. K. Ohira, B. Vayuvegula, M. Murakami, S. Gollapudi, E. Frohman, S. van den Noort, and S. Gupta, *J. Neuroimmunol. 31,* 43 (1993).
52. S. Kelic, T. Olsson, and K. Kristensson, *J. Neurol. Sci.* **114,** 62 (1993).
53. T. Yokota, K. Shimokado, C. Kosaka, T. Sasaguri, J. Masuda, and J. Ogata, *Arteriosclerosis Thrombosis* **12,** 1393 (1992).
54. P. W. Gray, S. Leong, E. H. Fennie, M. A. Farrar, J. T. Pingel, J. Fernandez-Luna, and R. D. Schreiber, *Proc. Natl. Acad. Sci. U.S.A.* **86,** 8497 (1989).
55. S. Hemmi, P. Peghini, M. Metzler, G. Merlin, Z. Dembic, and M. Aguet, *Proc. Natl. Sci. Acad. U.S.A.* **86,** 9901 (1989).
56. V. Balasingam, T. Tejada-Berges, E. Wright, R. Bouckova, and V. W. Yong, *J. Neurosci.* **14,** 846 (1994).
57. E. A. Goldmuntz, C. F. Brosnan, F.-C. Chiu, and W. T. Norton, *Brain Res.* **397,** 16 (1986).
58. S. K. R. Pixley and J. de Vellis, *Dev. Brain Res.* **15,** 201 (1984).
59. S. A. Meyer, C. A. Ingraham, and K. D. McCarthy, *J. Neurosci. Res.* **24,** 251 (1989).
60. A. C. H. Yu, Y. L. Lee, and L. F. Eng, *J. Neurosci. Res.* **34,** (1993).
61. T. Abo, C. A. Miller, G. L. Gardland, and C. M. Balch, *J. Exp. Med.* **157,** 273 (1983).
62. C. Y. Lu and E. R. Unanue, *Clin. Immunol. Allergy* **5,** 253 (1985).
63. I. Hannet, F. Erkeller-Yuksel, P. Lydyard, V. Deneys, and M. DeBruyere, *Immunol. Today.* **13,** 215 (1992).
64. B. Schmidt, G. Stoll, K. V. Toyka, and H.-P. Hartung, *Brain Res.* **515,** 347 (1990).
65. K. Unsicker, K. C. Flanders, D. S. Cissel, R. Lafyatis, and M. B. Sporn, *Neuroscience* **44,** 613 (1991).
66. W. L. Farrar, M. Vinocour, and J. M. Hill, *Blood* **73,** 137 (1989).
67. J.-L. Tchelingerian, J. Quinonero, J. Booss, and C. Jacque, *Neuron* **10,** 213 (1993).
68. P. A. Lapchak, D. M. Araujo, R. Quirion, and A. Beaudet, *Neuroscience* **44,** 173 (1991).
69. T. Olsson, K. Kristensson, Å. Ljungdahl, J. Maehlen, R. Holmdah, and L. Klareskog, *J. Neurosci.* **9,** 3870 (1989).
70. F. Eclancher, F. Perraud, J. Faltin, G. Labourdette, and M. Sensenbrenner, *Glia* **3,** 502 (1990).

[15] Immunocytochemistry in Brain Tissue

Hans Imboden and Dominik Felix

Introduction

Because of achievements in the area of immunocytochemistry, a large number of important results have been obtained in the field of neurobiology over the past few years. The sensitivity, specificity, and also simplicity of immunocytochemical techniques have made them useful tools which are used in nearly every routine histology laboratory. Since the discovery of the use of antibodies to localize previously undetectable components in histological sections, these techniques continue to improve.

In this chapter we describe the use of monoclonal and polyclonal antibodies in light microscopic immunocytochemistry and important methods and procedures used in combination with these techniques. Special emphasis is placed on peptides that play an important role as neuroactive substances (1).

Preparation of Immunogens

General Remarks

It is well known that peptides have a low immunogenicity, i.e., it is difficult to induce antibody formation against such small molecules. For this reason the peptide of investigation has to be coupled to a carrier protein in order to enhance immunogenicity. Bovine serum albumin (BSA), hemocyanin, and other proteins are used as carriers. The immunogenicity of the peptides used in our studies, in combination with the hemocyanin, is much higher than that with BSA.

Material and Solutions

Peptide of interest [e.g., human angiotensin II, an octapeptide, Sigma (St. Louis, MO); vasopressin, a nonapeptide, Sigma].

Hemocyanin from keyhole limpet (Sigma).

Methods in Neurosciences, Volume 24

Phosphate-buffered saline after Dulbecco [PBS-D: 8000 mg NaCl, 200 mg KCl, 1440 mg $Na_2HPO_4 \cdot 2H_2O$, 200 mg KH_2PO_4. Make up to 1 liter with distilled, deionized H_2O. Adjust pH to 7.4 with 1 N HCl (2). For use dilute 10 times with deionized H_2O (= diluted PBS-D)].

N-Ethyl-*N'*-(dimethylaminopropyl)carbodiimide hydrochloride (CDI; Fluka, Ronkonkoma, NY).

Sonicator.

Rotating apparatus.

Dialysis membrane tube with a molecular weight cutoff of 10,000.

Procedure

1. Add 20 mg of hemocyanin carefully to the surface of 3.6 ml cold diluted PBS-D (incubate for 20 min, then sonicate the solution in order to obtain good solubilization).
2. Add 3 mg of the peptide of interest and sonicate.
3. Add 66 mg of CDI to the peptide–hemocyanin–PBS-D solution and sonicate.
4. Adjust the pH of the solution to 5 with 0.1 *N* HCl.
5. Incubate the solution at room temperature for 24 hr while shaking (the transparent solution will turn milky).
6. Sonicate the milky solution and transfer it to a dialysis tube.
7. Incubate the dialysis tube with the solution for 24 hr at 4°C in 1 liter of diluted PBS-D on a magnetic stirrer. Change the PBS-D solution four times during this period.
8. Transfer the solution into a beaker, sonicate, and divide it into portions of 300 μl in small tubes.

Notes

The solubilized hemocyanin–peptide complexes (see Fig. 1) are now ready for injection into animals or can be stored in the freezer.

Production of Antibodies

General Remarks

In principle, two kinds of systems can be used for producing antibodies. Either polyclonal antibodies are produced in rabbits (collected from the

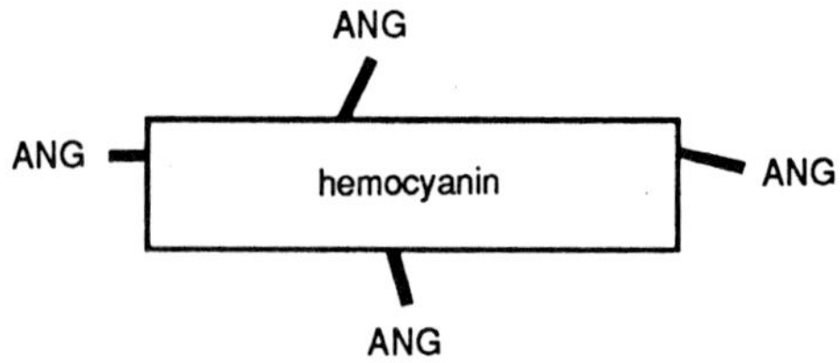

FIG. 1 Coupling of the peptide angiotensin II (ANG) to the carrier-protein hemocyanin by carbodiimide.

serum) or monoclonal antibodies are obtained from immunized mice (*in vitro* production). Here only the recipe for injecting solutions to immunize the animals is described.

Material, Animals, and Solutions

Hemocyanin–peptide complexes in solution as described above (see Preparation of the Immunogen).
Complete Freund's adjuvant (ACF; DIFCO laboratories, Detroit, MI).
Incomplete Freund's adjuvant (AIF; DIFCO laboratories).
Sonicator.
Syringes.
BALB/c mice.
New Zealand White rabbits.

Procedure

1. First injection: 300 μl of ACF (4°C) and 300 μl of the hemocyanin–peptide complex solution (4°C) are emulsified using the sonicator. Inject 300 μl of this solution intraperitoneally per mouse, 300 μl intramuscularly per rabbit.
2. Booster injections: same procedure as for the first injection but instead of ACF, AIF is used. Three booster injections at intervals of 3 weeks.

Notes

The presence of polyclonal antibodies against the peptide of interest in the serum of rabbits and mice is tested by using the nitrocellulose (NC) dot test (see Nitrocellulose Dot Test, below).

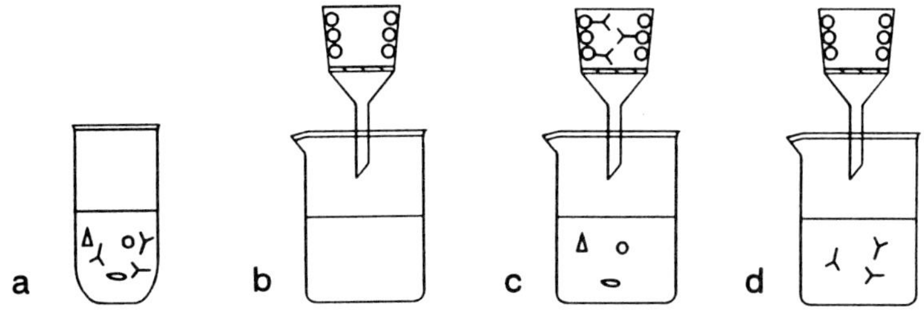

FIG. 2 Purification of monoclonal antibodies: (a) medium containing medium components and monoclonal antibodies, (b) protein G-Sepharose 4 column, (c) bound monoclonal antibodies to Protein G, and (d) elution of monoclonal antibodies.

To screen the medium of the clones for the presence of monoclonal antibodies the same NC dot test is used again.

Purification of Monoclonal Antibodies

General Remarks

Purification permits monoclonal antibodies synthesized in the incubation medium by the hybridoma cells to be isolated. Other substances contained in the incubation medium which might interfere with the immunocytochemical staining reaction are removed.

Material and Solutions

Protein G-Sepharose 4 fast flow column (Pharmacia; Piscataway, NJ) supplied ready for use.
Starting buffer: 20 m*M* sodium phosphate, pH 7.0.
Elution buffer: 0.1 *M* glycine hydrochloride, pH 2.7.
Collecting buffer: 1 *M* Tris–HCl, pH 8.5.

Procedure

1. Follow exactly the application manual of the supplier for equilibrating, packing, and loading the column.
2. The different steps for isolating monoclonal antibodies are shown in Fig. 2.

3. The bound antibodies are eluted with elution buffer and collected in tubes which contain collecting buffer (10% of the total elution volume).

Notes

Make small aliquots for storing the solution with the antibodies in the freezer. Avoid repeated freezing and thawing. If possible freeze-dry these aliquots before storing them in the freezer.

Purification of Polyclonal Antibodies

Preparation of Affinity Column

General Remarks

This purification permits the antibodies which are specific against the peptide of interest to be isolated from the serum. As an example we discuss the purification of antibodies against angiotensin II which are produced in a rabbit. All the other substances, especially all the other antibodies in the serum, which could interfere the immunostaining reaction are discarded.

Material and Solutions

CH-Sepharose 4B (Pharmacia). The free carboxyl groups at the end of 6-carbon spacer arms permit ligands containing primary amino groups to be coupled.

0.5 *M* NaCl.

Angiotensin II (ANG II; Sigma).

0.19 *M* *N*-ethyl-*N'*-(3-dimethylaminopropyl)carbodiimide hydrochloride (CDI; Fluka).

Blocking buffer: 0.1 *M* Tris–HCl, pH 8.

Washing buffers:

- 0.1 *M* acetate buffer, pH 4.0, containing 1 *M* NaCl (acid buffer).
- 0.1 *M* Tris–HCl buffer, pH 8.0, containing 1 *M* NaCl (alkaline buffer).

10 m*M* Tris–HCl, pH 7.6, containing 140 m*M* NaCl (TBS, Tris-buffered saline).

Rotating apparatus.

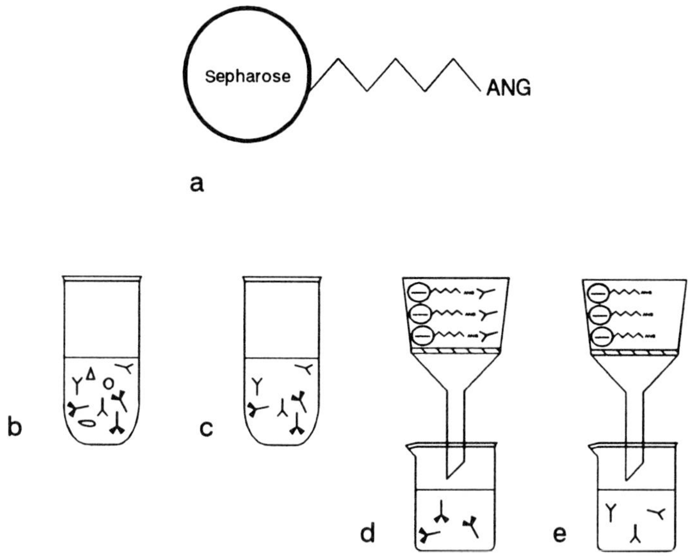

FIG. 3 Purification of polyclonal antibodies: (a) coupling of the peptide angiotensin II (ANG) to CH-Sepharose 4B using carbodiimide, (b) serum containing serum components and normal and specific antibodies, (c) partial purification of all the normal and specific antibodies by ammonium sulfate, (d) bound specific antibodies to ANG in the CH-Sepharose 4B column, and (e) elution of the specific antibodies.

Procedure

1. 1 g of freeze-dried resin (CH-Sepharose 4B) is suspended in 0.5 *M* NaCl, yielding approximately 3.5 ml swollen gel.
2. The gel is washed on a sintered glass filter with 300 ml 0.5 *M* NaCl to remove additives. Wash the gel with 500 ml H_2O to remove the NaCl.
3. 5 mg ANG II is dissolved in 2 ml H_2O and added to the gel.
4. While gently stirring the mixture at room temperature, add 5.5 ml 0.19 *M* CDI in drops. The pH is measured at the beginning of the incubation and adjusted to pH 5.0.
5. Allow the reaction to continue for 24 hr at room temperature while shaking.
6. The ANG II-linked gel is washed with five alternate cycles of 200-ml alkaline and acid buffer each.
7. The gel is then washed successively with 200 ml H_2O and 200 ml TBS.

Notes

This gel is ready to be used for affinity purification of polyclonal antibodies from the serum specific for ANG II (see Fig. 3a).

To purify antibodies against a peptide, a gel with a spacer arm is required for immobilizing the small hapten. Steric hindrance of the antibodies at the binding site means that Sepharose 4B cannot be used without spacer arms.

Precipitation of Polyclonal Antibodies from Serum

General Remarks

Immunoglobulins of most species can be precipitated with ammonium sulfate. This salt can therefore be used to achieve a crude separation of all antibodies in the serum before applying it to the affinity column.

Material and Solutions

Serum with antibodies of interest.
Diluted PBS-D (for recipe see the section Nitrocellulose Dot Test: Material and Solutions).
3.2 *M* $(NH_4)_2SO_4$.
Rotating apparatus.
Centrifuge.
10 m*M* Tris–HCl, pH 7.6, containing 140 m*M* NaCl (TBS).
Dialysis membrane tube.

Procedure

1. Add to 200 μl crude rabbit antiserum (see Fig. 3b) 200 μl diluted PBS-D at 4°C.
2. Precipitate the antibodies by adding dropwise 400 μl cold 3.2 *M* ammonium sulfate at 4°C.
3. Incubate the solution for 30 min at room temperature while stirring.
4. Centrifuge for 10 min (about 8000*g*) at room temperature.
5. Discard the supernatant.
6. Resuspend the pellet in 3 ml TBS (see Fig. 3c).
7. Transfer solution with the antibodies to a dialysis tube. The dialysis takes place at 4°C in 1 liter TBS while shaking for 24 hr. Change the solution three times over this period.

Affinity Purification of Polyclonal Antibodies with CH-Sepharose 4B-Hapten Column

Procedure

1. The resuspended pellet together with additional 5 ml TBS is added to the gel.
2. The suspension is gently stirred for 2 to 4 hr at room temperature.

IMPORTANT: Do not incubate more than 4 hr because antibodies with high affinity to the antigen will stick too strongly to it and cannot be eluted! This might cause negative results of the immunocytochemical staining procedure!

Notes

Protein G-Sepharose 4 (see Purification of Monoclonal Antibodies, above) or a similar gel cannot be used to isolate the specific polyclonal antibodies from the serum only.

Elution of Bound Antibodies

Material and Solutions

Glass column (e.g., 1.3 × 6 cm).
Peristaltic pump.
Spectrophotometer.
10 m*M* TBS, pH 7.6 (solution A; Precipitation of the Polyclonal Antibodies from the Serum: Materials and Solutions, above).
10 m*M* TBS, pH 7.6 containing 1 *M* NaCl (solution B).
0.1 *M* glycine hydrochloride, pH 2.8 (solution C).
1 *M* Tris–HCl, pH 8.5.

Procedure

1. The gel is loaded into the glass column and washed with solution A at a flow rate of about 3 ml/min, until 280 nm absorbance returns to baseline (usually 50 ml, see Fig. 3d).
2. Solution B which elutes low bound substances from the column is applied to the gel.
3. With solution A the high salt concentration of solution B is washed out.
4. The affinity-bound antibodies are eluted with three cycles of 4.5 ml of 0.1 *M* glycine hydrochloride, pH 2.8, and collected in tubes containing 0.5 ml of 1 *M* Tris–HCl, pH 8.5 (see Fig. 3e). A typical elution profile is shown in Fig. 4.
5. The three fractions are mixed together and aliquoted into small volumes for storage in the freezer.

Notes

Avoid repeated freezing and thawing of the antibody solution.
Preferably freeze-dry the samples and store them in the freezer.
These antibodies are now ready for specificity tests (NC dot test) and for immunocytochemical studies.

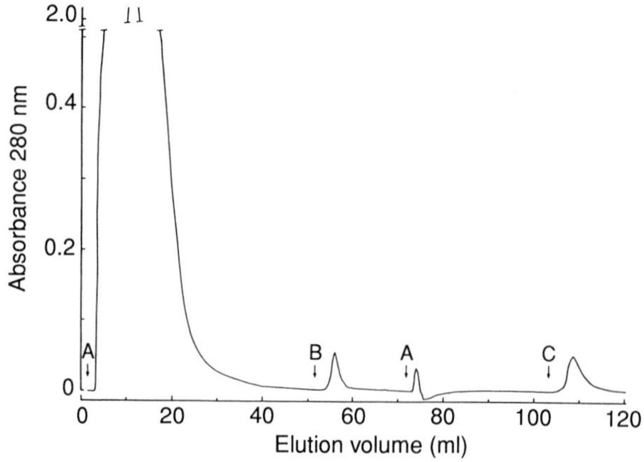

FIG. 4 A typical elution profile of the CH-Sepharose 4B column. Eluting solutions were as follows: (A) 10 m*M* TBS, pH 7.6, (B) 10 m*M* TBS, pH 7.6 + 1 *M* NaCl, (C) 0.1 *M* glycine hydrochloride, pH 2.8. The purified antibodies eluted between 105 and 115 ml of elution volume. Reproduced by permission from Imboden *et al.* (3).

Storage of CH-Sepharose 4B-Hapten Gel

1. The gel is transferred to a sintered glass filter and washed with 20 ml 10 m*M* HCl to elute any antibodies which remain bound.
2. Wash the gel with 100 ml solution A.
3. Store the gel in 10 m*M* TBS containing 1 *M* NaCl and 20 m*M* NaN_3, pH 6.8, at 4–8°C.

Purification of Second and Third Antibodies

General Remarks

The use of polyclonal antibodies as second antibodies (e.g., goat anti-rabbit as a link between the first and the third antibodies or goat anti-rabbit marked with peroxidase, gold, or a fluorescent dye, or any other antibodies) can result in unspecific background staining even in control experiments without the first antibodies. To reduce this unspecific binding of the second antibodies some immunocytochemists preincubate the sections with normal serum or other proteins to block nonspecific surface attachment of the reagents applied later. We found that this pretreatment is of little advantage and sometimes even enhances the background staining.

For the immunocytochemical incubation we therefore only used antibody solutions that should not bind to brain tissue. For this reason we prepared affinity columns with either brain homogenates or serum from rats and incubated the second antibodies with one of these column resins.

The application of such "purified" antibodies resulted in the absence of unspecific background staining in rat brain sections. Because there was no visible difference between the two columns used, we decided to use the serum column which is easier to prepare.

Material and Solutions

CNBr-activated Sepharose 4B (Pharmacia).
1 m*M* HCl.
Sintered glass filter.
Coupling buffer ($NaHCO_3$, 0.1 *M*, pH 8.3, containing NaCl, 0.5 *M*).
Blocking buffer, Tris–HCl buffer (0.1 *M*, pH 8.0).
Washing buffers:
  Acid buffer (0.1 *M* acetate buffer containing 0.5 *M* NaCl, pH 4.0).
  Alkaline buffer (0.1 *M* Tris buffer containing 0.5 *M* NaCl, pH 8.0).
Tris-buffered saline (5 m*M*, pH 7.6; see Immunocytochemistry: Materials and Solutions below).
Serum (serum of the species with which the immunocytochemical studies are performed!).
NaN_3.
Triton X-100.
Serum containing the second (goat anti-rabbit immunoglobulins, rabbit anti-mouse immunoglobulins with peroxidase) or third antibodies (PAP complexes, mouse or rabbit origin).

Procedure

1. Suspend 1 g freeze-dried powder of the Sepharose in 1 m*M* HCl. The gel swells immediately to a volume of about 3.5 ml.
2. Put the gel on a sintered glass filter and wash it for 15 min with 200 ml 1 m*M* HCl.
3. Wash the gel with 200 ml H_2O followed by 100 ml coupling buffer.
4. Dilute 100 μl rat serum with 10 ml coupling buffer.
5. Put the gel into the serum-coupling buffer solution.
6. Incubate this mixture on a rotating apparatus for 1 hr at room temperature.

7. Wash the gel with 200 ml coupling buffer.

8. Block any remaining active groups with Tris–HCl buffer (0.1*M*, pH 8) for 1 hr at room temperature.

9. Wash with three cycles of alternating acid and alkaline buffers (each 50 ml).

10. Wash again with 100 ml TBS, pH 7.6. This gel is ready for incubation with the second antibodies!

11. Transfer the gel into a beaker with TBS (5 m*M*, pH 7.6).

12. Add 1 ml serum containing the second antibodies.

13. Incubate for 4 hr at 4°C while rotating!

14. After incubation transfer the gel to a sintered glass filter. Elute the unbound antibodies with TBS (5 m*M*, pH 7.6). Add Triton X-100 and NaN_3 to the eluate to get a final concentration of 0.1% each.

15. Store this solution at 4°C. These antibodies can now be used for immunocytochemical studies.

Notes

Only the antibodies that did not bind to the serum column are used for immunocytochemistry.

The same procedure (Sepharose serum column) can be used for purifying polyclonal peroxidase–antiperoxidase (PAP) complexes.

Nitrocellulose Dot Test

General Remarks

The nitrocellulose (NC) dot test is a technique which is easy to apply and a very useful and important tool in combination with immunocytochemistry. It is normally the first step for testing antigenicity and is used to determine the specificity and the cross-reactivity of antibodies without brain tissue.

As none of the tested NC membranes bind peptides to a sufficient extent (only 5 to 30% binding) the choice of the binding technique is crucial. In the following we present a technique which yielded higher binding results (85 to 90%):

NC membranes are incubated with a protein solution. The peptide of interest (synthetic origin or from an extract) is applied to circles of membranes coated with this protein. After exposure to formaldehyde vapor (linking of the peptide to the protein) and washing, the circles are processed with the antibody solution of interest for immunostaining.

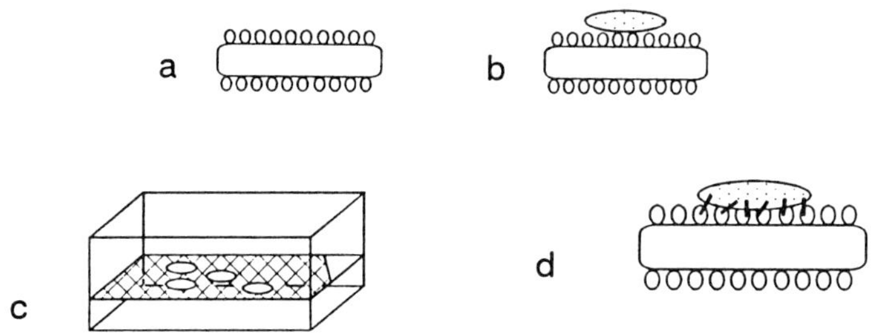

FIG. 5 Nitrocellulose dot test: (a) nitrocellulose (NC) coated with egg serum albumin (side view of a NC circle), (b) application of the peptide of interest to the center of the circle (side view), (c) incubation box with NC circles on the sieve, (d) binding of the peptides to egg serum albumin using formalin.

This procedure of fixing peptides to "artificial sections" (NC circles) mimics the fixation of the peptides in the brain during perfusion with paraformaldehyde. Subsequently they are processed the same way as the brain sections in immunocytochemistry.

Material and Solutions

0.45 NC membrane (Bio-Rad, Richmond, CA).
Peptide of interest, e.g., vasopressin (100 ng/μl H_2O; Sigma).
Formaldehyde solution, 35%.
Tris-buffered saline (20 m*M* Tris, 500 m*M* NaCl, adjusted to pH 7.5 with HCl).
Albumin solution; egg serum albumin (ESA; Ovalbumin, chicken egg, Grade V; Sigma). For a NC membrane of 8 × 8 cm prepare 50 ml protein solution (50 mg ovalbumin in 50 ml TBS).
Phosphate-buffered saline after Dulbecco, diluted 10 times (diluted PBS-D; for recipe see Preparation of the Immunogen: Materials and Solutions, above).
Fixation solution: 5% formalin in PBS-D (8.5 ml PBS-D+ 1.4 ml 35% formalin, adjusted to pH 7.4 with 0.5 *N* NaOH).
Incubation box, e.g., plastic slide box (9 × 5 × 5 cm with a tight cover) with a plastic sieve as illustrated in Fig. 5c.
An ordinary commercially available office hole puncher.

Procedure

1. Soak a NC sheet (8 × 8 cm) in PBS-D for 15 min.
2. For coating, incubate it in the ESA solution (50 ml) at room temperature for 1 hr while shaking.

3. Wash the NC twice with 50 ml diluted PBS-D at room temperature for 20 min, while shaking.
4. Allow the coated NC to dry at room temperature for 20 min.
5. Punch out circles from the NC-coated membrane with the hole puncher (circles with 5 mm diameter; see Fig. 5a).
6. Mark the circles with a pencil for later identification.
7. Apply vasopressin (in 1–2 μl volume) to the center of each circle (see Fig. 5b).
8. Place the circles on the plastic sieve in the incubation box (see Fig. 5c).
9. Warm the fixation solution to 40°C and pour it into the box (through the opening in the plastic sieve).
10. Close the box tightly with the cover immediately.
11. Incubate at room temperature for 16 to 20 hr.
12. Wash the NC circles three times in TBS. These NC circles with vasopressin (see Fig. 5d) are now ready to use for immunostaining and can be processed as described under Procedure for Nitrocellular Dot Test, below.

Notes

Egg serum albumin-coated NC circles with or without applied peptides can be stored in the freezer for at least 1 year!

Application of brain extracts to NC membranes and the use of hot formaldehyde vapor yields unsatisfactory results. The surface of the extract applied gets too hard during heating and the antibodies cannot react with the antigens.

Chemical Fixation of Brain Tissue

General Remarks

The chemical fixation of the tissue that contains the antigens of interest is one of the most critical points in immunocytochemical staining. Optimally fixed tissue displays good morphology and a high binding capacity for the specific antibodies. For each molecule of interest the most suitable conditions (kind of fixative, combinations and concentrations of fixatives, pH of the solution, temperature, time of treatments, etc.) have to be evaluated. Concerning the kind of fixation procedure to be used, perfusion fixation is preferable to immersion fixation.

Material, Animals, and Solutions

Rat.
Ringer's solution.
Heparin.
$MgCl_2 \cdot 6H_2O$.
Paraformaldehyde powder (Merck).
2.5% NaOH.
1 *N* HCl.
Diethyl ether.
Thiopentane sodium (Pentothal; Abbott).
Warming plate with magnetic stirrer.
Rinsing perfusion solution: 100 ml Ringer's solution containing 1000 U heparin and 1 g $MgCl_2 \cdot 6H_2O$, 37°C.
Phosphate buffer (buffer A, pH 7.4) to prepare the fixing perfusion solution: Dissolve 1.32 g $NaH_2PO_4 \cdot H_2O$ and 13.5 g $Na_2HPO_4 \cdot 7H_2O$ in deionized H_2O and fill up to 400 ml.
Perfusion fixative (2% paraformaldehyde, pH 7.3): Heat 50 ml H_2O to 60°C with adequate ventilation in a hood. Carefully add 6.7 g paraformaldehyde powder to the warm water while stirring and dissolve for 3 min. Add 2.5% NaOH dropwise to the milky solution until it becomes transparent (about 40 drops). Cool the solution to room temperature. Filter it into a cylinder and add 250 ml of buffer A. Measure the pH of this solution and adjust it with 1 *N* HCl to pH 7.3. Add more buffer A to make up a final volume of 333.3 ml. Cool the solution to 4°C.
The schematic illustration of the equipment for perfusion is shown in Fig. 6.

Procedure for Perfusion–Fixation

A schematic drawing of the manipulation at the heart for perfusing the brain is shown in Fig. 7.

1. After a short diethyl ether narcosis anesthetize the rat intraperitoneally with 100 mg/kg thiopentane sodium.
2. Open the chest of the rat and pinch off the descending aorta with a clip.
3. Insert a canula into the left ventricle of the heart.
4. Make an incision into the right atrium.
5. Open the valve for the rinsing perfusion solution and flush out the blood. After 2 to 3 min (about 100 ml solution) the circulatory system will be free of blood.

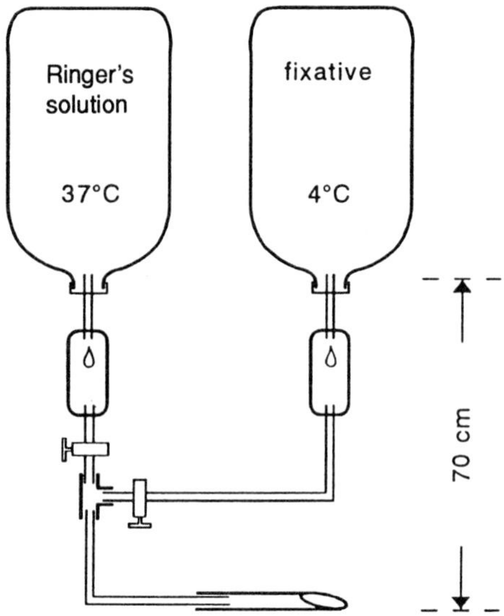

FIG. 6 Perfusion equipment.

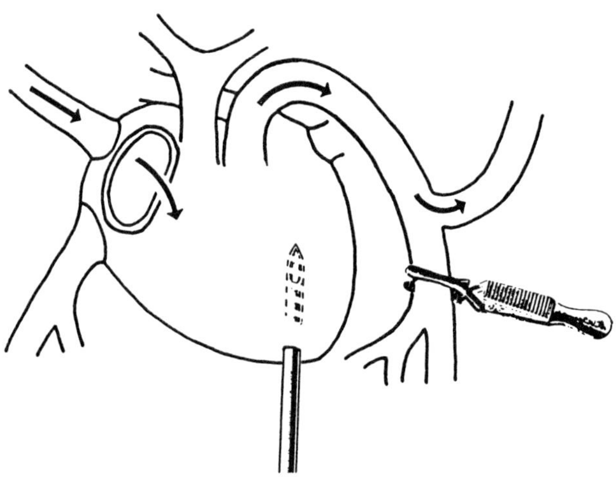

FIG. 7 Schematic drawing of the manipulation at the heart for perfusing the brain.

6. Close this valve and open the valve for the fixative; perfuse with 200 ml of this solution for 15 to 20 min.

7. Remove the brain carefully and chop it into appropriate pieces with a razor blade.

8. Immerse the pieces in 100 ml perfusion fixative for 28 hr at 4°C. Change the fixative solution once during this period.

Notes

An alternative to perfusion fixation is immersion fixation (for example, for postmortem tissue). In this case cut the tissue into pieces of maximum 5 mm in length. Due to endogenous peroxidase (especially in red blood cells) nonperfused tissue has to be treated specifically to destroy the enzyme (4, 5) before using the PAP method.

Cryostate Sectioning

General Remarks

A number of different sectioning methods (e.g., paraffin-embedded microtome sections, vibratome and cryosections) exist for light microscopy investigations involving paraformaldehyde-fixed brain tissue. The choice of method depends on the subject of the study. Note that cryosectioning is a relatively quick method and yields morphological and immunocytochemical results that are comparable with other procedures.

Material and Solutions

Diluted PBS-D (see Preparation of Immunogen: Materials and Solutions, above).
Sucrose (saccharose) extra pure (Merck).
Cryostat (cabin temperature −17°C, holder with the tissue −13°C).
CO_2 flask with an immersion tube.
M-1 embedding matrix for frozen sectioning (Lipshaw, Pittsburgh, PA).
Tris-buffered saline (5 mM Tris, pH 7.6; see Immunocytochemistry: Material and Solutions, below).
Triton X-100.

Procedure

1. After paraformaldehyde fixation (see Chemical Fixation of Brain Tissue: Procedure for Perfusion–Fixation, above), the tissue is washed for 14 hr in 100 ml diluted PBS-D containing 18% sucrose at 4°C.
2. Cover brain tissue with the embedding matrix and block it on the cryostat chuck by CO_2 freezing.
3. Cut 30-μm sections and put them indiluted PBS-D at 4°C.
4. Transfer each section with a paintbrush to diluted PBS-D at room temperature and wash them for 30 min.
5. Wash sections in TBS (5 m*M* Tris) at pH 7.6 containing 0.1% Triton X-100 for 30 min.

These sections are now ready for immunocytochemical incubation.

Notes

The sucrose immersion and the CO_2 freezing are very important steps for preventing the formation of ice crystals within the tissue which would destroy the cell structure.
Never allow the sections to dry out!
Under the conditions described here the use of M-1 embedding matrix yields better results than the use of comparable embedding media.

Immunocytochemistry

General Remarks

Different immunostaining methods exist for localizing antigens in histological sections at the cellular level. As examples we discuss below indirect methods using peroxidase as a ligand on the antibodies (6, 7).

Material and Solutions

Polyclonal or monoclonal affinity-purified first antibodies (see Purification of Monoclonal Antibodies and Purification of Polyclonal Antibodies, above).

Goat anti-rabbit immunoglobulins (GAR/IgG, H+L; Nordic Immunological Laboratories B.V., Tilburg, The Netherlands).
Peroxidase-conjugated rabbit immunoglobulins to mouse immunoglobulins (Dako, Glostrup, Denmark).
Peroxidase–antiperoxidase complex (PAP, rabbit origin; Sternberger Monoclonals, Inc., Baltimore, MD).
MILLEX-OR, 0.22-μm filter (Millipore, Bedford, MA).
MILLEX-GV, 0.22-μm filter (Millipore).
3,3′-Diaminobenzidine tetrahydrochloride (DAB · 4HCl; Polyscience, Inc.).
Imidazole buffer substance (Merck).
H_2O_2.
Ammonium nickel sulfate.
Tris buffer, 50 m*M*, pH 7.6: Add 7.68 ml 1 *N* HCl to 180 ml H_2O. Dissolve 1.12 g Tris in this solution and adjust the pH of the solution to 7.6. Make up to 200 ml with H_2O.
Tris-buffered saline (TBS, 5 m*M*, pH 7.6): Add 3.9 g NaCl to 50 ml Tris buffer (50 m*M* pH 7.6). Make up to 500 ml with H_2O.
5 m*M* TBS, pH 7.6, containing 0.1% Triton X-100 and 0.1% NaN_3.
5 m*M* TBS pH 7.6, containing 0.1% Triton X-100.
Substrate incubation solution (for staining the free-floating sections)
  8.1 ml Tris buffer, 50 m*M*, pH 7.6.
  420 μl DAB (1 mg/100 μl).
  150 μl 1% imidazole (in H_2O).
Filter this solution with a 0.2-μm filter (MILLEX-OR) and immediately before incubation add 240 μl cold 0.3% H_2O_2.
Substrate incubation solution (for staining with the NC dot test):
  8.1 ml Tris buffer, 50 m*M*, pH 7.6.
  420 μl DAB (1 mg/100 μl).
  150 μl 1% imidazole (in H_2O).
  150 μl 1% ammonium nickel sulfate (in H_2O).
Filter this solution with a 0.2-μm filter (MILLEX-OR) and immediately before incubation add 240 μl cold 0.3% H_2O_2.

Procedure for Free-Floating Sections

1. After washing, incubate the free-floating sections for 44 hr at 4°C while continuously shaking in a solution containing the affinity-purified ANG-II antibodies in TBS (5 m*M* Tris) at pH 7.6, 0.1% Triton X-100, and 0.1% NaN_3 (see Fig. 8a). After incubation this solution is discarded.

2. Wash four times for 15 min each with TBS containing 0.1% Triton X-100.

3. Subsequently incubate with GAR immunoglobulins (affinity purified,

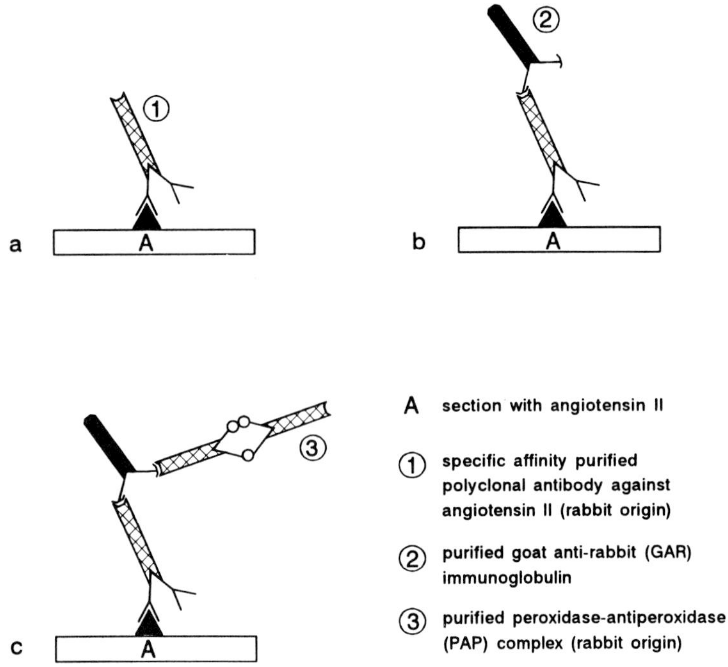

FIG. 8 Incubation steps for free-floating sections using the PAP method: (a) incubation of the free-floating sections with the first antibody, (b) incubation with excess GAR, (c) incubation with PAP. The last step is to add a substrate for the peroxidase to visualize indirectly the presence of angiotensin in the section.

see Purification of Second and Third Antibodies, above; Fig. 8b) in TBS at pH 7.6, 0.1% Triton X-100, and 0.1% NaN_3 for 45 min at room temperature (1 : 40; dilution depends on batch). This solution can be reused! Filter with MILLEX-GV and store at 4°C.

4. Wash three times with TBS Triton X-100 for 15 min each.

5. Incubate the section with the rabbit peroxidase–antiperoxidase complex (affinity purified, see Purification of Second and Third Antibodies, above; Fig. 8c) in TBS Triton X-100 solution for 45 min at room temperature (1 : 200; dilution depends on batch). After incubation this solution is discarded.

6. Wash twice in TBS Triton X-100, at room temperature, 15 min each.

7. Wash in TBS alone at room temperature for 15 min.

8. Incubate the sections with the peroxidase substrate solution (DAB solution for sections!) at room temperature for 5 to 10 min.

9. Wash twice in TBS at room temperature for 10 min each.

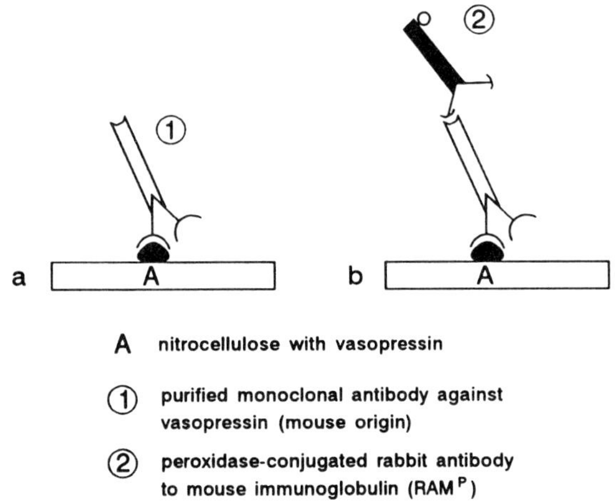

FIG. 9 Incubation steps for the nitrocellulose (NC) dot test: (a) incubation of the NC with vasopressin with the first antibody, (b) incubation with the RAM^{P}. The last step is to add a substrate for the peroxidase to visualize indirectly the presence of vasopressin on the NC.

10. Transfer the slice carefully with a fine paintbrush into a large petri dish containing warm tap water (about 45°C).

11. Hold the slice at the surface of the water with the brush and carefully guide the coated slide under the slice (recipe for preparing chrome–alum–gelatin-coated slides, see Slide Treatment, below).

12. Lift the slice out of the water and let it dry at room temperature for about 20 min. Do not use a hot plate or a hair dryer! It could cause morphological destruction if you allow the sections to dry completely.

Procedure for Nitrocellulose Dot Test

1. Incubate the NC circles with vasopressin (see Nitrocellulose Dot Test: Procedure, above) for 1 hr at room temperature in a solution containing monoclonal antibodies (affinity purified, see Purification of Monoclonal Antibodies, above; Fig. 9a) against vasopressin in TBS (5 m*M* TBS) at pH 7.6 and 0.1% Triton X-100. After incubation this solution is discarded.

2. Wash three times for 10 min each with TBS containing 0.1% Triton X-100.

3. Incubate the NC circles with peroxidase-conjugated rabbit immunoglobulins to mouse immunoglobulins (see Fig. 9b) in TBS containing 0.1% Triton X-100 (1 : 1000; dilution depends on batch). After incubation the solution is discarded.

4. Wash twice in TBS Triton X-100 for 10 min each.
5. Wash in TBS alone at room temperature for 10 min.
6. Finally incubate the NC membranes with the peroxidase substrate solution (DAB solution for the NC test!) at room temperature for 5 to 10 min.
7. Wash in TBS at room temperature for 10 min.
8. Wash in H_2O and let dry. The positive reaction product is a dark, stable color in the center of the white NC circle.

Notes

PRECAUTIONS: DAB · 4HCl if swallowed, inhaled, or absorbed through the skin may be harmful. Use with adequate ventilation in a hood. Follow the advice of the manufacturer!

The antibody dilution producing the best immunocytochemical staining has to be decided by testing. If possible only affinity-purified, specific polyclonal antibodies should be used (see Fig. 10).

For thick cryosections we only use free-floating sections. Using this incubation procedure the antibodies can penetrate from both sides into the sections. Because NaN_3 is an inhibitor of peroxidase, do not use sodium azide before, in combination with, or after incubation with peroxidase. Ammonium nickel sulfate in combination with free-floating sections is negative for morphological preservation. Imidazole in the substrate incubation solution markedly enhances the staining intensity (8).

Slide Treatment

General Remarks

As the sections do not stick well to untreated glass, the slides have to be pretreated. Different recipes exist and adhesive solutions for slides are also commercially available. We prepare our own slides coated with chrome–alum–gelatin.

Material and Solutions

Diethyl ether/ethanol (1 : 1)
Gelatin.
Chrome(III) potassium sulfate.

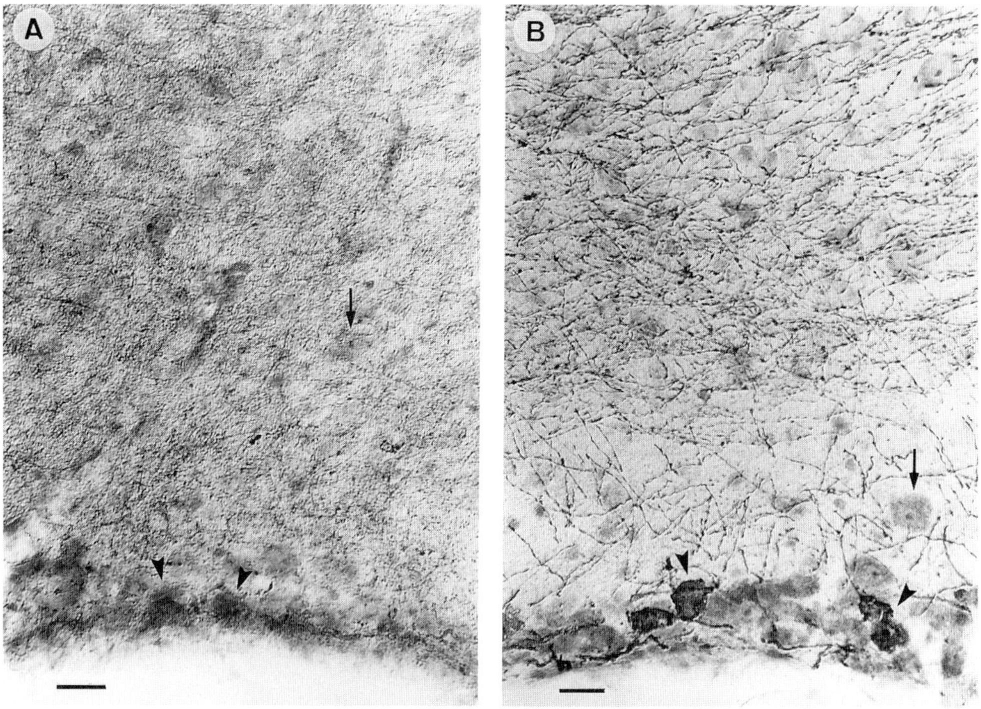

FIG. 10 Comparison of angiotensin II-like immunoreactive product in fiber tracts of the dorsal and ventral supraoptic commissure and in cells of the ventral base of the hypothalamus. Bars: 20 μm. (A) Staining with the crude antiserum. Only few cells at the hypothalamic border show faint and diffuse reaction (arrow heads). No clear fiber) pathways were observed in the commissure. (B) Staining with the affinity-purified antibody. Angiotensin II-like immunoreactive fiber pathways are clearly visible. Immunoreactive cells (arrowheads) can be distinguished from toluidine blue counterstained, nonreactive cells (arrows). Reproduced by permission from Imboden *et al.* (9) by courtesy of Marcel Dekker, Inc., N.Y. (1987).

Procedure for Preparing Chrome–Alum–Gelatin-Coated Slides

1. Prepare a solution by dissolving 750 mg gelatin in 150 ml H_2O at 40°C.
2. Add 75 mg chrome(III) potassium sulfate.
3. Clean the slides in the ether/ethanol solution.
4. Coat the clean slides by dipping them in the warm solution.
5. Dry slides vertically at 40°C for about 12 hr.

Notes

These coated slides can be stored at room temperature in a dust-free box for at least 6 months.

Counterstaining and Permanent Coverslipping

General Remarks

The DAB as a substrate for peroxidase permits permanent coverslipped sections, which can be restudied after years of storage.

Material and Solutions

Toluidine blue O (TB, zinc chloride double salt; Merck).
2.5% sodium carbonate (in H_2O).
Preparation of the TB solution: Prepare a 1% TB solution (1% TB) in H_2O. Add 50 ml 2.5% sodium carbonate and 16.5 ml 70% ethanol to 100 ml 1% TB. Add as a preservative 160 mg sodium azide. Filter before each use!
70, 80, 90, 96, and 100% ethanol.
Xylol (dimethylbenzene).
Mounting medium.

Procedure

1. Immerse the slides with the air-dried sections in 70% ethanol for at least 5 min.
2. Stain these sections at room temperature in TB for about 1 min.
3. Destain in 70% ethanol to get the desired staining intensity.
4. Dehydrate in 80, 90, 96, and twice in 100% ethanol, each for about 2 min.
5. Clear twice in xylol for at least 10 min each time and cover with a coverslide using mounting medium.

Notes

The toluidine solution can be used several times for about 1 month. Store at 4°C. Before each use filter it anew and warm it to room temperature. The intensity of TB counterstaining can be determined by changing the length of the different incubation steps. The counterstaining method enhances the morphological and immunocytochemical interpretation of the results. The brown DAB reaction product turns black with a high contrast in combination with the TB staining. Cells without the DAB reaction product are blue (see Fig. 10).

Controls for Immunocytochemistry

General Remarks

Preabsorption controls are produced with the purified first antibodies when they are incubated initially in a batch procedure with the peptide of interest which is covalently liked through its N terminals to CH-Sepharose 4B. When this column solution is used for incubation, no staining is observed. This means that all the purified antibodies are bound to the CH-Sepharose 4B with the corresponding antigen.

Further control tests are carried out either by incubating the first antibodies with the CH-Sepharose 4B without the antigens coupled to the resin before these antibodies are used for immunocytochemistry, or by applying preimmune serum or no first, second, or third antibodies to the sections.

Acknowledgments

This work was supported by Grant No. 31-40469.94 from the Swiss National Science Foundations and by the "Stiftung zur Förderung der wissenschaftlichen Forschung an der Universität Bern." We especially thank Susanne Gygax for technical assistance, Isabelle Maye and Jürg Pfister for helpful discussion, and Ruth Schweizer for typing the manuscript.

References

1. H. Imboden and D. Felix, *Regul. Pept.* **36,** 197–218 (1991).
2. R. Dulbecco and M. Vogt, *J. Exp. Med.* **99,** 167–182 (1954).
3. H. Imboden, J. W. Harding, R.H. Abhold, D. Ganten, and D. Felix, *Brain Res.* **426,** 225–234 (1987).
4. E. J. van Zwieten, R. Ravid, P. J. van der Sluis, A. A. Sluiter, Chr. W. Pool, D. Smyth, and D. F. Swaab, *Brain Res.* **550,** 263–267 (1991).
5. G. Torres, S. Lee, and C. Rivier, *J. Neurosci. Lett.* **146,** 96–100 (1992).
6. L. A. Sternberger, *in* "Immunocytochemistry." Wiley, New York, 1986.

7. F. Vandesande, *in* "Immunohistochemistry" (A. C. Cuello, ed.), pp. 101–119. Wiley, Chichester, 1983.
8. W. Straus, *J. Histochem. Cytochem.* **30(5),** 491–493 (1982).
9. H. Imboden, J. W. Harding, D. Ganten, and D. Felix, *Clin. Exp. Theory Practice,* **A9(7),** 1133–1139 (1987).

[16] Characterization of Neuronal Antigens and Antineuronal Antibodies

Josep Dalmau and Myrna R. Rosenfeld

Introduction

Paraneoplastic neurological syndromes are disorders of nervous system function that occur in association with cancer but are not a direct result of tumor mass or of metastasis to the nervous system. These disorders are the rarest neurological complications in cancer patients but they are important for two reasons. First, in one-half to two-thirds of patients, neurological symptoms precede the diagnosis of the tumor and, therefore, can direct the search for an occult and potentially curable cancer. Second, these syndromes provide a unique model to study the relationship between cancer and the nervous system at the biochemical and molecular level (1). In the past several years investigators have found that patients with some of these syndromes develop high titers of antibodies in their serum and cerebrospinal fluid (CSF) that specifically react with neuronal antigens that are also expressed by the tumor (2–5). Detection of a specific antibody is generally associated with a characteristic neurological syndrome and specific type of cancer. Therefore, detection of such antibodies confirms the paraneoplastic origin of a neurological syndrome and, in patients with unknown cancer, directs the search for a neoplasm to one or a few organs.

In addition to the antibody-associated paraneoplastic disorders, other antibodies directed against neuronal proteins have been identified in nonparaneoplastic neurological disorders including stiff-man syndrome (6, 7), immune-mediated autonomic disorders (8), and motor neuron syndromes (9).

The following protocols provide the methodology that has been developed and used to identify and characterize antineuronal antibodies associated with paraneoplastic disorders. These studies led to the isolation and cloning of the corresponding tumor and neuronal antigens (10–12). The recombinant antigens are used in serological testing for diagnostic purposes. The identification of these tumor antigens provides a unique opportunity to study the antitumor immune response in these patients and to isolate proteins that under normal conditions are uniquely expressed in the nervous system.

Methods in Neurosciences, Volume 24

Detection of Antineuronal Antibodies in Serum and Cerebrospinal Fluid

Basic immunohistochemistry and Western blotting can be used to determine if the serum or CSF of patients contains antibodies against neuronal tissue. These are simple techniques that allow for the rapid screening of multiple samples. Immunohistochemistry demonstrates the tissue distribution and cellular localization of antibody reactivity and offers the possibility to visualize a small population of reactive cells within a larger population of nonreactive cells. Western blot analysis provides the size of the protein antigen and can serve to distinguish between antibodies that have similar reactivity by immunohistochemistry but identify different antigens. For example, the anti-Hu (paraneoplastic encephalomyelitis) (13, 14) and anti-Ri (paraneoplastic opsoclonus) (15) antibodies have identical patterns of immunohistochemical reactivity on sections of cerebral cortex, but they identify different nuclear antigens by Western blotting (16).

Immunohistochemistry

Avidin–Biotin Peroxidase Method

Frozen tissue samples are preferred for this assay. Fresh tissue samples are embedded in Optimal Cutting Temperature Compound (Miles, Inc., Elkhart, IN), snap frozen in isopentane that has been chilled with liquid nitrogen, and stored at −70°C until use. To assay, cut 5- to 7-μm-thick tissue sections and allow to come to room temperature. Fix for 10 min in cold acetone (4°C), wash three times (5 min each) in phosphate-buffered saline (PBS), and then incubate for 10 min at room temperature with 0.3% hydrogen peroxide (to destroy endogenous peroxide activity) followed by several washes with PBS. Incubate sections for 30 min at room temperature with 10% normal serum (diluted in PBS) from the same animal species from which the secondary labeled antibody is made (to block nonspecific binding of the secondary antibody). Remove the blocking serum by aspiration, and incubate with the patient's serum (diluted 1 : 500 and 1 : 5000) for 1 hr at room temperature. Dilutions are made in 10% blocking serum. Remove the human serum and wash several times with PBS, then incubate for 1 hr at room temperature with a biotinylated anti-human immunoglobulin G (IgG) antibody (usually made in goat, from Vector, Burlingame, CA), diluted 1 : 2000. Dilutions can be made using the 10% blocking serum indicated above or 1% bovine serum albumin (BSA) in PBS. Wash several times with PBS, incubate for 30 min with avidin–biotin peroxidase complex (Vectastain Elite Kit, Vector), and wash again with PBS. Reactions are developed with 0.05% diaminobenzidine hydrochloride, 0.05% Triton-X 100, and 0.01% hydrogen peroxide in PBS. The developing time may vary from assay to assay; for sections of frozen tissue it usually takes 1 to 2 min, but if paraffin sections are used (see below) it may take 10–15 min. The reaction can be stopped at any time, by placing the slides in PBS; check the reactivity under the microscope, and continue developing with diaminobenzidine if needed. Sections may be counterstained with hematoxylin. After counterstaining, dehydrate by sequential 2-min washes with 70, 95, and 100% ethanol, followed by xylene, and mount with Permount (Fisher, Pittsburgh, PA). Tissue sections incubated with serum from normal individuals and from patients with antineuronal antibodies serve as negative and positive controls.

Some epitopes are preserved in formalin-fixed paraffin-embedded tissue. If paraffin tissues are used, 7-μm-thick sections of tissue are deparaffinized by heating to 60°C for 1 hr, followed by immediate immersion in xylene and rehydration with sequential 10-min washes with 100, 95, and 70% ethanol, then PBS. Sections are then treated as indicated for frozen tissues, skipping the fixation with acetone. Longer incubations (overnight) may be used for the primary serum (human serum), and the developing reaction with diaminobenzidine usually takes 10–15 min.

Immunofluorescence

The immunofluorescence method is faster than the immunoperoxidase method, but is less sensitive and has more background reactivity due to the presence of lipofucsin in neurons. The fixation and sequential incubations are identical; however, incubation with 0.3% hydrogen peroxide is not necessary. For the secondary labeled antibody we use fluorescein-labeled anti-human IgG antibody (usually made in goat, from Vector). The secondary antibody is diluted 1:400 in blocking serum or 1% BSA in PBS, and incubations are for 30 min at room temperature. Sections are then washed in PBS and mounted in aqueous media (Lipshaw Immonon, Pittsburgh, PA).

Preparation of Antigens for Western Blotting

Because several antineuronal antibodies with similar immunohistochemical reactivity, but different antigen specificity, have been reported (16), the antigen identified by these antibodies should always be characterized by Western blot analysis. Immunoblots of crude preparations of either cortical neurons or cerebellar Purkinje cells are sufficient for this purpose. Isolation of cerebral cortical neurons and Purkinje cells is carried out following modifications of the methods of Blomstrand and Hamberger (17) and Yanagihara and Hamberger (18). Both preparations are made on ice or in a 4°C cold room, from human tissue obtained within 16 hr of death. If necessary, tissue may be stored overnight at 4°C in RPMI 1640 (GIBCO, Grand Island, NY).

Cortical Neuron Preparation

Start with approximately 50 to 80 g of cerebral cortex. Trim the white matter, meninges and vascular tissue from the underlying cortex, weigh, and mince into a slurry. Mix with 2% Ficoll in 0.32 *M* sucrose, 10 m*M* Tris–HCl (pH 7.5), 50 m*M* NaCl, 0.5 m*M* EDTA (sucrose buffer) at 0.75 ml/g of original wet weight. Force the suspension through a 1000-μm nylon mesh (Tetko, Inc., Elmsford, NY) 15 times. Dilute the resulting suspension to 12 ml/g of original wet weight in 2% Ficoll (diluted in sucrose buffer) and pass sequentially through 330-μm ($\times$2), 120-μm ($\times$2), 73-μM ($\times$2), and 53-μm ($\times$2) nylon meshes. Centrifuge the resulting suspension at 1500 rpm for 20 min. Resuspend the pellet in sucrose buffer and repeat the centrifugation. Resuspend the pellet in 30% Ficoll and pass through the 53-μm mesh. Layer the suspension on a nonlinear Ficoll gradient, prepared as follows: 5 ml 2 *M* sucrose in 50 m*M* Tris–HCl (pH 7.4), 4 ml 40% Ficoll, 5 ml 30% Ficoll, 10–15 ml 20% Ficoll containing the cortical homogenate, 5 ml 15% Ficoll, 5 ml 10% Ficoll. All Ficoll solutions are diluted in sucrose buffer. Centrifuge in a SW 28 rotor at 17,000 rpm (54,000 *g*) for 120 min at 4°C.

The fraction containing neurons is collected from the 30% Ficoll and 40% sucrose layers, diluted with an equal volume of sucrose buffer, and centrifuged at 1500 rpm for 20 min. Resuspend the pellet in sucrose buffer and check for the presence of neurons and purity of the preparation by diluting a small volume with trypan blue and examining under a microscope. The cells may be recentrifuged, resuspended in PBS, protein determined, and then stored in aliquots at −70°C.

Purkinje Cell Preparation

Follow the above protocol for preparation of cortical neurons with these modifications. The slurry of minced cerebellum is passed through the 1000-, 330-, 120-, and 73-μm meshes only. Prior to layering on the Ficoll gradient, repass the suspension once through the 120- and 73-μm meshes. The nonlinear Ficoll gradient is prepared as follows: 5 ml 2 *M* sucrose in 50 m*M* Tris–HCl (pH 7.4), 3.5 ml 40% Ficoll, 3.5 ml 30% Ficoll, 5 ml 23% Ficoll, 10–12 ml 20% Ficoll containing the cerebellar suspension, 3 ml 15% Ficoll, 3 ml 12% Ficoll, 3 ml 10% Ficoll. Centrifuge in a SW 28 rotor at 21,000 rpm (81,000*g*) for 100 min. Purkinje cells will be found in the 30% Ficoll layer and the upper part of the 40% Ficoll layer. A red band just below this layer will contain some Purkinje cells mixed with capillaries. Granule cells with occasional Purkinje cells may be found in the 40% Ficoll/2 *M* sucrose interface. Collect the Purkinje cell fraction, dilute with an equal volume of sucrose buffer, and centrifuge at 1500 rpm for 20 min. Resuspend pellets in sucrose buffer and check for Purkinje cells and purity of the preparation as noted above for cortical neurons. Recentrifuge and resuspend pellet in PBS, measure protein, and store in aliquots at −70°C.

Western Blotting

Use approximately 15 μg of crude cortical neuron or Purkinje cell protein preparation per lane. Protein samples are boiled for 10 min in an equal volume of sample buffer [0.125 m*M* Tris–HCl (pH 6.8), 4% sodium dodecyl sulfate (SDS), 0.01% bromophenol blue, 10% 2-mercaptoethanol, and 20% glycerol]. Proteins are separated in a 10% SDS–polyacrylamide gel electrophoresis with a 5% polyacrylamide–SDS stacking gel and transferred to nitrocellulose as described by Towbin *et al.* (19). The nitrocellulose filter is blocked with 5% Blotto (5% Carnation evaporated milk in PBS) overnight at 4°C. After blocking, cut the nitrocellulose into strips and incubate with serum (1 : 1000) or CSF (1 : 10 to 1 : 50) for 2 hr at room temperature. Serum and CSF are diluted in 10 m*M* Tris–HCl (pH 7.4), 1% BSA, 0.9% NaCl, 0.5% Triton X-100 (TBST buffer). After incubation, filters are washed three times with TBST buffer for 15 min each, incubated with ^{125}I-labeled protein A (0.1 μCi/ml) for 1 hr at room temperature, washed again three times with TBST buffer, dried and exposed to Kodak XAR film at −70°C.

To determine if the protein antigen identified by Western blot is the same antigen visualized by immunohistochemistry, the serum IgG is immunopurified on nitrocellulose strips containing the immobilized antigen as shown in Fig. 1. Proteins are separated on a SDS–polyacrylamide gel and transferred to nitrocellulose as described above. Strips of nitrocellulose from both sides are made (Figs. 1A and 1B) and incubated with a high antibody titer serum to accurately identify the position of the antigen on the nitrocellulose. The remaining nitrocellulose is divided into two pieces and incubated with serum containing the antineuronal antibody (1) or a negative control serum (2). The segment of the nitrocellulose that contains the antigen is removed (Figs. 1C and 1D) and each divided into small pieces. The bound IgG is eluted with 0.1 *M* sodium citrate (pH 2.5), neutralized with Trizma base (pH 8.8), and dialyzed against PBS. After dialysis, the immunopurified antibody (from Fig. 1C) can be used undiluted for immunohistochemistry. Eluate from Fig. 1D serves as a negative control.

For laboratories wishing to avoid the use of radioactive chemicals Western

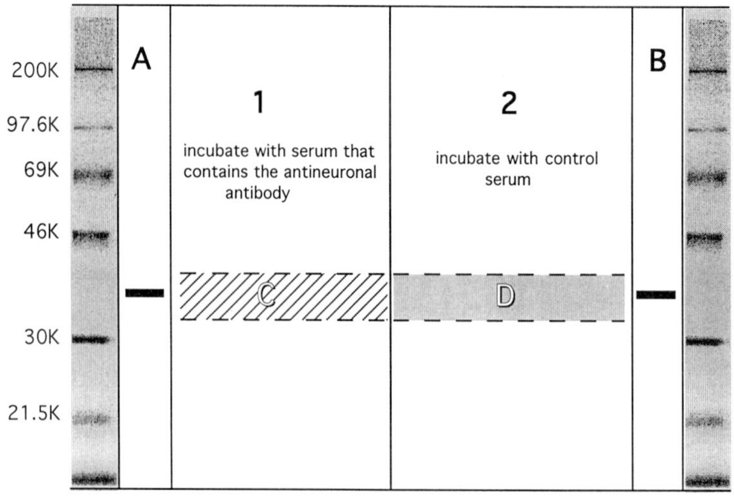

FIG. 1 Immunopurification of IgG from nitrocellulose.

blot filters may be developed using enhanced chemilluminescence (ECL, Amersham, Arlington Heights, IL), according to the manufacturer's specifications.

Measurement of Antibody Titer in Serum and Cerebrospinal Fluid by Western Blot Analysis

Quantitation and comparison of antibody titers in serum and CSF determine whether the antibody is synthesized intrathecally and allow for monitoring of titers.

Titers of antineuronal antibodies are determined by quantitative Western blotting. Increasing amounts of sera are incubated with nitrocellulose strips containing identical amounts of antigen. Conditions are established in which the amount of binding of IgG to the antigen is proportional to the amount of IgG used. The amount of ^{125}I-labeled protein A bound to the segment of the strip that contains the immobilized antigen is taken as a measure of antibody titer. The nonspecific binding of IgG is measured by determining the amount of ^{125}I-labeled protein A bound to the same segment of a strip incubated with serum obtained from a normal individual. The segment of the nitrocellulose strips corresponding to the antigen is cut out and 5 ml of scintillation solution (CytoScint, ICN Biomedicals, Inc., Costa Mesa, CA) is added. The strips are then counted in a liquid scintillation counter. We have defined 1 unit of antibody as the amount of antibody that yields 10,000 cpm of bound ^{125}I-labeled protein A. The normal serum value (usually less than 6 U) is subtracted from the value obtained for the strip incubated with the patient's serum.

Study of Expression of Paraneoplastic Antigens in Tissue

The expression of paraneoplastic antigens by normal human tissues and tumor tissues can be studied by immunohistochemistry and Western blotting (4, 14). At present, there are no monoclonal antineuronal antibodies available, so serum from patients with high titers of antineuronal antibodies must be used.

However, the use of human serum in immunohistochemical studies of human tissue is complicated by the presence of high concentrations of endogenous IgG in human tissue. This is not a problem in normal brain, which does not contain IgG other than IgG present in vessels. Therefore, conventional immunohistochemistry (as described under Detection of Antineuronal Antibodies in Serum and Cerebrospinal Fluid: Immunohistochemistry, above) in tissues other than brain is usually unsuccessful because the reaction of the secondary antibody (usually goat anti-human IgG) with endogenous IgG obscures the reactivity of the primary antibody. The isolation and biotinylation of the IgG from the serum of an individual with high titers of antineuronal (IgG) antibodies obviates the requirement for a secondary antibody, avoiding the reactivity with endogenous irrelevant IgG. Before use, the serum from which the IgG will be isolated should be studied in order to rule out the presence of other antibodies with nonneuronal reactivity.

Isolation and Biotinylation of Immunoglobulin G from Serum

Immunoglobulin G is isolated from serum by adsorption to a protein A-Sepharose gel. A column containing protein A-Sepharose beads is prepared according to the manufacturer's instructions. The volume of the column should be half the serum volume. After prewashing the column with 0.1% Nonidet P-40 in PBS, the patient's serum is added, and the column washed extensively (10 times the column volume with 0.1% Nonidet P-40 in PBS). The adsorbed IgG is eluted with sodium citrate (pH 2.5), neutralized with Tris, pH 8.8, and dialyzed against PBS. The purified IgG is reacted with biotin *N*-hydroxysuccinimide ester (Vector) for 2 hr at room temperature. The amount of biotin used in this reaction is $\frac{1}{10}$ the weight of the total amount of IgG. The reaction is terminated by the addition of 10 mg glycine. Free biotin is removed by dialysis against PBS.

Immunohistochemistry with Biotinylated Immunoglobulin G

Seven-micrometer-thick frozen tissue sections are fixed for 10 min in cold acetone and sequentially incubated with 0.3% hydrogen peroxide (to destroy tissue peroxidase activity) and 10% normal human serum (to block nonspecific binding of human IgG). The blocking serum is removed by aspiration, and sections are then incubated with 2.5–10 μg/ml of the biotinylated IgG containing the antineuronal antibody. Bound biotinylated antibody is visualized with the avidin–biotin peroxidase method described under Detection of Antineuronal Antibodies in Serum and Cerebrospinal Fluid: Immunohistochemistry. Incubation of the sections with the same amount of biotinylated IgG obtained from a normal individual serves as the negative control.

Since the biotinylated IgG used in this assay is total IgG isolated from the serum of a patient with a high titer of antineuronal antibodies, there is the possibility that other (non-antineuronal IgG may react with the tissue. A simple and rapid method to test this possibility is to preincubate the section of tissue with undiluted serum from another individual which contains the same antineuronal antibody. The antineuronal antibody contained in this serum will compete and block the reactivity of the biotinylated IgG isolated from the first individual, resulting in abrogation of the immunostaining.

If no other sera containing the same antibody are available the antineuronal IgG should be immunopurified from serum or total IgG. Total biotinylated IgG can be immunopurified by incubating with immunoblots that contain the neuronal antigen (see Detection of Antineuronal Antibodies in Serum and Cerebrospinal Fluid: Western Blotting and Measurement of Antibody Titer in Serum and Cerebrospinal Fluid by Western Blot Analysis). The biotinylated IgG bound to the segment of the immunoblot that contains the neuronal antigen is then eluted using 0.1 *M* sodium citrate (pH 2.5), neutralized with Trizma base (pH 8.8), and dialyzed against PBS. After dialysis, the biotinylated antineuronal antibody can be used undiluted for immunohistochemical studies.

Western Blot Analysis of the Expression of Antigens by Tissues

Fresh or frozen tissues samples are thawed at room temperature and after washing with PBS homogenized with 0.1% Nonidet P-40 in PBS. If frozen tissue blocks are available, serial 30-μm-thick frozen tissue sections are collected, washed in PBS, and then homogenized. Centrifuge homogenates at 15,000 rpm for 10 min at 4°C and measure the protein content of the supernatant. Aliquots of 60–80 μg are electrophoresed on 10% SDS–polyacrylamide gel and transferred to nitrocellulose. The nitrocellulose filter is then blocked with 5% Blotto overnight at 4°C. After blocking, incubate with a serum that contains high titers of the antineuronal antibody (diluted 1 : 500 in TBST buffer, see Detection of Antineuronal Antibodies in Serum and Cerebrospinal Fluid: Western Blotting). After incubation wash three times with TBST buffer for 15 min each, incubate with ^{125}I-labeled protein A (0.1 μCi/ml) for 1 hr at room temperature; wash again three times with TBST, dry, and expose to film overnight at −70°C. Immunoblots containing the same amount of protein, incubated with serum from a normal individual, serve as a negative control.

Analysis of Endogenous Immunoglobulin G

Since normal brain tissue (excluding vessels) does not contain IgG, the presence of abnormal deposits of IgG can easily be demonstrated by immunohistochemistry. The IgG found in the nervous system, along with IgG contained in other tissues and tumor, can be eluted and further characterized by quantitative Western blot analysis (20).

Immunohistochemical Analysis of Endogenous Immunoglobulin G in Brain Tissue

The goal of this assay is to study the presence of IgG in brain; therefore, the tissue substrate is usually sections of brain obtained at autopsy from a patient with a paraneoplastic disorder. The steps of this assay are identical to those described above under Detection of Antineuronal Antibodies in Serum and Cerebrospinal Fluid: Immunohistochemistry, omitting the incubation with the patient's serum. Only incubation with biotinylated anti-human IgG is used in this assay. Sections of brain obtained at autopsy from a neurologically normal individual serve as control tissue.

Quantitation of Immunoglobulin G

Quantitation of IgG is required for comparison of IgG antibody titers contained in samples obtained at different times or from different tissues of the same individual. Immunoglobulin G can be quantified by reaction with ^{125}I-labeled protein A in a dot-blot assay.

A nitrocellulose filter is moistened in double-distilled water and then air-dried. Aliquots of serum, CSF, or fractions with IgG eluted from tissues are dotted onto the dry nitrocellulose filters and blocked with 5% Blotto for a minimum of 2 hr at room temperature. Incubate with ^{125}I-labeled protein A (0.1 μCi/ml) for 1 hr at room temperature. After being washed three times for 15 min each with 0.1% Nonidet P-40 in PBS, the filters are dried and apposed to X-ray film. The radioactive dots are located and the radioactivity determined by liquid scintillation spectroscopy (see Measurement of Antibody Titer in Serum and Cerebrospinal Fluid by Western Blot Analysis). For each determination a standard curve is performed using known amounts of human IgG (Quantitrol, Kallestad, Chaska, MN).

Western Blot Quantitation of Extracted Antineuronal Antibody

Pieces of frozen tissue are thawed at room temperature, washed and homogenized in PBS, centrifuged at 15,000 rpm for 10 min, resuspended in PBS, and centrifuged again. The pellet is retained. Immunoglobulin G bound to tissue is extracted by resuspending the pellet with 0.5 ml of 0.1 *M* sodium citrate (pH 2.5) and centrifuging at 15,000 for 10 min at 4°C. The supernatant containing the eluted IgG is neutralized with Trizma base (pH 8.8). The concentration of total IgG in the eluates from tissues is measured as described under Quantitation of Immunoglobulin G, above.

The content of antineuronal antibody in the eluted fractions is then established by Western blot analysis using nitrocellulose strips containing immobilized neuronal antigen. For comparative analysis of the amount of antibody contained in different areas of brain, tumor, or other tissues (including serum and CSF), the same amount of total IgG eluted from each area should be used in the Western blot analysis. Quantitation of the antibody is based on the amount of ^{125}I-labeled protein A bound to the segment of the immunoblot which contains the immobilized antigen (see Measurement of Antibody Titer in Serum and Cerebrospinal Fluid by Western Blot Analysis, above). Immunoglobulin G eluted from the brain of a neurologically normal individual serves as a negative control.

Acknowledgment

We thank Dr. Jerome B. Posner for advice and support.

References

1. J. B. Posner, *Curr. Neurol.* **9,** 245 (1989).
2. F. Graus, K. B. Elkon, C. Cordon-Cardo, and J. B. Posner, *Am. J. Med.* **80,** 52 (1986).

3. J. E. Greenlee, and H. R. Brashear, *Ann. Neurol.* **14,** 609 (1983).
4. H. M. Furneaux, M. K. Rosenblum, J. Dalmau, *et al., N. Engl. J. Med.* **322,** 1844 (1990).
5. J. Dalmau, H. M. Furneaux, R. J. Gralla, M. G. Kris, J. B. Posner, *Ann. Neurol.* **27,** 544, (1990).
6. M. Solimena, F. Folli, S. Denis-Donini, *et al., N. Engl. J. Med.* **318,** 1012 (1988).
7. R. B. Darnell, J. Victor, M. Rubin, P. Clouston, and F. Plum, *Neurology* **43,** 114 (1993).
8. R. J. Polinsky, A. McRae, S. M. Baser and A. Dahlstrom, *J. Neurol. Sci.* **106,** 96 (1991).
9. R. G. Smith, S. Hamilton, F. Hofmann, *et al. N. Engl. J. Med.* **327,** 1721 (1992).
10. E. J. Dropcho, Y.-T. Chen, J. B. Posner, L. J. Old, *Proc. Natl. Acad. Sci. U.S.A.* **84,** 4552 (1987).
11. H. Fathallah-Shaykh, S. Wolf, E. Wong, J. B. Posner, and H. M. Furneaux, *Proc. Natl. Acad. Sci. U.S.A.* **88,** 3451 (1991).
12. A. Szabo, J. Dalmau, G. Manley, *et al., Cell (Cambridge, Mass.)* **67,** 325 (1991).
13. F. Graus, C. Cordon-Cardo, and J. B. Posner, *Neurology* **35,** 538 (1985).
14. J. Dalmau, H. M. Furneaux, C. Cordon-Cardo, and J. B. Posner, *Am. J. Pathol.* **141,** 881 (1992).
15. F. A. Luque, H. M. Furneaux, R. Ferziger, *et al., Ann. Neurol.* **29,** 241 (1991).
16. F. Graus, G. Rowe, J. Fueyo, R. B. Darnell, and J. Dalmau, *Neurosci. Lett.* **150,** 212 (1993).
17. C. Blomstrand and A. Hamberger, *J. Neurochem.* **16,** 1401 (1969).
18. T. Yanagihara and A. Hamberger, *Brain Res.* **59,** 445 (1973).
19. H. Towbin, T. Staehelin, and J. Gordon, *Proc. Natl. Acad. Sci. U.S.A.* **76,** 4350 (1979).
20. J. Dalmau, H. M. Furneaux, M. K. Rosenblum, F. Graus and J. B. Posner, *Neurology* **41,** 1757 (1991).

[17] Immunohistochemistry of Leukocyte Antigens in Rat Brain

Wolfgang J. Streit, Alexander G. Rabchevsky, Daniel P. Theele, and William F. Hickey

Introduction

The availability of monoclonal antibodies directed against immune system antigens, such as major histocompatibility complex (MHC) antigens, lymphocyte, and myelomonocytic markers, has contributed significantly to our understanding of cellular neuroimmunology in recent years. Antibodies against rat leukocyte antigens have been especially useful because rat models are widely used to study a variety of neuropathologic disease mechanisms. These antibodies, which became available in the 1980s, have been critical for defining a role of central nervous system (CNS) microglial cells as endogenous immunocompetent cells of the brain (1). Contrary to earlier studies conducted *in vitro* claiming a role for astrocytes as antigen-presenting cells (APCs) of the CNS (2), subsequent immunohistochemical work conducted *in vivo* failed to support this concept by showing that microglial cells, and not astrocytes, are the parenchymal cells of the CNS capable of expressing MHC antigens *in situ* (3, 4). The immunohistochemical detection of MHC antigens on microglia was a fundamental observation which changed the preexisting view of the brain as an immunologically privileged organ that is largely devoid of immunocompetent cells. Even though the immunohistochemical detection of MHC antigens cannot in itself prove that microglia are functional APCs causing lymphocytes to proliferate, it is now generally accepted that microglia, among the three glial cell populations, are the best candidates for indigenous APCs of the CNS. The present chapter is intended to provide a concise summary of our experiences with monoclonal antibodies against rat leukocyte antigens used for the monitoring of microglial activation during various neuropathological states.

Functional Plasticity of Microglia

The term *functional plasticity* is used to describe changes in microglial morphology and surface antigen expression that are observed to occur as a result of motor neuron injury (4). Axotomy of the rat facial or optic nerves is

Methods in Neurosciences, Volume 24

known to induce localized microglial proliferation and activation (5–7), and the consistent reproducibility of these types of acute lesions has provided good models to study the various stages of microglial activation. Microglia in the normal uninjured brain exist as *resting microglia* that are quickly transformed into the *activated* or *reactive* state as soon as neuronal injury occurs. If the injury is severe enough to cause neuronal degeneration, the reactive microglia may further transform into a *phagocytic* state, giving rise to microglia-derived brain macrophages. The transitions from resting to reactive and/or phagocytic are not only marked by characteristic changes in morphology, but also entail striking changes in immunophenotype, i.e., they either cause the *de novo* expression of previously absent surface antigens or induce the upregulation of previously existing surface antigens (see Fig. 1). The term *immunomolecules* is used here to refer to this group of antigens because the antigens expressed by microglia are usually found on immunologically active cells, such as blood mononuclear cells. Table I lists the various kinds of immunomolecules associated with microglial activation states, as well as the antibodies used to detect them. As can be seen from Table I, a number of immunomolecules are expressed constitutively by resting microglia in the normal brain. The strongest constitutive expression is seen with the C3bi complement receptor which is found on virtually all resting microglia (8). Leukocyte common antigen (LCA), the CD4 coreceptor, as well as MHC antigens are expressed only weakly by some scattered microglial cells in the normal brain. These weakly immunopositive microglia predominate in white matter regions (9, 10). When microglia become activated following an injury the expression of LCA, CD4, and MHC class II antigens does not involve all of the activated microglia, but only a select few. Presumably, these MHC class II positive microglia are the functional antigen-presenting cells. While resting microglia are not labeled with antibodies ED1, ED2, ED3, these antibodies do stain perivascular cells (macrophage-like cells associated with blood vessel walls) in the normal brain (11). The epitopes recognized by antibodies of the ED series do become expressed to some extent on activated microglia (12). Regarding the CD8 epitope, it is possible that this surface antigen becomes expressed weakly by some microglia in brain tumors (13), however, this will require further investigation.

Detection of Immunomolecules in Rat Brain

Fixation and Tissue Processing

Initial attempts to localize MHC antigens in the human and rodent CNS were largely unsuccessful and seemed to support the existing view of the brain as an immunologically privileged organ (14–16). It is likely that these

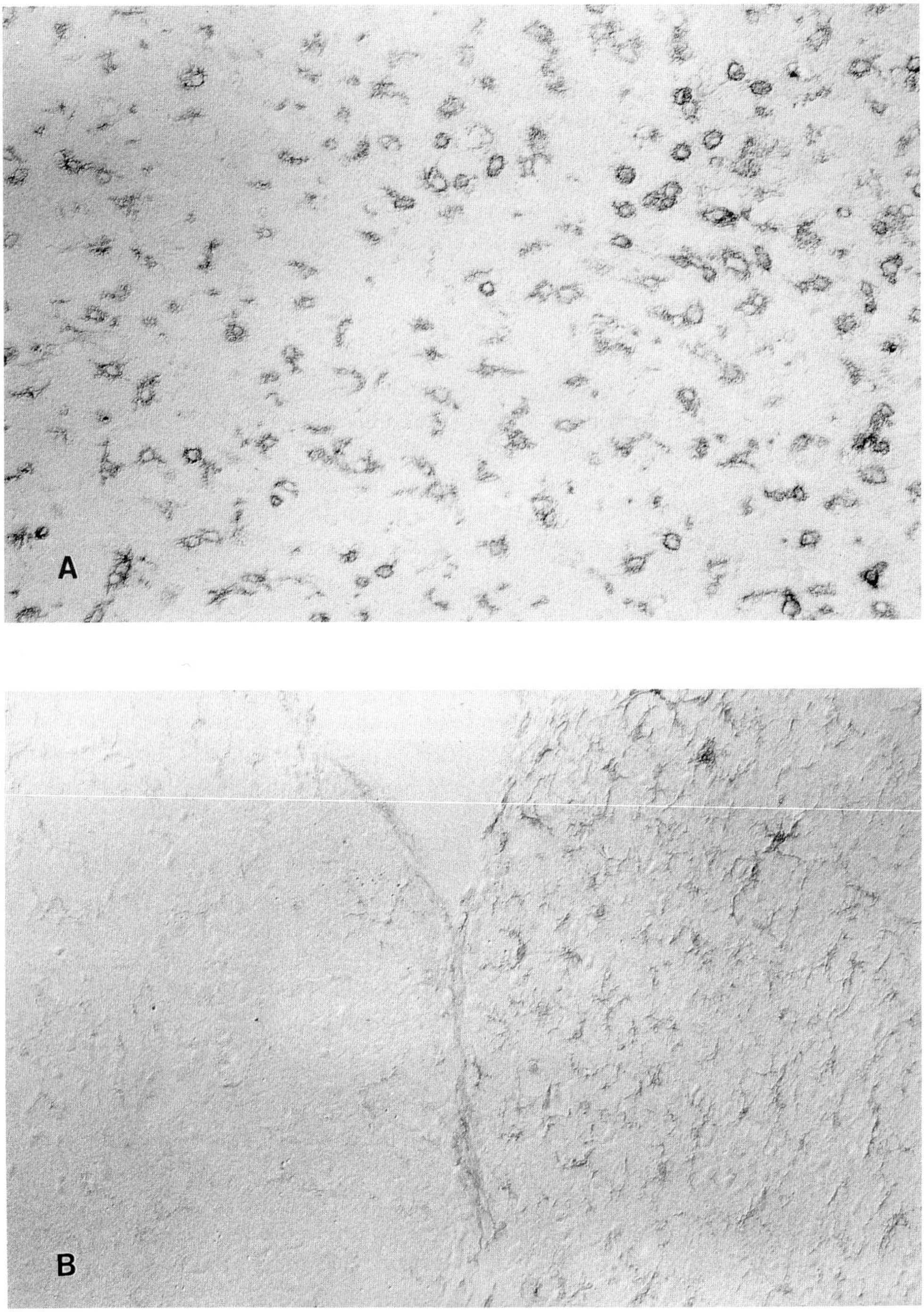
A
B

TABLE I Differential Expression of Immunomolecules on Rat Microglia during Resting, Activated, and Phagocytic States

Type of immunomolecule	Cluster of differentiation nomenclature	Antibody designation[a]	Microglial activation state[c]		
			Resting	Activated	Phagocytic
Leukocyte common antigen	CD45	OX-1	±	+	+
T-helper cell coreceptor	CD4	W3/25	±	+	+
T-suppressor/cytotoxic cell coreceptor	CD8	OX-8	−	±(?)	±(?)
Pan T lymphocyte	CD43	W3/13	−	−	−
MHC class I	—	OX-18	±	+	+
		OX-27[b]			
MHC class II	—	OX-6	±	+	+
		OX-17	±	+	+
		OX-3[b]			
C3bi complement receptor	—	OX-42	+	+	+
Brain macrophage antigen	—	ED1, ED2, ED3	−	±	±

[a] All antibodies are commercially available from Harlan Bioproducts for Science, Indianapolis, IN.

[b] These antibodies are directed against polymorphic determinants that are expressed only in certain rat strains. We have not evaluated the expression of these in the appropriate strains.

[c] Rating scale: (−) not expressed; (±) weakly expressed; (+) strongly expressed

negative findings were, at least in part, due to the extraordinary susceptibility of immunomolecules to conventional fixation procedures using aldehydes which quickly result in cross-linking of membrane antigens, and thus in a lack of epitope recognition by the monoclonal antibodies. Because the stability and degree of cross-linking by aldehyde fixatives varies with the type of fixative employed, e.g., glutaraldehyde (a dialdehyde) causes more stable and faster cross-linking than formaldehyde (a monoaldehyde), careful consideration should be given to the type and concentration of fixative to be used. Because rat leukocyte antigens are very sensitve to cross-linking by aldehydes, in those cases where perfusion fixation of the tissue is needed, such as immunoelectron microscopy, it is generally advisable to use low concen-

FIG. 1 (A) Brain parenchyma adjacent to the fibrous capsule of an experimental staphylococcal abscess. The hematogenously derived macrophages stain as dark rings while the activated, endogenous microglial cells are paler, arborizing cells (OX-42 immunohistochemistry). (B) MHC class I expression is induced on microglia of one superior colliculus (right-hand side) 4 days following contralateral optic nerve transection. No such MHC expression is noted in the normally innervated colliculus on the left (OX-18 immunohistochemistry). Magnification ×184.5.

trations of formaldehyde (2–4%) prepared freshly from paraformaldehyde, rather than glutaraldehyde. Furthermore, since the degree of cross-linking of the relevant antigens by a given fixation regimen cannot be predicted, short fixation times should be used (less than 24 hr). A number of published studies have reported successful immunolocalization of rat leukocyte antigens using paraformaldehyde-fixed tissue (17–26). As is often the case in ultrastructural immunohistochemistry, immunoreactivity can only be maintained at the expense of tissue preservation so that both good structure and robust immunostaining are difficult to obtain. We recommend the following protocol of tissue processing for immunostaining of fixed tissue:

1. Perfuse transcardially with 50–100 ml of phosphate-buffered saline (PBS) followed by 200–300 ml of 2% paraformaldehyde prepared freshly in 0.1 *M* phosphate buffer, pH 7.4.
2. Remove tissue of interest.
3. Postfix for 30–60 min in 2% paraformaldehyde.
4. Rinse with 0.2 *M* phosphate buffer, pH 7.4, until no obvious paraformaldehyde vapor persists.
5. Keep in 0.2 *M* phosphate buffer overnight at 4° C.
6. Cut sections on vibratome (50–60 μm), and process for immunostaining (see below).

Notes

Although the paraformaldehyde solution should be prepared fresh each time, the stock solution is stable at 4°C in the dark for several days. Use the granular (prill) form of paraformaldehyde, and prepare a 4% stock solution in water. Equal volumes of the stock and 0.2 *M* phosphate buffer can then be combined to make the perfusate. For details on the preparation of fixatives and buffers see Ref. 27. Tissue can be stored for extended periods in the 0.2 *M* phosphate buffer if a small amount of a 1% solution of sodium azide is added to the buffer. Storage should be at 4°C; however, note that slats will precipitate around the tissue. This does not damage the tissue, but should be dissolved at room temperature before the tissue is used. For vibratome sectioning it may be helpful to embed pieces of tissue in 2–4% agarose.

If electron microscopy is not desired and only light microscopy of perfusion-fixed tissue is needed, it is possible to use a cryostat for tissue sectioning instead of the vibratome. Prior to sectioning in a cryostat, the tissue must be cryoprotected in an aqueous solution of 30% sucrose (or a 20% solution of sucrose in PBS). Following overnight immersion in 30% sucrose at 4°C, the tissue may be embedded in OCT compound (Miles, Inc.) or a similar medium, if needed. The tissue is then frozen, preferably in isopentane cooled to −40 to −60°C by liquid nitrogen. If isopentane is unavailable, small pieces of tissue can also be frozen on glass slides that have been placed on blocks of dry ice. The ambient temperature inside the cryostat for cutting fixed frozen sections should be set at −18°C or lower.

In cases where tissue fixation by perfusion is not needed or wanted, i.e., if only light microscopy is desired, fresh frozen sections can be cut on a cryostat followed by brief fixation of the mounted sections. We recommend the following protocol (see also Refs. 8, 10–13, 28–32):

1. Remove tissue of interest and freeze as described above. The frozen tissue can be stored at −80°C; if it is to be cut immediately, the frozen tissue should be placed in the cryostat for 30 min allowing it to equilibrate to cryostat temperature prior to cutting.
2. Cut fresh frozen sections of 20–25 μm thickness on a cryostat at −12°C.
3. Mount sections on gelatin-coated (subbed) slides.
4. Air-dry sections for 20–30 min at room temperature.
5. Fix the sections by immersing slides consecutively in the following solutions at room temperature:
   3.7% (v/v) formaldehyde in 0.1 *M* phosphate buffer for 5 min
   50% acetone for 2 min
   100% acetone for 2 min
   50% acetone for 2 min
   PBS for 5 min (2×).

Notes

It is recommended that animals be perfused with 0.9% saline (or PBS) prior to dissection of the tissue in order to remove blood. This does not only expedite the dissection, but also results in the removal of peroxidase-containing erythrocytes from the vascular channels. The latter is of considerable advantage when using peroxidase-based detection techniques because it drastically reduces the nonspecific background staining due to endogenous peroxidase.

Cryostat sections can be cut thinner than 20 μm, if desired. However, this is not critical for obtaining good results, and the novice may find it easier to prepare 20-μm sections.

It is important to ensure that the sections are dried completely before proceeding with step 5, otherwise they may slip off the slides when placed into the solutions. The formaldehyde fixation step may be shortened or completely omitted if staining is not successful. An alternate way of processing the tissue is to fix the freshly cut and mounted sections in absolute methanol in a Coplin jar which has equilibrated to cryostat temperature. After 30 to 60 sec of methanol fixation the sections should be rinsed extensively in 0.5 *M* Tris, pH 7.6, and then placed for at least another 10 min in the same buffer prior to applying primary antibodies. The choice of fixative is always a critical issue relative to any single antigen. For fresh frozen tissue absolute methanol works well. Nevertheless, for the rat MHC class II molecule, diethyl ether is also an excellent (and some believe superior) fixative. For some antigens acetone or absolute ethanol work well, although they are not optimal for certain glycoprotein antigens like CD4. For any antigen it is best to try a number of fixatives to determine which fixation is optimal.

Both Tris and phosphate buffers have been used successfully for immunostaining, and it is difficult to say which one of these is the better choice.

Immunostaining Procedures

When reading published staining methods from various laboratories, it is apparent immediately that there is virtually an unlimited number of modifications that can be made in the staining protocol with regard to antibody concentrations, incubation times, choices of buffers, etc. Obviously, these are factors which will not make a difference if the tissue is processed improperly and immunoreactivity of the antigens to be localized has been destroyed. Conversely, if the tissue has been properly prepared the antibody concentrations, as well as the length and temperature of the incubation, can often be varied over a wide range of values without losing or gaining much in the final product. For example, monoclonal antibody OX-6 gives virtually identical results whether it is used at 1 : 100 or 1 : 2000 dilution, or whether the incubation period was 1 hr at room temperature or 18 hr at 4°C. In other words, if the antigen is preserved well enough for the antibody to recognize it, then the binding of antibody to antigen occurs rapidly and consistently. Thus, for the immunohistochemical detection of rat leukocyte antigens the greatest care has to be taken in the tissue preparation, and if this is done properly then the actual staining is easily accomplished. Accordingly, the staining method below is intended to serve only as a guideline rather than providing a detailed protocol that must be followed exactly.

1. Prepare a solution of 1% bovine serum albumin in PBS (PBS/BSA).
2. Incubate sections in PBS/BSA for 15 min at room temperature.
3. Dilute primary antibodies in PBS/BSA.
4. Incubate sections in primary antibodies at 4°C overnight.
5. Rinse with PBS (3×, 5 min each).
6. Incubate sections in biotinylated secondary (linking) antibody, diluted in PBS, for 1 hr at room temperature.
7. Rinse with PBS (3×, 5 min each).
8. Incubate sections in the appropriately diluted avidin conjugate of the

desired detection reagent (e.g., avidin–peroxidase or avidin–fluorochrome) for 45 min at room temperature.

9. Rinse with PBS (3×, 5 min each).
10. Carry out substrate reaction (for enzyme-based detection) or view under fluorescent microscope.

Notes

The PBS/BSA should always be made fresh. If an antibody is to be used for the first time, we strongly recommended a dilution series; that is, try various dilutions of the primary antibody, e.g., 1 : 100, 1 : 500, 1 : 1000, 1 : 2000. The addition of detergents, such as Triton X-100, to the PBS/BSA is optional, but not critical for the detection of rat leukocyte antigens.

The secondary biotinylated antibody (linking antibody) should be preabsorbed with normal serum from the rat strain in which the staining is done in order to reduce nonspecific background staining. This is accomplished by mixing equal volumes (10–100 μl) of the undiluted biotinylated antibody and strain-specific serum in a microcentrifuge tube and letting it sit at room temperature for 15 min. The mixture is then diluted with PBS, based on the volume of linking antibody only, not the total volume! Typical dilutions for secondary antibodies are 1 : 200 or 1 : 400, but again, a dilution series is recommended. Various substrates yielding differing colored reaction products are available for peroxidase-based detection systems. Among these, 3,3′-diaminobenzidine (DAB) is perhaps the most commonly employed, and it is prepared as follows: dissolve 3–5 mg of DAB per 10 ml of buffer, add 10 μl of 3% H_2O_2 for every 10 ml of DAB solution, and incubate slides in DAB–H_2O_2 medium for a maximum of 10 min.

References

1. M. B. Graeber and W. J. Streit, *Brain Pathol.* **1,** 2 (1990).
2. A. Fontana, W. Fierz, and H. Wekerle, *Nature (London)* **307,** 273 (1984).
3. W. F. Hickey and H. Kimura, *Science* **239,** 290 (1988).
4. W. J. Streit, M. B. Graeber, and G. W. Kreutzberg, *Glia* **1,** 301 (1988).
5. G. W. Kreutzberg, *Acta Neuropathol. (Berlin)* **7,** 149 (1966).
6. M. B. Graeber, W. Tetzlaff, W. J. Streit, and G. W. Kreutzberg, *Neurosci. Lett.* **85,** 317 (1988).
7. M. C. Molleston, M. L. Thomas, and W. F. Hickey, *Adv. Neurol.* **59,** 333 (1993).
8. M. B. Graeber, W. J. Streit, and G. W. Kreutzberg, *J. Neurosci. Res.* **21,** 18 (1988).
9. V. H. Perry and S. Gordon, *J. Exp. Med.* **166,** 1138 (1987).
10. W. J. Streit, M. B. Graeber, and G. W. Kreutzberg, *Exp. Neurol.* **105,** 115 (1989).

11. M. B. Graeber, W. J. Streit, and G. W. Kreutzberg, *J. Neurosci. Res.* **22,** 103 (1989).
12. M. B. Graeber, W. J. Streit, R. Kiefer, S. W. Schoen, and G. W. Kreutzberg, *J. Neuroimmunol.* **27,** 121 (1990).
13. T. Morioka, T. Baba, K. L. Black, and W. J. Streit, *Acta Neuropathol. (Berlin)* **83,** 590 (1992).
14. M. Oehmichen, H. Wiethölter, and M. F. Greaves, *J. Neuropathol. Exp. Neurol.* **38,** 99 (1979).
15. D. N. Hart and J. W. Fabre, *J. Exp. Med.* **153,** 347 (1981).
16. L. A. Lampson, *Trends Neurosci.* **10,** 211 (1987).
17. K. Rao and R. D. Lund, *Brain Res.* **488,** 332 (1989).
18. K. T. Yee, A. M. Smetanka, R. D. Lund, and K. Rao, *Brain Res.* **530,** 121 (1990).
19. E. A. Ling, C. Kaur, T. Y. Yick, and W. C. Wong, *Anat. Embryol.* **182,** 481 (1990).
20. H. Konno, T. Yamamoto, H. Suzuki, H. Yamamoto, Y. Iwasaki, Y. Ohara, H. Terunuma, and N. Harata, *Acta Neuropathol. (Berlin)* **80,** 521 (1990).
21. H. Lassmann, F. Zimprich, K. Vass, and W. F. Hickey, *J. Neurosci. Res.* **28,** 236 (1991).
22. W. F. Hickey, K. Vass, and H. Lassmann, *J. Neuropathol Exp. Neurol.* **51,** 246 (1992).
23. B. R. Finsen, M. B. Jørgensen, N. H. Diemer, and J. Zimmer, *Glia* **7,** 41 (1993).
24. J. Gehrmann, R. Gold, C. Linington, J. Lannes-Vieira, H. Wekerle, and G. W. Kreutzberg, *Glia* **7,** 50 (1993).
25. V. H. Perry, M. K. Matyszak, and S. Fearn, *Glia* **7,** 60 (1993).
26. P. G . Popovich, W. J. Streit, and B. T. Stokes, *J. Neurotrauma* **10,** 37 (1993).
27. A. M. Glauert, "Fixation, Dehydration and Embedding of Biological Specimens." North-Holland/American Elsevier, New York, 1975.
28. Y. Matsumoto, K. Kawai, and M. Fujiwara, *Immunology* **66,** 621 (1989).
29. M. Poltorak and W. J. Freed, *Exp. Neurol.* **103,** 222 (1989).
30. W. J. Streit, M. B. Graeber, and G. W. Kreutzberg, *J. Neuroimmunol.* **21,** 117 (1989).
31. T. Morioka and W. J. Streit, *J. Neuroimmunol.* **35,** 21 (1991).
32. W. J. Streit and M. B. Graeber, *Glia* **7,** 68 (1993).

Section III

Neuroimmune System: Effects of the Brain on the Peripheral Immune System

[18] Measuring Immune Responses to Brain Manipulation in Rat

M. Ian Phillips and Lewis D. Fannon

Introduction

Neuroimmunology has a double meaning. On the one hand, it is recognized that the brain has its own immune system and is by definition a neuroimmune system. On the other hand, the central nervous system (CNS) and the autonomic nervous system have effects which alter the peripheral immune system. These effects are therefore also neuroimmune. Since the brain is immune privileged, the two systems might work independently of each other in the absence of feedback and cojointly in the presence of feedback from lymphokine endocrine and neural signals. The brain is in a position to control the peripheral immune system through sympathetic innervation of the thymus, spleen, and lymphoid tissue and by the release from the pituitary of immune signaling peptides. Stress, sensory inputs, and experimentally injected peptides into the brain are all factors which produce disturbances in the population of lymphocytes in blood and it is the lymphocytes which orchestrate the specific immune response. For experiments involving studies on manipulations of the rat brain and their effects on the peripheral immune system, this chapter describes a straightforward method for measuring lymphocyte subpopulations from plasma samples in the rat. The method follows methods used in humans but requires specific monoclonal antibodies to rat antigen receptors. Lymphocytes are derived either from the thymus (T cells) or from the bone marrow in adults (B cells) (1–3). Because the most important function of lymphocytes in the initial response to invasion of nonself molecule is recognition, the lymphocytes can be defined by what they recognize. The T-cell antigen receptors (TCR) recognizes antigen–peptide fragments, presented to the membrane receptor as specialized molecules (major histocompatibility complex molecules, MHC) of which there are two classes: MHC class 1 and MHC class 2 molecules. The T cells are subdivided into two general classes by the MHC class molecules they bind. The T-helper cells (T_H, which in humans are labeled $CD4^+$ cells) recognize the MHC class I molecules and the T-nonhelper or cytotoxic/killer/suppressor cells (which in humans are labeled $CD8^+$ cells) recognize MHC class 2 molecules. The T-helper cells determine what the response to an antigen will be and the T-nonhelper cells carry out the effector response of the immune system. Al-

Methods in Neurosciences, Volume 24

though there are further subdivisions of the T cells into T-helper cell type 1 which produces predominately interleukin 2 (IL-2) and γ-interferon cytokines and T-helper cell type 2 which produces interleukins 4, 5, and 6, much information can be gained by measuring the proportions of $CD4^+$ T cells and $CD8^+$ T cells. In addition, the method described below measures B cells. B cells recognize intact solule antigens and have immunoglobulins as the receptors (in mature B cells these are IgG, IgA, IgE, and occasionally IgM. The B lymphocytes produce antibodies and the T lymphocytes facilitate and potentiate the immune response by first recognizing nonself molecules and, via the T-nonhelper cells, directly killing invading cells. Since both T and B lymphocytes secrete lymphokines which include the interleukins, they exert an effect on local tissue and it is believed that the interleukins and other lymphokines can feedback directly onto the CNS. The method below is accurate and rapid for measurement of ratios of T cells and B cells using fluorescence-activated cell-sorting (FACS) analysis.

Methods

Measurement of Immune System in the Rat

Blood Sampling

Rats are anesthetized with metofane anesthesia. The area of skin covering the left femoral vein is prepared and cleaned with a 70% ethanol solution. A 2-cm incision is made and the femoral vein exposed using minor dissection. Using a 25-gauge, butterfly scalp vein infusion set (Abbott Hospitals, Inc., North Chicago, IL), venipuncture is performed and 1 ml of blood obtained. A cotton swab is used to apply direct pressure to the vessel on removal of the needle. Wound clips are used to close the incision and the blood is placed in sterile vacutainer tubes (Becton–Dickinson, Rutherford, NJ). This method is a fast and efficient mode of blood collection as well as venous drug delivery. It is also useful when repeated samples are needed from the same animal over time, as the same incision and vessel can be used. With practice, blood samples can be collected from 7 to 10 animals in an hour. Also, this method has many advantages over venous catheterization.

Lymphocyte Preparation

The 1-ml whole-blood sample is combined with 1 ml of chilled phosphate-buffered saline (PBS) with 0.1% (w/v) NaN_3. This solution is layered on top of 3 ml of lymphocyte separation medium (LSM, Organon-Teknika, Durham, NC) in a 14-ml conical tube that has been lightly coated with fetal bovine serum (FBS). The tubes are centrifuged at 400*g* for 30 min at 12°C. Following centrifugation, the white layer found between the plasma and LSM is predominantly composed of lymphocytes. This layer is aspirated and placed in a tube coated with FBS and containing 1 ml of chilled PBS with 0.1% NaN_3. All subsequent tubes are lightly coated with FBS to prevent adhesion of cells to the surface of the plastic tubes. The lymphocyte suspension is washed twice with chilled PBS with 0.1% NaN_3 prior to staining with monoclonal antibodies. The cells are washed by adding the PBS and centrifugating at 400*g* for 5 min at 4°C. This is followed by aspiration of most of the supernatant, vortexing the pellet, and the addition of the next 3 ml of chilled PBS.

Four lymphocyte populations are examined: T cells, T-nonhelper cells, T-helper cells, and B cells. Mouse anti-rat monoclonal antibodies (Accurate Chemical, Westbury, NY) are used as primary antibodies and a goat anti-mouse fluorescein isothiocyanate (FITC)-conjugated reagent (Accurate Chemical, Westbury, NY) is used as a secondary antibody. As a control, mouse IgG is used.

For each sample, approximately 1.5×10^6 cells in a 300-μl volume are placed in each of five, labeled, 12×75, clear plastic tubes. The tubes are labeled as follows: control, T cell, T nonhelper, T helper, and B cell. The appropriate concentration of mouse IgG or monoclonal antibody is added to each tube and the tubes are incubated for 30 min at 4°C. Our laboratory has obtained good results by adding 3 μl of the stock antibody solution (the ascites fluid form) to the 300-μl lymphocyte suspension. Following this initial incubation, the cells are washed three times with 3 ml of PBS with 0.1% NaN_3.

After the third wash, the tubes are aspirated to approximately 300 μl and then 100 μl of a 1 : 100 dilution of the secondary FITC-labeled antibody is placed in each tube. The cells are again incubated for 30 min at 4°C. After an additional three washes with 3 ml of PBS with 0.1% NaN_3, each tube is adjusted to a final volume of approximately 500 μl prior to FACS analysis. A summary of these steps is shown in Fig. 1.

The FACS analysis involves hitting a thin stream of the cell suspension with a laser and then utilizing light detectors to collect the scattered light. All samples are run on a FACStar Plus (Bector–Dickinson, Rutherford, NJ). Information regarding cell size and granularity can be obtained and utilized to study selectively a single population of cells, such as lymphocytes in this case (Fig. 2). Fluorescently labeled cells can also be quantified by this method (Fig. 3).

Results

The method has been used to test effects of hypothesized overactivity of brain peptides by using genetically hypertensive rats (SHR) and by direct

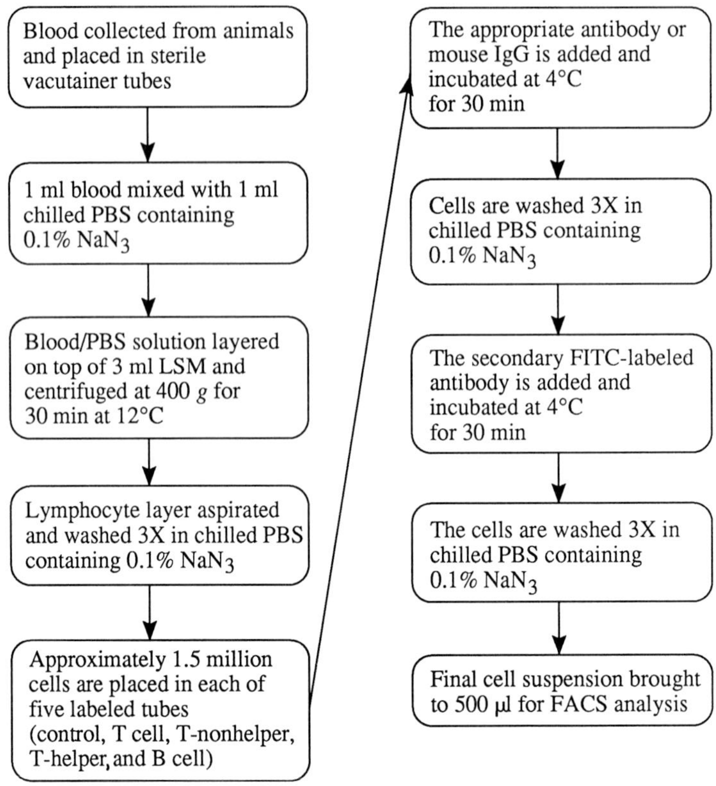

FIG. 1 Summary of lymphocyte preparation steps. Reproduced from ref. 5.

infusion of peptide into the brain (4, 5). An example is given in Fig. 4. In this case the peptide was angiotensin II which induces blood increases and drinking behavior. Overactivity of Ang II in the brain has to be postulated to trigger hypertension (9) and dysfunctional immune system (4). The data in Fig. 4 indicates that icv infusion of Ang II to mimic overactivity in the brain produces changes in the lymphocyte population distribution similar to those seen in the SHR (4).

Discussion

In the normal situation the balance between the different lymphocyte populations is carefully controlled. Lymphocytes are capable of producing chemical mediators. Other lymphoid cells such as macrophages also secrete chemical

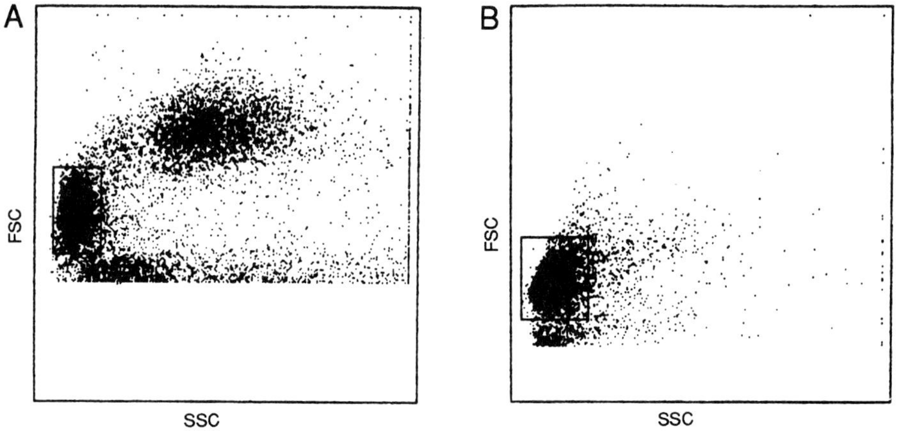

FIG. 2 Fluorescent-activated cell sorting (FACS) of rat blood. Side scatter is an indication of cell granularity, while forward scatter tends to be an indication of cell size. (A) Whole blood that has had red blood cells lysed. Populations of lymphocytes, monocytes and macrophages can be seen. (B) Whole blood that was separated using lymphocyte separation media. Note the relative purity of the lymphocyte population. In both cases the lymphocyte population has been boxed in.

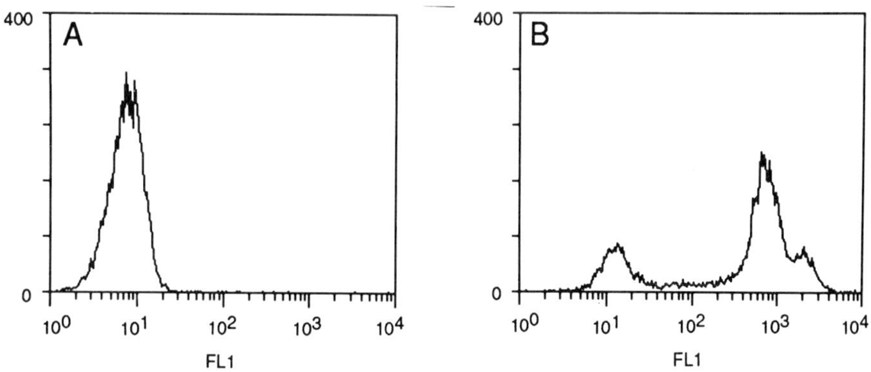

FIG. 3 Fluorescent-activated cell sorting (FACS) analysis of rat blood. (A) Background fluorescence in unstained cells. (B) Cells that have been fluorescently labeled to identify T cells. Background fluorescence can be deleted and the percentage of labeled cells quantified.

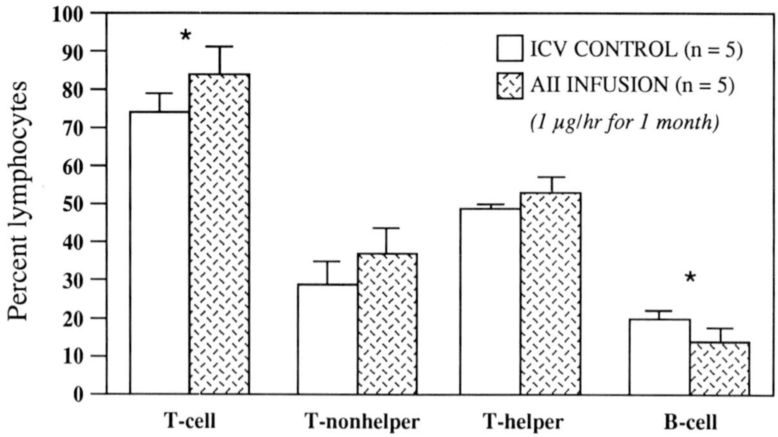

FIG. 4 Example of the immune measurement technique used in rat infused with a peptide in the brain. In this case the peptide is the octapeptide angiotensin II (Ang II), which was infused into the brain ventricle for 1 week at 0.1 $\mu g/\mu l$ per hr via osmotic minipumps implanted under the dorsal skin and connected by a catheter to a steel cannula on the skull. Percentage differences in lymphocyte populations in Ang II-infused rats versus artificial CSF controls. $^*p < 0.05$. All values are expressed as means ± SEM. Reproduced, by permission, from "Chronic ICV infusion of neuropeptides alters lymphocyte populations in experimental rodents," *Regulatory Peptides,* Vol. 34(3), 189–195, 1991.

mediators. It is through these messengers that the various cells of the immune system interact with one another. Because the chemical mediators released by one cell type may have a profound effect on the proliferation and differentiation of another cell type, it is possible that very subtle changes in certain cell types may have large effects throughout the entire immune system. Both T and B lymphocytes are capable of lymphokine secretion (6). Included in the lymphokine category are a variety of substances including osteoclast-activating factors (OAF), PMN migration inhibitory factors (MIF), and adrenocorticotropin (ACTH)-like substances, as well as others not fully explored (6–8). These substances are capable of acting at local sites as well as acting centrally. From this it is possible to hypothesize that an imbalance in various cells of the immune system may lead to the over or underproduction of various lymphokines that may exert numerous effects through peripheral and central action. In this particular case a decrease in the amount of suppressor cells may be releasing the brake on the action and activity of the other cell types. The finding of central peptide induction of changes in the immune system offers a method to approach the question of what mechanisms link emotional stress and disease.

By changing the B-cell and T-cell ratios, many aspects of the immune response are altered affecting a variety of body functions. The spontaneously hypertensive rat exhibits increased brain levels of Ang II (9) and increased sympathetic nerve activity (10). Several investigators have suggested changes in the immune system as at least a partial course of the hypertensive state (11–14) in the model. These changes involve alterations in the B-cell to T-cell ratio which appear to be significant in the pathogenesis of hypertension (12, 15). Bulloch (16) has shown that the ANS sends fibers to the immune organs. These fibers richly innervate areas high in T-cell concentration and avoid areas that contain developing B-cells. Thus, catecholamines act similarly to cortisol in that they inhibit cell-mediated immunity more than humoral immunity. The T-suppressor cells in the SHR are especially depressed (17). These cells are an important regulator of lymphokine secretion. Lymphocytes can also secrete as a lymphokine an interferon-like substance as well as an ACTH-like substance that will cause adrenal cortisol secretion (18).

A simplified mechanism of action may be initiated by a chronic stress (bacterial invasion, social stress, emotional and physiological disharmony) situation. In a chronic stress situation, an adaptation response will occur for cortisol and the increased levels will eventually diminish. This is not the case with catecholamines. On repeated stresses, the catecholamine levels will still increase (19). This stress can induce activation of the sympathetic nervous system to various parts of the body, including peripheral immune organs. This decreases the number of T cells, especially T-suppressor cells, relative to B cells, and, thus, removes control of B-cell and remaining T-cell lymphokine secretion provided by the T-suppressor cells. The unchecked B cells and remaining T cells are then able to increase secretion of lymphokines such as ACTH-like substances interferon-like substances, as well as others (OAF, MIF, etc.) which can act locally in tissues, as well as directly on the hypothalamus and other structures to further potentiate ANS activity. It is the B-cell to T-cell ratio that is important. During certain stress situations, it may be lymphocyte-derived ACTH rather than pituitary-derived ACTH that mediates increased cortisol secretion (7, 18).

Acknowledgments

Special thanks go to Dr. Raul Braylan and Melissa Chen of the Interdisciplinary Center for Biotechnology Research for help with the flow cytometry. Supported by NIH Grant HL27334

References

1. M. Hoffman, *Science* **255,** 531–534 (1992).
2. C. A. Janeway, *Sci. Am.* **Sept.** 73–79 (1993).
3. G. J. V. Nossal, *N. Engl. J. Med.* **316,** 1320–1325 (1987).
4. L. D. Fannon, R. C. Braylan, and M. I. Phillips, *J. Hypertens.* **10(7),** 629–634 (1992).
5. L. D. Fannon and M. I. Phillips, *Methods Neurosci.* **6,** 147–157 (1991).
6. D. Grant, I. Stern, and F. Everett, *in:* "Periodontics," 5th Ed., p. 233. Mosby, St. Louis, 1979.
7. J. Blalock, W. Meyer, and E. Smith, *Science* **218,** 1311 (1982).
8. E. Smith and J. Blalock, *Proc. 1st Int. Works. Neuroimmunomod.* 65 (1985).
9. M. I. Phillips and B. Kimura, *J. Hypertens.* **6,** 607–612 (1988).
10. W. Judy, A. M. Watanabe, D. P. Henry, H. R. Besch, W. R. Murphy, and G. M. Hockel, *Circ. Res.* **38** (Suppl. II), 21–29 (1976).
11. N. Takeichi, D. Ba, and H. Kobayashi, *J. Hypertens.* **4**(Suppl. 3), S433–S435 (1986).
12. A. Khraibe, R. Norman, and D. Dzielak, *Am. J. Physiol.* (*Heart Circ. Physiol.* **16)274,** H722–H726 (1984).
13. N. Takeichi, K. Suzuke, and H. Kobayashi, *Eur. J. Immunol.* **11,** 483–487 (1981).
14. G. Fernandes, R. Marius, and D. Troyer, *J. Hypertension* **4**(Suppl. 3), S469–S474 (1986).
15. A. Bendich, E. Belisle, and H. Strausser, *Biochem. Biophys. Res. Commun.* **99,** 600–607 (1981).
16. K. Bulloch, *in* "Neural Modulation of Immunity" (R. Guillemin *et al.,* eds.), p. 11. Raven, New York, 1985.
17. R. A. Norman and D. J. Dzielak. *Proc. Soc. Exp. Biol. Med.* **182,** 448–453 (1986).
18. J. Blalock, *J. Immunol.* **132**(No. 3), 1067 (1984).
19. R. Rose, *Phychiatr. Clin North Am.* **3**(No. 2), 251 (1980).

[19] Methods in Neuroimmunomodulation of Macrophage Function

Bruce S. Zwilling

Introduction

The macrophage is a phagocytic leukocyte that serves several important functions in host resistance. The macrophage has traditionally been thought of as a scavenger cell that eliminates tissue debris. The macrophage phagocytizes and destroys invading microorganisms. However, a large number of human pathogens have evolved so that they are capable of subverting initial antimicrobial defense mechanisms and can grow within the macrophage.

Despite their ability to subvert macrophage antimicrobial mechanisms, some of the organisms will die and be digested by lysosomal enzymes within phagolysosomes and be processed for presentation to antigen-specific T lymphocytes. Thus, the macrophage performs a central role as an initiator of the immune response because it can process and present antigens. The nature of the antigen will determine whether the macrophage will present antigen to a major histocompatibility complex (MHC) class II restricted $CD4^+$ T cell or to MHC class I restricted $CD8^+$ T cells. Generally, antigens that are derived exogenously, such as bacteria, are processed to associate with MHC class II glycoproteins. Antigens that are derived endogenously, that is, synthesized within the macrophage (e.g., viral proteins) will be processed to associate with MHC class I. All cells express MHC class I and can process and present viral peptides. However, the expression of MHC class II is more limited and presentation to $CD4^+$ T cells is limited to these cells. The macrophage and the B lymphocyte express MHC class II and serve as antigen-presenting cells.

Finally, the macrophage is an important effector cell of the immune response. Thus, the production of several cytokines by $CD4^+$ T cells as well as by the macrophage itself leads to macrophage activation. During the activation process the macrophage acquires the ability to suppress the growth of intracellular microorganisms that previously grew within the cell. Two books provide excellent reviews of macrophage biology and macrophage–pathogen interactions (1, 2).

The purpose of this chapter is to describe the methodology to assess macrophage function and to determine the role of the hypothalmic–pituitary–adrenal (HPA) axis and the sympathetic nervous system in modulating

Methods in Neurosciences, Volume 24

the functional capacity of the macrophage. Generally, the methods that are described have been adapted by us and have been described by others and are also detailed in macrophage methodology books edited by Herscowitz *et al.* (3) and Adams *et al.* (4).

Activation of Hypothalamic–Pituitary–Adrenal Axis

We activate the HPA axis by restraint stress (5–7). To accomplish this the mice are placed in 50-ml conical centrifuge tubes that have multiple ventilation holes. The holes can be made by heating the end of a 0.25-inch cork borer or by using an inexpensive soldering iron. We have found that the soldering iron works best. The mice should be about 6–8 weeks old. Younger mice are small and can turn within the tubes. The mice are stressed for 16 to 18 hr. The stress period should begin just as the mice enter their active period, from 4 to 6 p.m. Depending on the end point, a single or multiple restraint period may be used. For example, a single restraint period suppresses MHC class II expression (6), while suppression of antimicrobial resistance requires multiple restraint cycles (7) (see below). During restraint the mice are deprived of food and water. This does not appear to have an adverse effect on macrophage function.

While restraining the mice, it is best to place groups of mice together, each in their own tube, rather than separating the mice. A single standard mouse cage will usually accommodate five centrifuge tubes. Separation also results in stress and will result in some suppression of macrophage function. Control mice should also be group housed, but without food and water, during the stress period. When removing the mice after the stress period they will appear dirty but as soon as they are returned to normal housing they will resume eating and drinking and will groom themselves.

Multiple restraint cycles will eventually result in habituation of the corticosterone response. This will require at least 10 consecutive cycles. Thus, catecholamine levels will remain elevated while corticosterone levels will be lowered. When the mice are restrained for five cycles, rested for 2 days, and then restrained for five additional cycles, the corticosteroid response is not habituated (7).

In order to measure corticosterone levels following stress it is important that the mice be sacrificed immediately following the last stress cycle. Ether anesthesia affects the mice in about 30 sec. The mice are then sacrificed by cervical dislocation and the blood is collected from the incision site. It is important that the mice be sacrificed immediately once they have been anesthetized. Injection of 25 μl of a 60% : 40% mixture of ketamine (100 mg/ml)/xylacine (20 mg/ml) and bleeding by cardiac puncture takes too long and corticosterone levels will rise to abnormal levels in control mice. Corticosterone levels in control mice should be at or just below the level of detection of the assay kit (25 ng/ml) (Amersham, Chicago, IL) while corticosterone levels in stressed mice are as high as 500 ng/ml of plasma.

Macrophage Populations

Peritoneal Macrophages

Peritoneal macrophages can be obtained from the peritoneal cavity of mice by lavage. Several different populations can be obtained. Resident cells are present in the peritoneal cavity and represent older, unstimulated macrophage populations. Elicited macrophages can be obtained by injecting a variety of sterile irritants into the peritoneal cavity. This can include sterile medium containing 10% (v/v) fetal bovine serum (FBS), 4% fluid thioglycolate (Difco, Detroit, MI) that has been prepared at least 7 days in advance, mineral oil, starch, and proteose peptone. One to two mililiters is sufficient to induce an infiltration of cells into the peritoneal cavity within 3–5 days. These cells are considered to be inflammatory cells and are newly arrived from the blood but different from blood monocytes. The macrophage populations that are induced by the different irritants will differ. For example, thioglycolate will induce a population of elicited cells, consisting of about 70% macrophages, that are more metabolically active than those induced by the injection of peptone. In part this is because of the differences in bacterial lipopolysaccharide that are found within the eliciting agents. Thus, thioglycolate medium contains LPS while most preparations of peptone are devoid of LPS. Since LPS activates macrophages this may be an important consideration. The content of LPS in reagents can be determined using a *Limulus* amebocyte lysate assay available from BioWhittaker (Walkersville, MD). Preparations containing less than 0.03 ng/ml are acceptable. Fetal bovine serum can be obtained that routinely contains levels at or below this amount from Hyclone Laboratories (Logan, UT) but is also available from other vendors. Activated macrophages can be obtained following the injection of activating agents such as *Mycobacterium bovis, Corynebacterium parvum,* muramyl dipeptide, or other bacterial preparations (3, 4).

Prior to removal of the macrophages from the peritoneal cavity the mice are anesthetized with ether and then sacrificed by cervical dislocation. The fur is thoroughly saturated with 70% ethanol (v/v) and the skin is removed by making a lateral incision along the midline. Care must be taken to peel away the dermal layer and not to violate the integrity of the peritoneal cavity by cutting into the muscle wall. The macrophages are removed from the peritoneal cavity by injecting about 10 ml of ice-cold Hanks' balanced salt solution, massaging the muscle layer, and withdrawing the fluid using a 10-cm^3 syringe with an 18-gauge needle. All of the peritoneal macrophage populations must be purified prior to assessing macrophage function. This is usually accomplished by adherence onto plastic surfaces. Since the majority of cells within the peritoneal populations will be macrophages this can be done concomitantly with setting up the assay (see below).

Alveolar Macrophages

Alveolar macrophages are obtained by lung lavage. We use the method described by McCarron *et al.* (8), but modified by us. The mice are anesthetized by injection of ketamine/xylacine as above. The inferior vena cava is severed to remove blood from the heart and lungs. A midline incision is made in the neck and the trachea is exposed by dissecting away the fat layer. A blunted 25-gauge needle is attached to 0.020-inch i.d. × 0.037-inch o.d. silastic medical-grade tubing (Cat No. 602-135, Dow Corning, Baxter Health Care, McGaw Park, IL) and the needle inserted into the trachea at the level of the thyroid cartilage. About 1 to 1.5 cm is carefully threaded into the trachea until some "resistance" is experienced. This usually occurs as the needle reaches the major bifurcation of the trachea. The trachea is tied with the tubing in place using surgical square knots (4.O silk) at two places, one just below the point of insertion and the second 0.5 cm below the first, to prevent leakage. The tubing is then attached to a three-way stopcock that is attached to a 10-ml syringe containing a medium [Iscove's modified Dulbecco's medium (IMDM) containing 0.1% lidocaine] reservoir and another syringe that is used to remove medium from the lung. One-half milliliter of lavage medium is injected into the lung and then removed. This process is repeated 10 times and approximately 1×10^5 alveolar macrophages are removed.

Splenic Macrophages

To obtain splenic macrophages, the spleens from 10 animals are passed through 40-mesh tissue sieves into Hanks' balanced salt solution (HBSS) supplemented with 20% defined fetal bovine serum (Hyclone, Logan, UT) and subsequently passed through sterile needles with successively decreasing bore size (18-, 21-, and 25-gauge) in order to achieve a single-cell suspension. The cells are washed by centrifugation at 900*g* for 15 min. at 4°C and resuspended in IMDM (GIBCO/BRL, Gaithersburg, MD) supplemented with 20%

FBS, glutamine, penicillin, and streptomycin. The splenic macrophages are enriched by adding 70 × 10^6 cells to 100 × 20-mm tissue culture dishes (Falcon, Lincoln Park, NJ) in 5 ml IMDM. The cells are allowed to adhere during overnight culture at 37°C in an atmosphere containing 5% CO_2. The nonadherent cells are removed by gently washing with HBSS released from a 10-ml pipette and removing the medium by suctioning through an 18-gauge needle attached to a vacuum line. It is important to wash the cells so that the nonadherent cells are removed but the adherent cells are not washed away. This is only a problem with splenic macrophages which do not adhere as avidly as alveolar or peritoneal macrophages. The adherent cells are then removed by using a cell scraper (Bellco, Vineland, NJ, Cat. No 7731-22005, small blade). The medium must be precooled in an ice-cold water bath. Care must be exercised in removing the adherent cells. Any pressure will cause damage to the cells and significantly reduce yields. We try to drag the cell scraper carefully along the surface so that the weight of the scraper is sufficient to remove the cells. The initial adherence results in an enrichment of the macrophages; only about 50% of the cells will be macrophages. A second overnight adherence step is performed when adding macrophages to culture wells for determination of function. The second adherence step results in a population of cells that contains greater than 90% macrophages. We routinely use nonspecific esterase staining to identify the macrophages (9).

Determination of Major Histocompatibility Complex Class II Expression

Major histocompatibility complex class II is constitutively expressed by splenic (30–40%) and alveolar macrophages (30–40%). Only about 10 to 15% of peritoneal macrophages express MHC class II. In contrast, MHC class II is not expressed by murine monocytes. Major histocompatibility complex class II expression can be induced *in vivo* or *in vitro*. To induce or increase the level of MHC class II expression *in vivo*, mice can be injected intravenously via the tail vein with a suspension containing 10^5 colony-forming units (cfu) of *M. bovis* [strain Bacillus Calmette-Guérin (BCG) (ATCC Rockville, MD No. TMC 1029)] or intraperitoneally with 1 × 10^6 cfu. After about 7 days, more than 90% of the cells will express MHC class II.

To induce MHC class II expression *in vitro*, peritoneal macrophages are treated with 1 to 100 U of recombinant γ-interferon (rIFN-γ) for 48 hr. While the expression of I–A can be measured within about 8 hr, maximal expression by the cells requires 48 hr. Cells (5 × 10^4) can be cultured onto the surface of Lab-Tek (Nunc, Naperville, IL) slides and treated with rIFN-γ, and the percentage of cells expressing I–A can be assessed by indirect fluorescence (see below). For analysis by flow cytometry the peritoneal macrophages can be cultured on 35-mm petri dishes. Each dish contains 5×10^6 cell in 1 ml of Dulbeccos modified Eagle's medium (DMEM) containing 10–2500 U of rIFN-γ. After 48 hr the cells are removed from the monolayers by gentle scraping as described above. These cells are washed and stained for MHC class II expression.

Evaluation of Major Histocompatibility Complex Class II Expression

Class II MHC expression is evaluated by indirect immunofluorescence. The macrophages, either in suspension or as adherent monolayers on Lab-Tek slides, are first treated with 10% (v/v) heat-inactivated rabbit serum at 4°C for 30 min, in order to block Fc receptor binding. The monolayers are washed and then treated with a monoclonal antibody that reacts with the MHC class II haplotype of the mouse strain. The somatic cell hybrids that are producing the desired monoclonal antibodies are all available from the American Type Culture Collection (ATCC). We produce our own antibody and test the supernatant fluids for antibody activity and titer. Undiluted supernatant fluids can be used or the antibody can be purified by using protein A-Sepharose columns (Pierce, Rockville, IL). After the cells are reacted with the supernatant fluid for 40 min at 4°C, the cells are washed to remove unbound antibody and then treated with FITC-conjugated $F(ab')_2$ goat anti-mouse immunoglobulin (Zymed, South San Francisco, CA) for an additional 30 min. The cells are fixed with 1% (w/v) paraformaldehyde after staining by incubating the cells for 15 min at room temperature in the dark. After washing, the number of fluorescent cells per 200 cells is determined by epifluorescence and the percentage of macrophages expressing MHC class II is calculated. This is done by using coded slides to eliminate bias. Control cultures, stained with monoclonal antibody reacting with a different MHC haplotype, are included. Peritoneal cells from BCG-injected animals contain numerous B cells that also express MHC class II glycoproteins. Most of these wash away after the adherence step but care must be taken to distinguish these cells from the macrophages. This confusion can be avoided when using flow cytometry since the B cells are much smaller than the macrophages and can be gated out. Other advantages of using flow cytometry are that macrophages can be identified using monoclonal antibodies that react with proteins that are expressed primarily on macrophage surfaces (such as MAC-1 or CD14) and the cells analyzed for the expression of MHC class II and MAC-1 or CD14 by dual-parameter flow cytometry (10).

Hypothalamus–Pituitary–Adrenal Axis and Major Histocompatibility Complex Class II Expression

We have detailed the methodology required to affect MHC class II expression by peritoneal macrophages (5). A single 18-hr restraint experience is sufficient to suppress MHC class II expression by macrophages from mice that have been injected 7 days previously with BCG (5). The effect of restraint on the induction of MHC class II expression can be assessed by restraining mice on the same day as the injection of BCG. If the animals are not restrained within several hours following the injection of BCG, then no suppression will be observed (5). Class II expression can also be suppressed *in vitro* by treating macrophages that have been induced to express I–A, with corticosterone or with adrenocorticotropin (ACTH) (11). Both are effective at a range of doses around $10^{-6}M$.

Antimicrobial Activity of Macrophages

We have assessed the ability of macrophage preparations to kill mycobacteria, primarily *Mycobacterium avium* and *M. bovis* BCG, as well as *Mycobacterium tuberculosis*. The methodology described was adapted from that described by Flesch and Kaufman (12) and is applicable to other microorganisms except that the numbers of microorganisms as well as the duration of the assay period will have to be determined because the generation time of the microorganisms is different. For example, *M. avium* divides about once in 8 hr, *M. tuberculosis* about once every 24 hr, and *Listeria monocytogenes* about once every 30 min. Thus, an assessment of the effects of macrophages on *Listeria* growth can be completed within 24 hr, while other times will be required for other microorganisms. See Ref. 4 for details of antimicrobial assays for other microorganisms.

An additional consideration is the source of the macrophages used to assess antimicrobial activity. For example, thioglycolate-elicited peritoneal macrophages inhibit the growth of mycobacteria, but peptone-elicited peritoneal macrophages do not. Thus experiments must be performed using peptone-elicited cells, or on splenic or alveolar macrophages in order to determine the effect of various cytokines or hormones, etc., on macrophage function. Similarly, peptone-induced macrophages will kill *Listeria,* but thioglycolate-elicited macrophages will not (13).

In order to determine the antimicrobial activity of macrophages (7, 12), 1×10^5 macrophages are added to 96-well microtiter plates and allowed to adhere during overnight culture. The macrophages should be cultured in medium without antibiotics, but containing 20% FBS. The adherence of different cell preparations will differ and it is important to determine the cell differential and to determine the adherence of the different populations. We do this by determining the number of macrophages that have adhered to a random sample of wells by counting the adherent cells after washing the wells to remove the nonadherent cells. This is done using an ocular micrometer and is described in detail by Dolf Adams (14).

After adherence of the macrophages, the cultures are infected with bacteria. We use 4×10^5 cfu of *M. avium* (4 : 1, bacteria to macrophage ratio). The bacteria are suspended in Iscove's modified Dulbecco's medium without antibiotics and without serum and 0.2 ml is added to each well. The cultures are incubated overnight at 37°C to allow for phagocytosis of the bacteria and washed to remove unphagocytized bacteria. The cultures of infected macrophages are incubated for 5 days to allow intracellular growth of the ingested bacteria. After this time the macrophages are lysed to release the mycobacteria and the cultures pulsed with [^{3}H]uracil (5 μCi/ml, Amersham, Chicago, IL., specific activity 40–60 Ci/m*M*). This is accomplished by carefully removing 0.1 ml of the medium from each well and adding a lysing solution which consists of 7H9 Medium (Difco) containing 0.2% saponin (w/v) and label. The bacteria are incubated overnight and harvested onto glass fiber filter strips using a PhD Cell Harvester (Cambridge Technology, Inc., Watertown, MA). The radioactivity incorporated by the bacteria is determined by liquid scintillation spectrometry. In order to assess the effect of cytokines on the growth of the bacteria, rIFN-γ can be added to the macrophages prior to the ingestion of the bacteria.

Cytokine Production

Macrophages make inflammatory cytokines interleukin(IL)-1, tumor necrosis factor (TNF) α, IL-6, GM-colony stimulating factor, transforming growth factor β, and IL-10, as well as other locally and systemically active hormones. Their production can be stimulated by treating macrophages with bacterial lipopolysaccharide (LPS) alone at concentrations ranging from 10 ng to 10 μg/ml. Additionally, TNF-α can be stimulated by a combination of rIFN-γ and LPS or rIFN-γ and bacteria. The cytokines can be measured in the supernatant fluid of the cultures by enzyme-linked immunosorbant assay. Kits are available from Genzyme (Cambridge, MA), Endogen (Boston, MA), or Pharmagen (San Diego, CA).

Production of Reactive Nitrogen Intermediates

Nitric oxide is formed from arginine by an inducible nitric oxide synthase (NOS). Nitric oxide plays a role in the relaxation of vascular endothelium, as a neurotransmitter, and accounts for some of the antitumor and antimicrobial activities of macrophages. The production of NO, which is not stable, is assessed by measuring the level of NO_2 and NO_3 in the culture medium using the Griess reagent (7, 15). Macrophages are stimulated with 100 U of rIFN-γ, together with 100 ng of LPS (Difco) or 10^5 cfu BCG for at least 72 hr. The supernatant fluid (50 μl) is mixed with an equal volume of Griess reagent (1% sulfanilamide in 5% H_3PO_4, 0.1% *N*-1-naphthylethlyenediamine dihydrochloride in water). The mixture is incubated at room temperature for 10 min. To determine the amount of NO produced the optical density is measured at 550 nm and plotted using the optical density obtained with $NaNO_2$ as a standard.

Acknowledgments

The author thanks David Brown, Cary Yang, Mary Hilburger, Beth Miles, Thanh Nguyen, Kim Wilcox, and Fouza Yusuf for helpful discussions of the methodology. Thanks arc also extended to Jennifer Zwilling for synopsis of methods and to Ron and Jan-Kiecolt Glaser, Bill Malarkey, John Sheridan, and Caroline Whitacre for discussions. This work is supported by NIH Grants MH54679 and AA09321.

References

1. R. Van Furth, "Mononuclear Phagocytes." Kluwer Academic, Dordrecht, Netherlands, 1992.
2. B. S. Zwilling and T. K. Eisenstein, "Macrophage-Pathogen Interactions." Dekker, New York, 1993.
3. H. B. Herscowitz, H. T. Holden, J. A. Bellanti, and A. Ghaffar, "Manual of Macrophage Methodology." Dekker, New York, 1981.
4. D. O. Adams, P. Edelson, and H. Koren, "Methods for Studying Mononuclear Phagocytes." Academic Press, New York, 1981.
5. B. S. Zwilling, D. Brown, R. Christner, M. Faris, M. Hilburger, M. McPeek, C. Van Epps, and B. A. Hartlaub. *Brain Behav. Immun.* **4,** 330 (1990).
6. B. S. Zwilling, D. Brown, and D. Pearl, *J. Neuroimmunol.* **37,** 115 (1992).
7. D. H. Brown, J. Sheridan, D. Pearl, and B. S. Zwilling, *Infect. Immun.* **61,** 4793 (1993).
8. R. M. McCarron, D. K. Goroff, J. E. Luhr, M. A. Murphy, and H. B. Herscowitz, *Methods Enzymol.* **108,** 124 (1984).
9. I. R. Koski, D. G. Poplack, and R.M. Blaese, *in* "*In Vitro* Methods in Cell-Mediated and Tumor Immunology" (B. R. Bloom and J. R. David, eds.), p. 359. Academic Press, San Diego, 1976.
10. Z. Darzynkiewicz and H. A. Crissman, "Flow Cytometry." Academic Press, New York, 1990.

11. B. S. Zwilling, W. P. Lafuse, D. Brown, and D. Pearl, *J. Neuroimmunol.* **39,** 113 (1992).
12. I. E. A. Flesch and S. H. E. Kaufman, *Infect. Immun.* **59,** 3213 (1991).
13. C. E. Alford, T. E. King, Jr., and P. A. Campbell, *J. Exp. Med.* **174,** 459 (1991).
14. D. O. Adams, *in* "Methods for Studying Mononuclear Phagocytes" (D. O. Adams, P. J. Edelson, and H. Koren, eds.), p. 325. Academic Press, New York, 1981.
15. L. C. Green, D. A. Wagner, J. Glogowski, P. L. Skipper, J. S. Wishnok, and S. R. Tennenbaum, *Anal. Biochem.* **126,** 131 (1982).

[20] Stressor-Induced Immune Alterations in Rodents

Donald T. Lysle

There is a growing body of evidence indicating that various forms of stressful stimuli can compromise immunologic function. The investigation of stressor-induced immune alterations is important to the understanding of health problems, especially given that studies with human subjects have reported that common life events such as spousal bereavement, marital disruption, and first-year medical school examinations can induce a decrease in lymphocyte function (1–5). The presentation of a stressor induces the activity of many neural and hormonal factors that can interact with the immune system. Thus, the investigation of stress-induced immune alterations can also be used to determine the mechanisms of interaction between the central nervous and immune systems.

Animal research has shown that stressful stimulation can have pronounced effects on immune status and the pathogenesis of disease (6, 7). This area of research has used a plethora of stressor paradigms such as electric shock, loud noise, crowded and isolated housing conditions, handling, forced swimming, extreme temperatures, social conflict, rotation, forced exercise, and restraint. However, surprisingly little attention has been given to the qualitative and quantitative differences among these stressor procedures or to the relevance of these procedures to the human stress situation. My colleagues and I have been involved for a number of years in the examination of stressor-induced immune alterations in rodents. In the course of this work, we have identified some important parametric and procedural issues relating to the presentation of stimulation in the investigation of stressor-induced immune alterations. Furthermore, we have developed a stressor paradigm that is well-suited for the investigation of stressor-induced immune alterations in rodents.

Given the relatively large number of stressor procedures, one obvious question is whether different types of stressors influence the immune system in a similar manner. Furthermore, one can ask what characteristics of a particular stressor (i.e., frequency of stressor presentations within and across days) are important to the induction of immune alterations. There are few, if any, studies within the same laboratory directly comparing the effects of different stressor procedures. An initial study by Lysle and colleagues employed Lewis rats and electric footshock as the stressor (8). In this study, rats were presented with 4, 8, or 16 signaled shocks on a 4-min variable-

Methods in Neurosciences, Volume 24

time schedule for 1, 3, or 5 successive daily sessions in a standard rodent chamber. Each presentation of electric shock was 5.0 sec in duration. Immediately following the last shock experience, the subjects were sacrificed and the spleen and a sample of peripheral blood were removed. Lymphocytes from both tissues were evaluated for their responsiveness to the T-cell mitogen concanavalin A (Con A). The results indicated that following a single session of 16 shocks the spleen and peripheral blood lymphocytes showed only 6 and 12% of the normal response to Con A, respectively. However, the suppression of responsiveness of the spleen lymphocytes completely diminished with the increase in the number of shock sessions. In contrast, the peripheral blood lymphocytes showed no attenuation of suppressed mitogenic responsiveness with the increase in the number of shock sessions. Similar effects were obtained for the groups that received 8 shocks per session, whereas those groups that received 4 shocks per session showed little change from nonshocked controls. These results show that presentation of a stressor can have a dramatic effect on the status of the immune system, but the magnitude of the effect is dependent on the compartment of the immune system assayed, as well as the frequency of the stressor presentations both within and across days.

To determine whether a different stressor with similar parameters would produce comparable immunomodulatory effects, the effect of the chemical stressor, 2-deoxy-D-glucose (2-DG), was examined (9). The injection of 2-DG, an antimetabolic glucose analog, produces an acute intracellular glucoprivation. Acute glucoprivation is a metabolic condition which shows the physiological hallmarks of a physical stressor (10–14). Glucoprivation is an interoceptive condition and induces behavioral responses that are different from the behavioral responses induced by exteroceptive stressors such as footshock. Footshock produces an increase in locomotor activity and escape responses, whereas glucoprivation produces a decrease in motor activity (13). Thus, the behavioral consequences indicate that the effect of 2-DG is distinctly different from that of electric shock; however, the neural and endocrine patterns indicate that 2-DG administration is stressful.

In this study, different groups of Sprague–Dawley rats received one, three, or five injections of 2-DG (500 mg/kg, sc) or the phosphate-buffered saline vehicle. The injections were separated by 72 hr. The subjects were sacrificed 1 hr following the last injection, and blood and spleen lymphocytes were subjected to a mitogen stimulation assay. The results showed that a single injection of 2-DG decreased reactivity in both blood and spleen lymphocytes, as determined by mitogenic stimulation to Con A. The suppressed reactivity for the spleen lymphocytes attenuated with repeated injections, but the blood lymphocytes did not show any attenuation. The results of this investigation demonstrate a pattern of immunologic alteration identical to that obtained with electric shock.

In a preliminary study, Dykstra, Watts, and Lysle (unpublished data, 1992) investigated the effect of administration of morphine, an opioid-receptor agonist, on the status of the immune system using Fisher-344 rats. Morphine administration induces activation of the hypothalamic–pituitary–adrenal axis and the sympathetic nervous system which are characteristic of a stress response (15, 16). In this study, different groups of rats received one, three, or five injections of morphine (25 mg/kg, sc) or the phosphate-buffered saline vehicle. Injections were separated by a 72-hr period. The animals were sacrificed 1 hr after their last injection. The results showed that a single injection of morphine induced a pronounced reduction in the responsiveness of lymphocytes to Con A in both blood and spleen. The suppressed reactivity for the spleen lymphocytes was attenuated with repeated injections of morphine, but the blood lymphocytes did not show any attenuation. The results of this study demonstrate that morphine induced a pattern of immunologic alteration comparable to that found using electric shock and 2-DG.

Collectively, these studies show that different types of stressors can have similar effects on immune status provided that comparable temporal and quantitative aspects of the stressors are used. When similar presentation schedules are used there are comparable effects for electric shock, 2-DG, and morphine, even through these are very different types of stimulation and different strains of rats were used in each study. These studies also indicate that the restriction of immunologic assessments to certain compartments of the immune system and particular stressor parameters can lead to only partial conclusions regarding the effect of a stressor on immune status.

The investigations of stress-induced alterations in animals have almost exclusively relied on physically aversive stimulation as the stressor. The major concern about these types of studies is whether the observed alterations in immune status or disease resistance are the result of neuroendocrine processes or simply the result of the physical characteristics of the stimulus being used as the stressor. For example in rodent studies, the immunologic alterations induced by physical restraint may be related to an elevation in body temperature or to alterations in blood gases resulting from a lack of availability of oxygen in the restraining devise or a restriction of respiratory intake in the restrained animal. Moreover, the immunomodulatory effects of 2-DG may be the result of a direct effect of glucoprivation on the lymphocytes. Likewise, several stressor procedures such as social conflict and crowded housing conditions can cause physical injury, (i.e., bites and scratches from conspecifics) which induces a cascade of immunologic events that confound the neuroendocrine processes under investigation.

The concern about the physical confounds of stressor procedures prompted the development of a stressor paradigm that involves the assessment of a "psychological" stressor, a Pavlovian conditioned aversive stimulus. A conditioned aversive stimulus is an environmental event, such as an auditory, visual, or contextual stimulus, that is not inherently aversive or stressful, but acquires that property by being predictive of an event (such as electric shock) that is inherently aversive. Accordingly, this methodology allows an assessment to be made of the effect of stress induced by a conditioned aversive stimulus, without the concomitant effect of the aversive physical (or unconditioned) stimulus used to establish the conditioned stimulus.

To assess the immunomodulatory effect of a conditioned aversive stimulus, Lysle and colleagues (17) placed male Lewis rats in a standard rodent conditioning chamber (BRS/LVE Model RTC-020). The chambers were individually housed in sound-attenuating cubicles (BRS/LVE SEC-002). Timer circuitry to the output of a shock generator and scrambler (BRS/LVE Models SG-903 and SC-902) was used to provide an aversive unconditioned stimulus: a 5.0-sec, 1.6-mA, footshock. During each of two 40-min sessions in the conditioning chamber, the rats received 10 presentations of footshock on a 4-min variable-time schedule. This procedure is sufficient to establish the conditioning chamber as a learned stressor or a conditioned aversive stimulus. In a test session 12 days following conditioning, the rats were reexposed to the conditioning chamber (without the shock) prior to their sacrifice and the immunologic assessment. This experimental group was compared to a group of unmanipulated home cage subjects, and to two additional control groups of subjects to assure that the immune alterations were not the result of the shock experience itself during training, handling, or mere exposure to the stimulus used as the conditioned stimulus, i.e., the standard rodent chamber.

The results showed that exposure to the conditioned aversive stimulus induced a pronounced suppression of the mitogenic responsiveness of splenic lymphocytes to the T-cell mitogen Con A, and to the B-cell mitogen lipopolysaccharide (LPS). There was also a reduction in splenic natural killer cell activity for the experimental group relative to each control group. The conditioned stimulus also induced a pronounced suppression in the mitogenic responsiveness of blood lymphocytes to Con A. Subsequent studies have shown that these conditioned effects are pronounced and reproducible (18, 19). This conditioning model offers definite advantages over approaches that assess the direct effects of a physical stressor, for it eliminates the direct effects of the physical stimulation on the immune system. The model is also more representative of the human stress situation, which is typically psychological in nature and more often characterized as a state of anxiety or fear without physical adversity.

In addition to providing evidence of stressor-induced immunomodulatory effects, the above studies demonstrate that immunomodulatory effects can result from a relatively brief exposure to a stressor. Although some of the classic work in the field (20) used stressor procedures of 18 hr, it has become evident that procedures of a shorter duration are quite effective immunomodulatory stimuli. This consideration is very important in that long stressor procedures are plagued with additional confounds such as alterations in nutritional status and circadian rhythms.

Another advantage to the use of short stressors is that their use affords the opportunity for the investigation of time-sensitive neuroimmune interactions. The normal immune response is not static but involves many different cellular and humoral processes, each with a specific effect and precise timing. Some responses may take place in hours whereas other may occur over several days. For example, the immune response to a specific antigen typically involves the early processing of antigen by macrophages, the subsequent help of T lymphocytes, and finally the production of antibody by B lymphocytes after several days of exposure to the antigen.

To illustrate the importance of timing of the presentation of the stressor, we have examined the effect of a conditioned aversive stimulus on the development of an antibody response to keyhole limpet hemocyanin (KLH) and the development of adjuvant-induced arthritis (18, Lysle, Luecken, and Maslonek, unpublished data, 1992). For the antibody study, male Lewis rats were randomly assigned to five groups. Three groups of rats (conditioned) received 2 days of training in the conditioning chambers (BRS/LVE RTC-020) that involved 10 daily presentations of an aversive unconditioned stimulus. Two groups of rats received the same exposure to the conditioned chamber, but did not receive electric shock (control). Following their conditioning or control treatment, the rats were kept in their home cages for 12 days. On the following day (Day 0), all subjects received a subcutaneous injection containing 200 μg of KLH (Calbiochem, La Jolla, CA). Subjects designated Day 0, 2, 4 received a 40-min exposure to the conditioning chamber (without the shock) on Days 0, 2, and 4. Subjects designated Day 10, 12, 16 received a 40-min exposure to the conditioning chamber (without the shock) on Days 12, 14, and 16. The group designated HC was not reexposed to the conditioning chamber but remained in the home cages. Thus, conditioned and control groups received the same duration of exposure to the conditioning chamber at different times following the injection of antigen. On Day 15, all subjects were sacrificed and serum samples were collected.

Figure 1 shows the results of an enzyme-linked immunosorbent assay for the detection of KLH-specific IgG in serum using a biotin–streptavidin detection system. Dilutions of 1 : 320, 1 : 640, and 1 : 1280 of the serum samples were evaluated and the results expressed as absorbance. The results showed that presentations of the conditioned stimulus on Days 0, 2, and 4

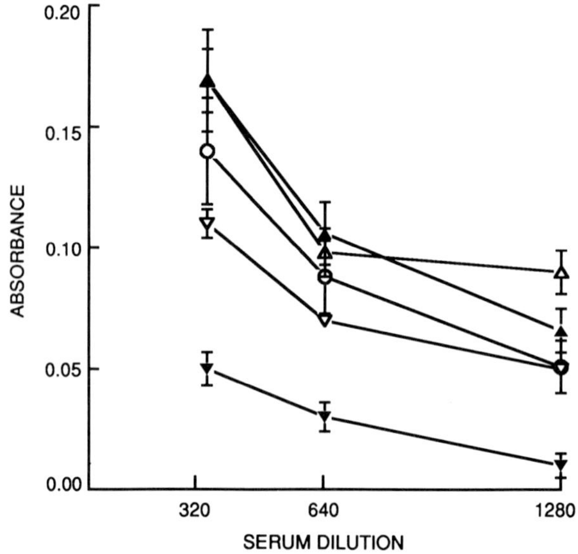

FIG. 1 Detection of KLH-specific IgG in serum using biotin–streptavidin deletion system. (△) Control, Days 0, 2, 4; (▽) control, Days 10, 12, 14; (▲) conditioned, Days 0, 2, 4; (▼) conditioned, Days 10, 12, 14; (○) HC.

following immunization had no effect on the KLH-specific IgG antibody production. In contrast, presentations of the conditioned stimulus on Days 10, 12, and 14 following immunization induced a significant decrease in the production of KLH-specific IgG antibody in the serum. This finding indicates that a conditioned aversive stimulus can modulate the immune response to specific antigen, but that the effect is dependent on the temporal relationship between antigen administration and presentation of the conditioned stimulus.

In a comparable study, we employed an animal model of rheumatoid arthritis, adjuvant-induced arthritis (18). Arthritis can be induced in rats by the injection of Freund's incomplete adjuvant containing killed *Mycobacterium tuberculosis*. In approximately 14 to 16 days, Lewis rats begin to develop arthritis in one or more paws. The severity of the disease can be scored, based on swelling, redness, and deformity of the ankles. A 14-point rating scale developed by Amkraut and colleagues (21) rates each forepaw, giving 1 point for beginning swelling and 2 points for severe swelling. Each hindpaw is also rated with 1 point being given for beginning swelling, 2 points for clear swelling, 3 points for severe swelling, and 4 points for extreme swelling with immobility of limb. One additional point is given for the occurrence of balanitis, and 1 point for the occurrence of a marked deterioration of general

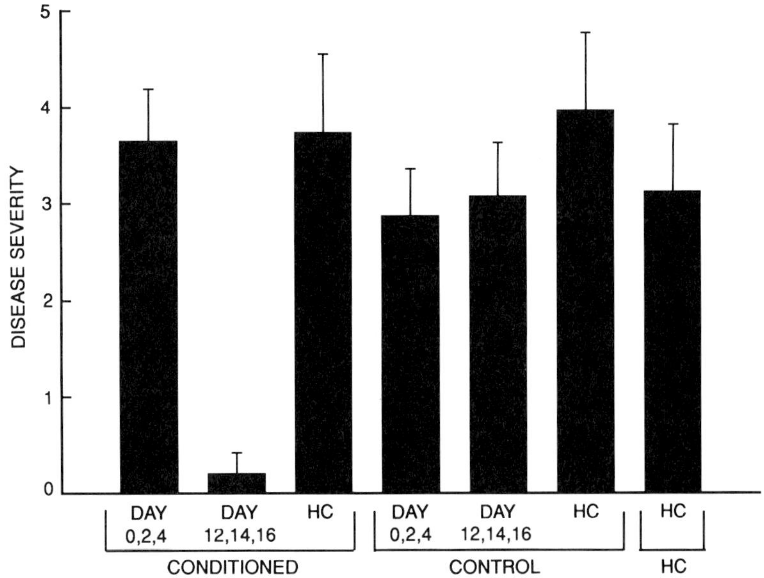

FIG. 2 Disease severity rating.

condition as judged by mobility, vigor, and condition of fur. Amkraut and colleagues (21) found this rating scale to be extremely consistent across consecutive days and between blind and nonblind raters with a standard error of 1 point.

In our study, male Lewis rats were randomly assigned to seven groups. Three groups of rats were given 2 days of conditioning as previously described, and following their conditioning the subjects were kept in their home cages for 12 days. On the following day, all subjects received a subcutaneous injection at the base of the tail of 0.2 ml of the adjuvant containing 5.0 mg/ml killed *M. tuberculosis* (Difco). One group of subjects (conditioned, Day 0, 2, 4) received a 40-min exposure to the conditioning chamber (without the shock) on Days 0, 2, and 4 following the injection. The second group of subjects (conditioned, Day 12, 14, 16) received a 40-min exposure to the conditioning chamber (without the shock) on Days 12, 14, and 16 following the injection. The third group was not reexposed to the conditioning chamber but remained in the home cages (conditioned, HC). Thus, two groups received the same duration of exposure to the conditioning chamber at different times following the injection of adjuvant. The third group was not reexposed to the conditioning chamber and thus served as a conditioned control group. To control for handling and exposure to the conditioning apparatus, three additional groups (control) were given the same training, injection, and chamber exposure as the three groups described above, except that the shock was never presented. The seventh group served as a general control and was kept in the home cages throughout the experiment (HC-HC). Following their injection with adjuvant, all rats were rated on a daily basis for the development of arthritis by an experimenter uninformed of the treatment of the subject using the 14-point rating scale developed by Amkraut and colleagues (21).

Figure 2 shows the results of the disease severity rating averaged across Days 11 to 40 for each group. The results clearly show that presentation of the conditioned aversive stimulus on Days 12, 14, and 16 following injection with adjuvant containing *M. tuberulcosis* greatly reduced the development of the autoimmune disease state. In contrast, presentation of the conditioned stimulus on Days 0, 2, and 4 had no significant influence on the course of disease. These results confirm that the immunomodulatory effect of a stressor is critically dependent on the timing of the antigen exposure and the presentation of the stressor.

The aim of this chapter has been to identify some of the important methodological issues involved in the investigation of stressor-induced alteration of immune status in rodents. The findings described in this chapter make it clear that researchers in this area must carefully consider their selection of a stressor paradigm and include in their assessments a range of parameters of varying frequency and duration. Furthermore, investigators must consider the relative timing of the stressor presentation and the types of immune processes involved in the investigation.

Acknowledgment

The writing of this chapter and some of the reported studies were supported by a grant from the National Institute of Mental Health (MH46284).

References

1. R. W. Bartop, E. Luckhurst, L. Lazarus, L. G. Kiloh, and R. Penny, *Lancet* **1,** 834–836 (1977).
2. J. K. Kiecolt-Glaser, W. Garner, C. Speicher, G. M. Penn, J. Holliday, and R. Glaser, *Psychosom. Med.* **46,** 7–14 (1984).
3. J. K. Kiecolt-Glaser, R. Glaser, E. C. Strain, J. C. Stout, K. L. Tarr, J. E. Holliday, and C. E. Speicher, *J. Behav. Med.* **9,** 5–21 (1986).
4. J. K. Kiecolt-Glaser, L. D. Fisher, P. Ogrocki, J. C. Stout, C. E. Speicher, and R. Glaser, *Psychosomat. Med.* **49,** 13–34 (1987).

5. R. Glaser, J. Rice, C. E. Speicher, J. C. Stout, J. K. Kiecolt-Glaser, *Behav. Neurosci.* **100,** 675–678 (1986).
6. P. K. Peterson, C. C. Chao, T. Molitor, M. Murtaugh, F. Strgar, and B. M. Sharp, *Rev. Infec. Dis.* **13,** 710–720, (1991).
7. B. S. Rabin, S. Cohen, R. Ganguli, D. T. Lysle, and J. E. Cunnick, *Crit. Rev. Immunol,* **9,** 279–312 (1989).
8. D. T. Lysle, M. Lyte, H. Fowler, and B. S. Rabin, *Life Sci.* **41,** 1805–1814 (1987).
9. D. T. Lysle, J. E. Cunnick, R. Wu, A. R. Caggiula, P. G. Wood, and B. S. Rabin, *Brain Behav. Immun* **2,** 212–221 (1988).
10. J. Brown, *Metabolism* **11,** 1098–1112 (1962).
11. R. L. Himsworth, *J. Physiol.* **198,** 451–465 (1968).
12. R. C. Ritter, and M. Neville, *Fed. Proc.* **35,** 642 (1976).
13. G. P. Smith, and A. N. Epstein, *Am. J. Physiol.* **217,** 1083–1087 (1969).
14. G. P. Smith, and A. W. Root, *Endocrinology* **85,** 963–966 (1969).
15. N. M. Appel, J. A. Kiritsy-Roy, and G. R. Van Loon, *Brain Res.* **378,** 8–20 (1986).
16. R. George and E. L. Way, *Br. J. Pharmacol.* **10,** 260–264, (1955).
17. D. T. Lysle, J. E. Cunnick, B. J. Kucinski, H. Fowler, and B. S. Rabin, *Psychobiology* **18,** 220–226 (1990).
18. D. T. Lysle, L. J. Luecken, and K. A. Maslonek, *Brain Behav. Immunity* **6,** 64–73 (1992).
19. D. T. Lysle, L. J. Luecken, and K. A. Maslonek, *Brain Behav. Immun.* **6,** 179–188 (1992).
20. E. S. Keller, J. M. Weiss, S. J. Schleifer, N. E. Miller, and M. Stein, *Science* **213,** 1397–1400 (1981).
21. A. A. Amkraut, G. F. Solomon, and H. C. Kraemer, *Pyschosomat. Med.* **33,** 203–214 (1971).

[21] Measurement of the Immune System in Response to Psychological Intervention

Beree R. Darby and Lewis D. Fannon

Introduction

Over the past several years there has been an explosion of studies in the field of psychoneuroimmunology. This field attempts to examine how the brain and behavior can influence health and the susceptibility to disease through the immune system. For decades a cause-and-effect relationship between emotional state and disease has been suspected. Solomon and Amkraut (1) have described numerous clinical observations that psychological and emotional factors alter resistance to infectious diseases. Also, Ader (2, 3) has shown conditioning to influence the immune system. Recent reviews have focused on neurotransmitter influences on immune function (4), hormones and receptors common to the central nervous system and the immune system (5–7), neuroanatomic wiring of lymphoid organs (8), immune-related brain syndromes (9), and the role of stress and psychiatric morbidity on immune dysfunction (10–12).

Lymphocytes are a major effector cell in the immune system. There are two major types: T lymphocytes and B lymphocytes. T cells can be further subdivided into T-helper cells, or those cells that facilitate and potentiate the immune response, and T-nonhelper cells, which are involved in such things as direct killing of invading cells, destruction of virally infected cells, and possibly inhibition of immune action. B lymphocytes are in charge of antibody production. Both T and B lymphocytes are capable of secreting lymphokines which include interleukins. These chemical mediators can act locally at tissue sites of immune system activity and directly or indirectly feed back on the central nervous system.

There are several different ways of measuring the activity of the immune system. The method described here was developed for human blood lymphocyte measurement. The method provides an overview of changes in the immune system in an accurate and rapid way. The ratios of T cells, T-nonhelper cells, T-helper cells, and B cells are given by this method.

Hypnosis has been suggested as a means of studying the cognitive and psychological factors that affect the immune system during stressful events. Recently, researchers have directed their attention toward the psychological and cognitive factors involved in hypnosis that influence the recovery from

Methods in Neurosciences, Volume 24

illness. Bowers and Kelley (13) and Jemmott and Locke (14) have written reviews discussing the case examples showing the influence hypnosis has on the immune system. There is a strong possibility that hypnosis may influence the activity of the immune system through central nervous system involvement. However, more scientific studies which include control groups and sophisticated measurements of the immune system need to be conducted in this area.

In this chapter a method is described in which human subjects in the experimental group received four individual sessions of self-hypnosis training during a 3-week period. Subjects in the control group did not receive the self-hypnosis training. Blood samples are obtained from subjects in both groups before the sessions begin and after the training has ended. Quantification of different lymphocyte populations is carried out using fluorescense-activated cell sorting (FACS) analysis. The results suggest that hypnosis may provide an effective means of stabilizing the immune system during stressful life events.

Methods

Subjects

Twenty-eight subjects are included in the study: 22 females and 6 males. Both the experimental and the wait list control group have 11 females and 3 males. The average age of the subjects in the wait list control group is 31.43 with a range of 22 to 49. The average age of the experimental subjects is 33.07 with a range of 23 to 50.

Design and Procedures

This project was approved by the university's institutional review board. Subjects are randomly assigned to one of two groups: an experimental group that receives self-hypnosis training and a wait list control group. Each group has blood samples drawn for determination of total lymphocyte number, Total T-cell levels, helper T-cell levels, nonhelper T-cell levels, natural killer T-cell levels, and B-cell levels. The blood samples are drawn 3 weeks apart for both groups and assessed on a pretest, post-test basis using six monoclonal antibodies that detect antigens on human lymphocytes. The monoclonal antibody test for lymphocytes contains a monoclonal antibody linked to a fluorescent dye. This conjugate specifically binds to lymphocytes which

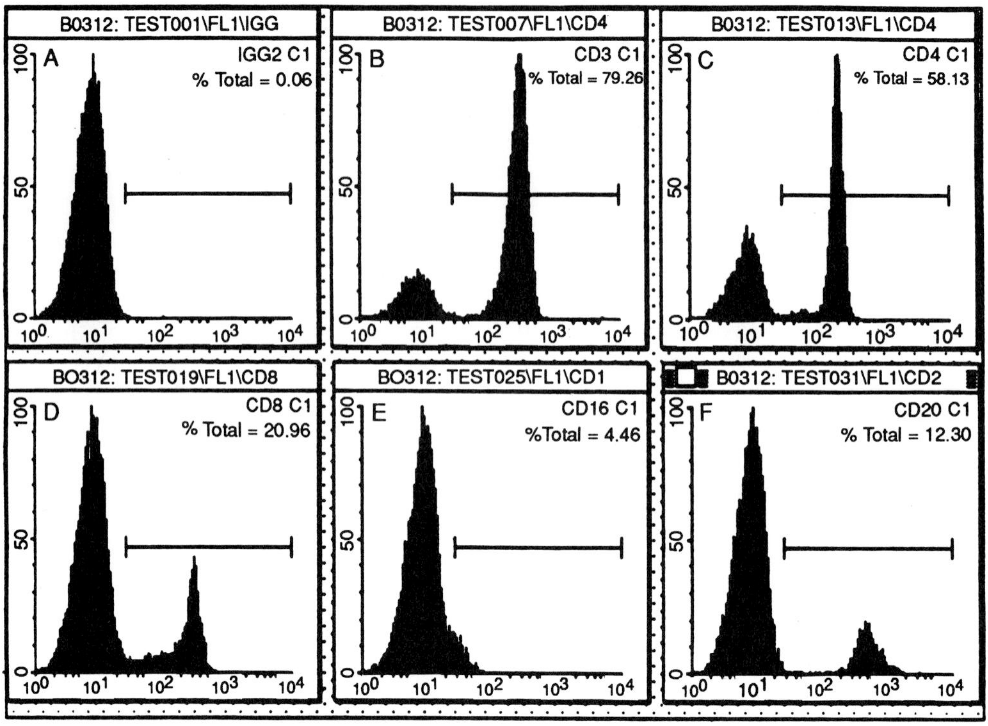

FIG. 1 Fluorescence-activated cell sorting (FACS) analysis of human blood. (A) Mouse Ig fluorescence control. (B) Total T lymphocytes. (C) T-helper cells. (D) T-nonhelper cells. (E) Natural killer cells. (F) B cells.

can be detected when the dye is excited by light from a FACS. The FACS analysis involves hitting a thin stream of the cell suspension with a laser beam and then utilizing light detectors to collect the scattered light. Fluorescently labeled cells can be quantified accurately by this method of analysis. All samples are run on the FACStar Plus (Becton–Dickinson, Rutherford, NJ).

The six antibodies used in this experiment are the following: Anti-Leu-4 (CD3) labeled total T lymphocytes; Anti-Leu-3a (CD4) labeled T-helper cells; Anti-Leu-2a (CD8) labeled T-nonhelper cells; Anti-Leu-11a (CD16) labeled natural killer cells; Anti-Leu-16 (CD20) labeled B-lymphocytes; and a mouse IgG control. All antibodies are purchased from Becton–Dickinson, (Rutherford, NJ). Figure 1 is an example of the fluorescence-activated cell sorting analysis of the six monoclonal antibodies used in this study.

Blood Collection

Blood is drawn by a registered nurse using sterile technique into a vacutainer collection tube containing the anticoagulant ethylenediaminetetraacetic acid (EDTA) to prevent clotting. The blood is mixed well and taken to the hemotology laboratory for analysis on the Coulter Counter-STKS to determine the number of total lymphocytes present.

Direct Monoclonal Antibody Staining

The following day, 200 μl of well-mixed anticoagulated peripheral blood is added to 200 μl of PBS with 0.1% sodium azide. Ten microliters of the appropriate monoclonal antibody is added to each blood sample, and each tube is vortexed. The tubes are placed in the refrigerator to incubate for 30 min. After 30 min, the tubes are removed from the refrigerator and 3 ml of lysing buffer are added to each tube. The blood samples are mixed thoroughly and incubated at room temperature for 10 min.

Following incubation the samples are centrifuged at 1500 revolutions per minute (rpm) for 7 min at 4°C to maintain discrete cell clusters. After centrifugation, most of the supernate is aspirated from each tube. A small amount of liquid is left in each tube to ensure that each cell pellet is not disturbed. The cell pellets are vortexed, and 2 ml of cold phosphate-buffered saline (PBS) is added to each tube. The samples are centrifuged again and the supernates are removed following the same procedure.

Cells are resuspended in 250 μl of PBS and mixed well. To each tube 250 μl of 2% paraformaldehyde is added, and the samples are incubated for 30 min in the refrigerator. After the incubation, the cells are washed twice with 1 ml cold PBS with 0.1% sodium azide and resuspended in 500 μl PBS. The cell suspension is then filtered through a 20-μm mesh filter before being run on the fluorescence-activated cell sorter.

Self-Hypnosis Training

Four individual self-hypnosis training sessions are conducted for each experimental subject over a 3-week period. The sessions covered: (i) the definition, misconceptions, and applications of self-hypnosis, (ii) self-hypnosis training, (iii) research findings in immunology, (iv) biochemical details of the immune response, and (v) direct and indirect suggestions for increased self-confidence and improved immune response.

Self-Report Measures

The Beck Depression Inventory (BDI) is administered each time the blood is drawn to both the experimental and control subjects. The BDI is a 21-item questionnaire constructed to assess the depth and severity of depression. Subjects that scored 17 or higher on the BDI are assessed as clinically depressed. Since research has shown that depression suppresses the immune system, subjects who scored in the clinically depressed range are not included in the analysis. Also, subjects who experienced highly stressful events during the study are not included in the results.

The Strain Questionnaire (SQ) is administered at each blood drawing to both the experimental and control subjects. This self-report instrument measures the everyday manifestations of the stress response on the physical, behavioral, and cognitive levels. Subjects that scored above 111 on the SQ are excluded from the study.

At the blood drawings, subjects are asked to complete a pretest and post-test background questionnaire which askes about chronic health problems, acute health problems, average alcohol intake in 1 week, average number of beverages containing caffeine per day, average hours of sleep at night, and amount of smoking per week.

An additional post-test questionnaire is administered which asks subjects to describe any unusual stressful situations that occured in the 3 weeks during the study. This form also asks for a subjective determination of any change in the subjects self-confidence, self-reliance, self-acceptance, self-esteem, feeling relaxed, and concentration during the study. Each subject rates his/her change on a 5 point Likert scale (1 = significant decrease, 2 = some decrease, 3 = no change, 4 = some increase, 5 = significant increase). The subjects are asked if they have decided to change any health-oriented aspects of their life since the study began. Finally, the experimental subjects are asked to describe any benefits they received from the training.

Results and Discussion

This study investigated the relationship between self-hypnosis training and the immune response. The baseline comparisons of the subjects revealed no significant differences between the no-treatment control group and the experimental group on the amount of ethanol intake per week, caffeine intake per week, or in the hours of sleep per night. No subject reported any acute or chronic health problems which might have a significant immunological component, aside from mild allergies. No subject reported taking any medica-

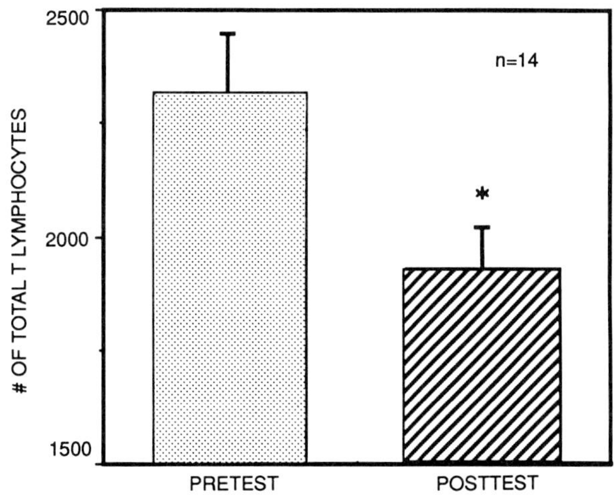

FIG. 2 Control group mean of total T lymphocytes. All values are expressed as mean + SEM. $^*p < 0.05$.

tion which had known immunological consequences. Each subject was in the normal range of the Strain Questionnaire and Beck Depression Inventory.

Results of this study suggest that self-hypnosis training may alter immune system functioning. Figure 2 shows T-lymphocyte mean levels for the control group at each blood drawing 3 weeks apart. These subjects experienced a significant decline in their total T-lymphocyte levels. Figure 3 also demonstrates the T-helper cell mean levels of the control subjects. These subjects also experienced a significant drop in their T-helper cells. These results are consistent with the literature reports that psychosocial factors which stress an individual's adaptive capacity are associated with alterations of specific immune functions which tend to suppress the immune system. The research by Kiecolt-Glaser and co-workers (15, 16) showed that medical students had significantly lower percentages of helper T lymphocytes during stressful exam periods and a significant decline in natural killer cell activity.

Figure 4 illustrates that the experimental subjects who received the self-hypnosis training did not experience a significant decline in their mean level of total T lymphocytes. Also, Fig. 5 shows that the subjects who received the self-hypnosis training did not have a significant decrease in their T-helper cells. Perhaps the self-hypnosis training prevented the significant decline in the immune system that graduate students typically experience. Table I summarizes the comparison of results in a repeated measures analysis of variance. The students who received self-hypnosis training were significantly different from the control group in the change in level of total T lymphocytes,

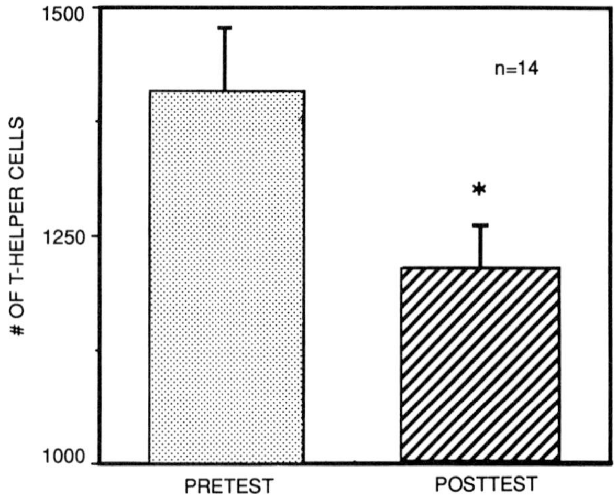

FIG. 3 Control group mean of T-helper cells. All values are expressed as mean + SEM. $*p < 0.05$.

helper T cells, total number of lymphocytes, natural killer T cells, and non-helper T lymphocytes. There was no significant effect in the B lymphocytes as a function of the group membership and change over time. This suggests that psychological intervention may prevent the significant decline in the level of immune cells in graduate students as they progress into the semester.

The subjects were asked to rate their level of self-confidence, self-assurance, self-reliance, self-esteem, feeling relaxed, and level of concentration as compared to when they first began the study. Each subject rated his/her levels on a 5-point Likert scale where 1 = significant decrease, 2 = some decrease, 3 = no change, 4 = some increase, 5 = significant increase. A Wilcoxson Rank Sums procedure was used to analyze the information. There was a significant increase in the level of reported self-confidence ($p < 0.001$), self-assurance ($p < 0.001$), self-reliance ($p < 0.009$), self-esteem ($p < 0.001$), feeling relaxed ($p < 0.0002$), and concentration ($p < 0.008$) between the no-treatment control group and the experimental group. These results suggest that the self-hypnosis training also had a significant enhancement in the students perceived psychological states.

The belief that psychological states and life circumstances have an effect on the health of an individual has been a repeated theme in medical theory (17). However, experimental attempts to study the impact of such effects on health did not occur until the recent beginning of the psychoneuroimmunology field. Numerous experiments have now been conducted to study the

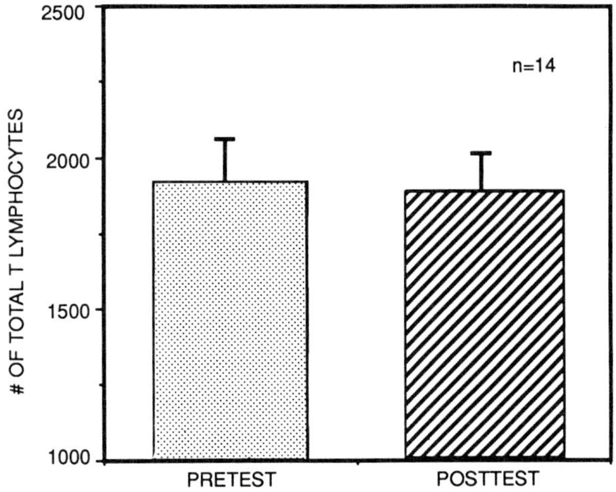

FIG. 4 Experimental group mean of total T lymphocytes. Values are expressed as mean + SEM. No significant difference.

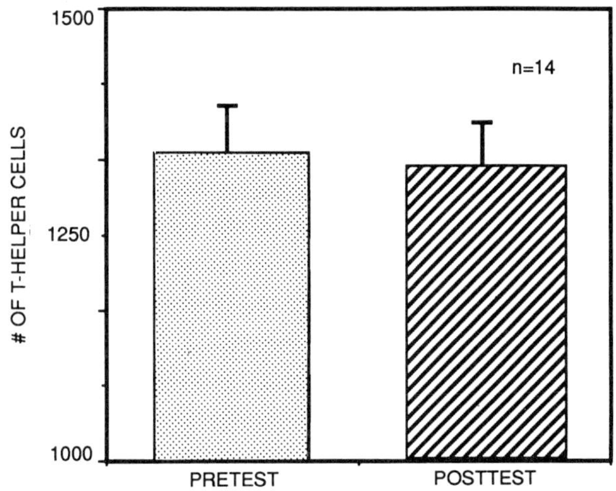

FIG. 5 Experimental group mean of T-helper cells. Values are expressed as mean + SEM. No significant difference.

complex interactions between disease and psychological states characterized by negative affect, stressful life events, and social circumstances (18–23).

Furthermore, evidence exists that demonstrates psychosocial factors directly affect immune function (24). Research has consistently found de-

TABLE I Repeated Measures Analysis of Variance: between Subjects/Interaction Effect

Measurement	F value	PR > F^a
Total T lymphocytes	12.74	0.002**
Helper T lymphocytes	11.67	0.003**
Total number of lymphocytes	14.43	0.001***
Nonhelper T lymphocytes	9.04	0.007**
Natural killer T cells	4.50	0.047*
B lymphocytes	1.51	0.235

[a] Key to p values: $***p = 0.001$; $**p < 0.01$; $*p < 0.05$.

creased immune function in patients experiencing severe depression (25, 26); in individuals who experience stressful life events, such as the loss of a job (27), death of a spouse (28–30), illness in the family (31), or divorce (32); and in students undergoing exams (15, 16). Thus, these psychosocial factors may have the potential to influence a wide range of disorders, including allergies (33), autoimmune diseases (34), infections (13), and tumors (10).

Allergic responses are mediated through a humoral immunity involving immunoglobulins (IgE, IgG, IgA, and IgM). Several clinical case studies have partially examined the influence of hypnosis on various allergic conditions. Clarkson (35) demonstrated the use of hypnosis to inhibit an allergic skin reaction in an 18-year-old girl. The subject reacted with a wheal to the injection before treatment. The girl was deeply hypnotized the next day and given the suggestion that there would be no reaction to the inoculation. Then the subject was inoculated while she was still hypnotized and no wheal was seen. The same inoculation given the next day without hypnosis produced a wheal. Mason and Black (36) reported on the use of hypnosis to inhibit the allergic symptoms associated with asthma and hay fever. This case study involved a woman who had a history of unsuccessful medical treatment for asthma. One week before the woman's usual yearly attacks the hypnotic treatment was started, and for the first time in 12 years the woman did not experience her asthmatic attacks. Kroger (37) employed hypnosis in successfully treating a 12-year-old boy who was allergic to cats, weeds, and candy. After the first hypnotic session the subject reported no allergic reactions. Also, in a 1-year follow-up the subject reported no incidents of allergy attacks.

Hypnosis has been a treatment employed in a variety of skin disorders. Since many dermatological conditions are mediated by underlying immunological mechanisms, the following clinical case studies provide indirect evidence for the relationship between hypnosis and the immune response. Immunoglobulin E is thought to cause a hypersensitive immune condition that underlies urticaria. Kaneko and Takaishi (38) used hypnosis in the treatment of urticaria and showed improvement in 80% of the subjects. Mason (39) has also shown hypnosis to improve other incurable skin conditions. Therefore, the mechanisms of the immune system appear to be affected in some way by the use of hypnosis.

The purpose of this study centered on attempts to stabilize, or enhance, the immune system. Many research studies have been conducted on the effects of stress on the suppression of the immune system, but relatively few have focused on how to enhance the immune system. This study describes an accurate and precise procedure to measure the lymphocytes in the immune response and suggests that hypnosis may be an effective technique to stabilize the immune system during stressful life events.

References

1. G. Solomon and A. Amkraut, *Annu. Rev. Microbiol.* **35,** 155 (1981).
2. R. Ader, *in* "Psychoneuroimmunology." Academic Press, New York, 1981.
3. R. Ader, L. J. Greta, and N. Cohen, *Ann. N. Y. Acad. Sci.* **497,** 532 (1987).
4. T. Roszman, J. Jackson, R. Cross, M. Titus, W. Markesbery, and W. Brooks, *J. Immunol.* **135(Suppl.),** 769s (1985).
5. D. Weigent and J. Blalock, *Immunol. Rev.* **100,** 79 (1987).
6. C. Pert, M. Ruff, R. Weber, and M. Herkenham, *J. Immunol.* **135(Suppl.),** 820s (1985).
7. J. Blalock, D. Harbour-McMenamin, and E. Smith, *J. Immunol.* **135(Suppl.),** 858s (1985).
8. D. Felten, S. Felten, S. Carlson, J. Olschowka, and S. Livnat, *J. Immunol.* **135(Suppl.),** 755s (1985).
9. B. Jankovic, *J. Immunol.* **135(Suppl.),** 853s (1985).
10. V. Riley, *Science* **212,** 1100 (1981).
11. Y. Shavit, G. Terman, F. Martin, J. Lewis, J. Liebeskind, and R. Gale, *J. Immunol.* **135(Suppl.),** 834s (1985).
12. J. Calabrese, M. Kling, and P. Gold, *Am. J. Psychiatry* **144,** 1123 (1987).
13. K. S. Bowers and P. Kelly, *J. Abnormal Psychol.* **85,** 490 (1979).
14. J. B. Jemmott and S. E. Locke, *Psychol. Bull.* **95,** 78 (1984).
15. J. Kiecolt-Glaser, W. Garner, C. Speicher, G. Penn, J. Holliday, and R. Glaser, *Psychosomat. Med.* **46,** 7 (1984).
16. J. Kiecolt-Glaser, R. Glaser, E. Strain, J. Shout, K. Tarr, J. Holliday, and C. Speicher, *J. Behav. Med.* **9,** 5 (1986).
17. Z. Lipowski, *Psychosomat. Med.* **46,** 153 (1984).
18. J. Goodwin, W. Hunt, and C. Key, *J. Am. Med. Assoc.* **258,** 3125 (1987).
19. K. Helsing, G. Comstock, and M. Szklo, *Am. J. Epidemiol.* **116,** 524 (1982).

20. J. House, K. Landis, and D. Umberson, *Science* **241,** 540 (1988).
21. S. Kasl, A. Evans, and J. Neiderman, *Psychosomat. Med.* **41,** 445 (1979).
22. S. Kobasa, S. Maddi, and S. Kahn, *J. Person.Soc. Psychol.* **42,** 168 (1982).
23. V. Persky, J. Kempthorne-Rowe, and R. Shekelle, *Psychosomat. Med.* **49,** 435 (1987).
24. R. Ader, *Psychosomat. Med.* **42,** 307 (1980).
25. S. Locke, L. Kraus, J. Leserman, M. Hurst, J. Heisel, and M. Williams, *Psychosomat. Med.* **46,** 441 (1984).
26. S. Schleifer, S. Keller, and A. Meyerson, *Arch. Gen. Psychol.* **41,** 484 (1984).
27. B. Arnetz, J. Wasserman, B. Petrini, and S. Brenner, *Psychosomat. Med.* **49,** 3 (1987).
28. R. Bartrop, L. Lazarus, E. Luckherst, L. Kiloh, and R. Penney, *Lancet,* **1,** 834 (1977).
29. M. Irwin, M. Daniels, T. Smith, E. Bloom, and H. Weiner, *Brain Behav. Immunity,* **1,** 98 (1987).
30. S. Schleifer, S. Keller, M. Camerino, J. Thornton, and M. Stein, *J. Am. Med. Assoc.* **250,** 374 (1983).
31. J. Kiecolt-Glaser, R. Glaser, E. Shuttleworth, and B. Dyer, *Psychosomatic Med.* **49,** 523 (1987).
32. J. Kiecolt-Glaser, L. Fisher, P. Ogrocki, J. Shout, and R. Glaser, *Psychosomat. Med.* **49,** 13 (1987).
33. P. Buisseret, *Sci. Am.* **247,** 86 (1982).
34. Y. Shoenfeld and R. Schwartz, *N. Engl. J. Med.* **311,** 1019 (1984).
35. A. Clarkson, *Br. Med. J.* **2,** 845 (1937).
36. A. Mason and S. Black, *Lancet* **1,** 887 (1958).
37. W. Kroger, *Ann. Allergy* **22,** 123 (1964).
38. Z. Kaneko and N. Takaishi, *Folia Psychiatr. Neurol. Japon.* **17,** 16 (1963).
39. A. Mason, *Br. Med. J.* **2,** 122 (1959).

[22] Cloning and Sequencing Immunoglobulin and T-Cell Receptor Variable Regions Involved in Neuroimmune Disorders

Curtis C. Maier and J. Edwin Blalock

Introduction

The polymerase chain reaction (PCR) is a powerful tool which has greatly facilitated the rapidity and ease of cloning and sequencing variable (V) regions of immunoglobulins (Igs) and T-cell receptors (TCRs). However, the extraction and isolation of RNA for first-strand cDNA synthesis can still be a time-consuming and costly venture, generally requiring at least 10^5 to 10^6 cells for a workable RNA yield. In this report we describe a rapid and inexpensive method for the generation of cDNA from very low numbers of lymphocytes involved in neuroimmune disorders. The method involves lysing as few as 10 cells in a 0.5% Nonidet P-40 (NP-40) detergent solution which should release cytoplasmic RNA yet not disrupt the nuclear membrane. Thus, most contaminating DNA and immature mRNA are easily removed with the cellular debris by centrifugation while the mature target mRNA remains in the supernatant. The cytoplasmic mRNA is then converted to cDNA and used as template in the amplification of the V regions of Igs and TCRs. This methodology was first worked out by amplifying V regions of Igs produced by hybridomas specific for encephalitogenic epitopes of myelin basic protein (MBP) and has now been applied to TCRs from encephalitogenic T-cell lines and clones as well as Ig V regions expressed by lymphocytes which have infiltrated the central nervous system (CNS) of multiple sclerosis (MS) patients.

Materials and Methods

Cells

All cells used in this study have been donated by Drs. John N. Whitaker and Shan-Ren Zhou (UAB, Birmingham, AL). The hybridoma, denoted 845D3, secretes IgG_1/κ and is specific for human MBP peptide 80–89 (1). RT1 is a T-cell line established from Lewis rats immunized with guinea pig

Methods in Neurosciences, Volume 24

(gp) MBP and specifically responds to the encephalitogenic antigen gpMBP 68–88. Cerebral spinal fluid (CSF) cells are obtained by spinal taps and are processed as quickly as possible following the tap.

Oligonucleotide Primers

Oligonucleotide primers are synthesized in this laboratory on a Dupont Coder 300 DNA synthesizer (Dupont, Wilmington, DE) and purified on Nensorb Prep columns (NEN, Boston, MA) or purchased from Oligos Etc. (Wilsonville, OR), unless otherwise noted. The random hexamers used to prime first-strand synthesis have a 3′-C and all four nucleotides at the remaining five positions. Sequences of primers used to amplify mouse and human Ig and rat TCR V regions are given in Table I.

Rapid Method for cDNA Synthesis

Cultured and primary lymphocytes are processed in the same manner. Cells are washed two times with 1 ml cold phosphate-buffered saline (PBS) and are pelleted by centrifugation in an Eppendorf tabletop microcentrifuge at 5000 rpm for 1 min at room temperature. After the last wash the cells are counted in a hemacytometer and the percent viability is determined by trypan blue exclusion. We have found that first-strand cDNA synthesis will proceed successfully even at only 50% viability. The number of cells lysed for first-strand synthesis can vary from 10 to 10^6 with best yields generally in the 10^4 range. Transfer the desired number of cells to a fresh microfuge tube and pellet as above. Remove all residual PBS (recentrifuge, if necessary, to remove PBS on the sides of the tube). It is very important to do the following lysis and centrifugation at 4°C (i.e., move to the cold room) to impair any ribonuclease activity. Resuspend the pellet in ice-cold 20-μl lysis mix containing 1× superscript reverse transcriptase first-strand buffer (GIBCO BRL, Gaithersburg, MD) [50 m*M* Tris–HCl (pH 8.3), 75 m*M* KCl, 3 m*M* $MgCl_2$], 10 m*M* dithiothreitol (DTT) (GIBCO BRL), 0.5% NP-40 (molecular biology grade, Sigma, St. Louis, MO; due to the high viscosity of NP-40, it is easier to manipulate if a large volume, such as 500 μl, of a 10% solution is made as a stock), and 40 U recombinant RNasin (Promega, Madison, WI) as a ribonuclease inhibitor. Pipette the pellet several times to ensure it is resuspended and centrifuge 2 min, 12,000 rpm at 4°C. Add 10 μl of the supernatant to a fresh microfuge tube containing 11 μl of first-strand mix. First-strand mix consists of 1× superscript reverse transcriptase first-strand buffer (GIBCO BRL; see above), 1 m*M* dATP, 1 m*M* dCTP, 1 m*M* dGTP, 1 m*M*

TABLE I PCR Primers for Amplifying Antigen Receptor V Regions

Primers	Sequences[a]	Corresponding amino acid[b]
Mouse Ig Vκ	5′-CCG GTC GAC GA(C/T) ATT (C/G)(A/T)G CT(A/G) AC(C/T) CAG TCT CCA-3′	1–8
Human Ig Vκ[c]	5′-CCG GTC GAC CAT (C/T)(C/G)(A/T) G(A/T)T GAC (C/G)CA GTC (C/T)CC-3′	1–8
Mouse and human Ig Cκ	5′-CCG GTC GAC ATG GAT ACA GTT GGT GCA GC-3′	111–117
Mouse Ig VH[d]	5′-CGG TCG ACC GAG GT(G/C) (A/C)A(A/G) CTG CAG (C/G)AG TC(A/T) GG-3′	1–8
Mouse Ig Cγ[e]	5′-CCG GTC GAC CAG GGG CCA GTG GAT AGA C-3′	121–127
Human Ig VH[f]	5′-CCG GTC GAC CGC AGG TGC AGC TGC AG(C/G) AGT C(A/G/T)C-3′	1–8
Human Ig J_HCγ[f]	5′-CCG GTC GAC CGC TTG GTG GA(A/G) GCT GA(A/G) GAG ACG GTG ACC-3′	108–117
Human Ig Vλ[g]	5′-CCT CCT CA(C/T) (C/T)CT C(G/T)G C(A/G)(C/T) AG-3′	(−1)–(−5)
Human Ig Cλ[h]	5′-CGG GTC GAC CGA GTG TGG CCT TGT TGG CTT G-3′	126–132
Rat TCR Vα	5′-GTG GTC GAC AGC AGG TGA A(A/G)C AGA G(A/C/T)C C-3′	(−1)–6
Rat TCR Cα	5′-GAA TCA AAG TCG ACG AAC AGG CAG-3′	141–148
Rat TCR Vβ8	5′-AAA GTC GAC GCT GCA GTC ACA CAA AGC CC-3′	2–8
Rat TCR Cβ	5′-CCT GTC GAC CAA GCA CAC GAG GGT AGC-3′	143–148

[a] Underlined sequences have been modified or added to create a *Sal*I restriction site. Parentheses indicate the sites in the primers with more than one nucleotide at that position. Sequences of primers have been derived from E. A. Kabat, T. T. Wu, H. M. Perry, K. S. Gottesman, and C. Foeller, "Sequences of Proteins of Immunological Interest," 5th Ed., U.S. Dept. Health and Human Services, National Institutes of Health, Bethesda, MD, 1991, unless otherwise noted.

[b] Positions are numbered as determined by Kabat *et al.*, "Sequences of Proteins of Immunological Interest," 5th Ed. U.S. Dept. of Health and Human Services, National Institutes of Health, Bathesda, MD, 1991.

[c] Designed from J. D. Marks, M. Tristem, A. Karpas, and G. Winter, *Eur. J. Immunol.* **21,** 985 (1991).

[d] Modified from R. Orlandi, D. H. Güssow, P. T. Jones, and G. Winter, *Proc. Natl. Acad. Sci. U.S.A.* **86,** 3833 (1989).

[e] C. C.Maier, R. D. LeBoeuf, S.-R. Zhou, J. N. Whitaker, M. A. Jarpe, and J. E. Blalock, *J. Neuroimmunol.* **46,** 235 (1993).

[f] Generous gift from R. D. LeBoeuf, UAB, Birmingham, AL.

[g] Generous gift from D. R. Shaw, UAB, Birmingham, AL.

[h] Modified from E. Paul, A. Livneh, A. J. Manheimer-Lory, and B. Diamond, *J. Immunol.* **147,** 2771 (1991).

dTTP (Ultrapure dNTPs, Pharmacia LKB Biotechnology, Piscataway, NJ), 50 pmol random hexamers, and 50 U superscript RNase H^- reverse transcriptase (GIBCO BRL). Incubate this first-strand reaction at 42°C for 1 hr. Heat the reaction mix to 95–100°C for 5 min to destroy the superscript and dislocate it from the cDNA template. Reactions have been stored for a couple of months at −20°C, avoiding multiple freeze–thaws, and can still be used as template for PCR; however, after several months the template will degrade unless otherwise purified.

The same care taken to avoid template contamination in PCR (i.e., a set of pipettes for primers and buffers separate from those used for template and cells, using autoclaved doubly distilled H_2O, microfuge tubes, and pit tips) must also be followed when setting up the first-strand reaction. A sham control first-strand reaction is run simultaneously to determine if any contaminating template was introduced during the procedure. This simply consists of 10 μl of lysis mix combined with 11 μl of first-strand mix in the absence of any cells. This reaction is used later as template in the primer control PCR.

Polymerase Chain Reaction Amplification

The V region cDNA generated in the first-strand reaction is specifically amplified by PCR using the primers from Table I with either Amplitaq (Perkin-Elmer Cetus, Norwalk, CT) or cloned *Pfu* DNA polymerase (Stratagene, La Jolla, CA). Amplifications performed with Amplitaq are done in 10 m*M* Tris–HCl, pH 8.3, 50 m*M* KCl, 2.0 m*M* $MgCl_2$, 0.2 m*M* dATP, 0.2 m*M* dCTP, 0.2 m*M* dGTP, 0.2 m*M* dTTP, 1.25 U Amplitaq, 50 pmol of each of the appropriate primers, and 0.1 or 1.0 μl of the first-strand reaction. Cloned *Pfu* is supplied with a different buffer (10× reaction buffer No. 3); at the working concentration it contains 20 m*M* Tris–HCl, pH 8.75, 10 m*M* KCl, 10 m*M* $(NH_4)_2SO_4$, 20 m*M* $MgCl_2$, 0.1% Triton X-100, and 0.1 mg/ml bovine serum albumin (BSA). Polymerase chain reaction amplifications done with *Pfu* DNA polymerase are carried out in this buffer and also include 0.2 m*M* dATP, 0.2 m*M* dCTP, 0.2 m*M* dGTP, 0.2 m*M* dTTP, 2.5 U cloned *Pfu*, 50 pmol of each of the appropriate primers, and 1.0 μl of the first-strand reaction.

The PCR conditions for Amplitaq and cloned *Pfu* are similar except higher annealing temperatures are generally more permissive with Amplitaq (we routinely amplify Ig V regions with Amplitaq at annealing temperatures of 62°C); however, for the results presented in this paper, mouse Ig and rat TCR V regions are amplified with cloned *Pfu* and annealed at 58°C, while human Ig V regions are amplified with Amplitaq and cloned *Pfu* and annealed at 54°C. All V regions are subjected to 40 cycles of amplification in a thermal cycler (Perkin-Elmer Cetus DNA thermal cycler) under the following conditions: denature 96°C for 1 min (the first 5 cycles to minimize primer dimers, 94°C for the remaining 35 cycles), anneal at the temperatures mentioned above for 1 min, and extend at 72°C for 2 min. Five to 10 μl of the reaction product is electrophoresed on a 1.2% (w/v) agarose gel, stained with ethidium bromide, visualized under UV light, and photographed. The expected size of the amplified V regions is 350–450 bp for these primer combinations. First-strand reactions can also be amplified with β-actin (2) or GAPDH primers to ensure successful first-strand synthesis and correct PCR conditions.

Cloning and Sequencing of V Regions

The oligonucleotide primers used for PCR are designed to include *Sal*I restriction sites to facilitate cloning of the PCR products. The V region PCR products are cloned into the *Sal*I restriction site of the sequencing vector, M13mp18, by the following protocol. Polymerase chain reaction products are extracted with phenol/chloroform, followed by a chloroform extraction and then precipitated with 0.5 volumes of 7.5 *M* ammonium acetate and 2.5 volumes of ethanol. When DNA loss is a concern, the organic phases are back extracted with an equal volume of doubly distilled H_2O and the aqueous phases combined. The PCR products are recovered by centrifugation at 12,000 rpm for 30 min, washed with 70% ethanol, and digested with 8 U *Sal*I (Promega), 37°C for 16 hr (overlay the reaction mix with mineral oil).

The restriction digestion mix is loaded directly onto 5% Nusieve GTG agarose (FMC BioProducts, Rockland, ME) containing 0.5 μg/ml ethidium bromide and run in 1× TAE buffer. The DNA band at the correct molecular weight is excised from the gel, keeping the exposure time to UV light and the amount of gel excised to the bearest minimum, and the agarose digestesd with GELase (Epicentre Technologies, Madison, WI), following the manufacturer's fast protocol. The recovered PCR products are quantitated on an ethidium bromide-stained gel. If one 100-μl PCR is used as starting material, a yield of approximately 100–200 ng can be expected.

Ten to 50 ng of V region PCR products is combined with 50 ng M13mp18 and this mixture digested with 0.8 U *Sal*I for at least 6 hr at 37°C. The amount of *Sal*I is reduced in this reaction to avoid cleavage at inappropriate sites. The reaction is extracted and organic phases are back extracted and precipitated as above.

The digested V region PCR product and M13mp18 is then ligated with 0.3 U T4 DNA ligase (Promega) in a 10-μl volume for 4 hr at 16°C. During this reaction, JM109 strain *Escherichia coli* are made competent for transfection following the protocol outlined in Promega's "Protocols and Applications

Guide'' (3), except volumes are reduced 10-fold and the trituration buffer contains 50 m*M* $CaCl_2$ rather than 100 m*M* $CaCl_2$. The ligation mix is diluted 10-fold and 2 and 8 μl are transfected into 200 μl of competent cells. This generally yields 200–800 plaques/plate, 1% of which are recombinant (clear rather than blue).

Clear plaques are grown 5 hr in 4 ml 2XYT and assayed for carrying the correct size insert by PCR. Three microliters of selected plaque purified recombinants are added directly to PCR mix containing M13 forward and reverse primers (sequences can be obtained from New England Biolabs, Beverly, MA) and subjected to 30 cycles of amplification. Nonrecombinant clear plaques will yield a PCR product of 100 bp, while recombinant plaques will be 100 bp larger than the V region PCR product. Single-stranded recombinant M13 DNA is purified from 3 ml of selected recombinant M13 clones following the protocol provided by Sambrook *et al.* (4).

Three to five isolates are then sequenced using a Sequenase 7-deaza-dGTP sequencing kit (United State Biochemical, Cleveland, OH) and the reactions electrophoresed on both 6 and 4% acrylamide wedge gels (0.4–1.2 mm, BRL, Gaithersburg, MD). This allows the entire sequence to be clearly read and any discrepancies in isolate sequences determined. We routinely perform multiple, identical PCRs starting with the same first-strand reaction as template and then sequence recombinant M13 isolates from each, to ensure nucleotides are not misincorporated during the amplifications. Following this protocol, starting with cells, we obtain complete sequence information on V regions in 1 week.

Sensitivity of Method

Hybridoma cells, 845D3, secreting an antibody specific for the human MBP peptide 80–89 (1), are used to determine the minimum number of cells necessary to amplify Ig V regions. Figure 1 shows that both heavy-chain and light-chain V regions can be amplified from as few as 10 cells, but not 1 cell. This experiment was repeated three times with similar results. To verify that the PCR product amplified was the target sequence of interest, the PCR products were cloned into M13 and sequenced. Figure 2 shows the sequences of the 845D3-VH PCR products which indeed are heavy-chain V regions. Actually two populations of sequences exist in the PCR product, one is derived from the mRNA of the productively rearranged allele, while the other contains a frameshift at codon position 100d due to N-sequence additions, resulting in a nonproductive transcript encoded by the other allele. The sequence of the light-chain PCR product also comes from a nonproductively rearranged allele (data not shown); however, neither of the sterile transcripts are encoded by

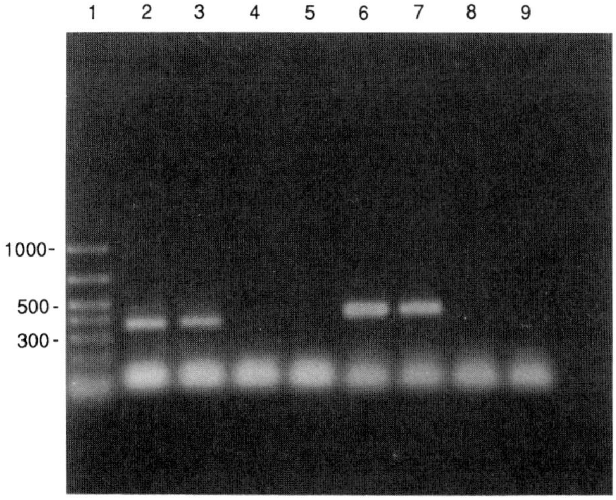

FIG. 1 Polymerase chain reaction products of 845D3 VL and VH amplified from low numbers of cells. Lane 1, molecular weight marker [1000, 700, 500, 400, 300, 200, 100, and 50 base pairs (bp) 50 ng of each; Biomarker Low, Bioventures, Inc., Murfreesboro,TN]. Bands at 1000, 500, and 300 bp are indicated on the left-hand side. Lanes 2–5 and 6–9 are PCR products of cDNA generated from 100, 10, 1 and 0 hybridoma 845D3 cells, respectively. The cDNA was amplified with primers mouse Ig Vκ and mouse and human Ig Cκ in lanes 2–5 to yield 360 bp products, while lanes 6–9 show the 400-bp PCR products from cDNA amplified with primers mouse Ig VH and mouse Ig Cγ.

the myeloma fusion partner, SP2/O, which commonly arises when cloning V regions from hybridomas. Avoiding cloning of the myeloma sterile transcript was accomplished by designing the Vκ and VH degenerate primers to have the most 3′ nucleotide of the primer mismatched with the myeloma sequence, thereby preventing the amplification of myeloma V region cDNA.

Amplification of Rat T-Cell Receptor Regions

The majority of T cells from Lewis rats specific for the encephalitogenic gp MBP peptide 68–88 express the V region gene Vβ8.2 (5, 6). Using a Vβ primer which is designed to specifically amplify Vβ8 family members we can amplify a PCR product of the expected size from 350 T cells of a T-cell line (as well as T-cell clones established from the line) specific for gp MBP 68–88 (Fig. 3). Analysis of the sequences of the PCR product verified that it is Vβ8.2 (data not shown).

```
                                                           10
                                                       Ala Glu Leu Val Arg Pro Gly Ala Ser Val
845D3 VH      GAG GTG CAA CTG CAG CAG TCT GGG GCT GAG CTG GTG AGG CCT GGG GCT TCA GTG
Sterile VH    --- --- --- --- --- G-- --A --A C-- -GC --- --- -AA --- TCT CAG --T C--

    20                                      30      CDR 1      35a
Lys Leu Ser Cys Lys Ala Leu Gly Tyr Thr Phe Thr Asp Tyr Glu Met His     Trp Val Lys
AAG CTG TCC TGC AAG GCT TTG GGC TAC ACA TTT ACT GAC TAT GAA ATG CAC *** TGG GTG AAG
TCC --C A-- --- -CT -TC ACT --- --- T-C A-C --C AGT G-- T-T GCC TGG AAC --- A-C CG-

    40                                      50          52a         CDR 2
Gln Thr Pro Val His Gly Leu Glu Trp Ile Gly Ala Ile His Pro Gly Ser Gly Gly Thr Ala
CAG ACA CCT GTG CAT GGC CTG GAA TGG ATT GGA GCT ATT CAT CCA GGA AGT GGT GGT ACT GCC
--- TTT --A -GA A-C A-A --- --G --- --G --C TAC --A AGC *** TAC --- --- ACC --- AG-

    60                                      70
Tyr Asn Gln Lys Phe Lys Gly Lys Ala Thr Leu Thr Ala Asp Lys Ser Ser Ser Thr Ala Tyr
TAC AAT CAG AAG TTC AAG GGC AAG GCC ACA CTG ACT GCA GAC AAA TCC TCC AGC ACA GCC TAC
--- --C -CA TCT C-- --A A-T CGA AT- T-T A-C --- CG- --- -C- --- AAG -A- CAG TT- -T-

80          82a 82b 82c                         90
Met Glu Phe Ser Ser Leu Thr Ser Glu Asp Ser Val Val Tyr Tyr Cys Ile Arg Lys Gly Leu
ATG GAG TTC AGC AGT CTG ACA TCT GAG GAC TCT GTT GTC TAT TAC TGT ATA AGA AAG GGG CTT
C-- C-- --G *** *** *** -AT --- -T- ACT A-- -AG -A- ACA GCC AC- T-T TAC TGT -CA ACG

CDR 3  100  a   b   c   d   e  101                               110
Tyr Gly Ser Ser Ser         Leu Ala Tyr Trp Gly Gln Gly Thr Leu Val Thr Val Ser Ala
TAC GGT AGT AGT TCC *** *** CTT GCT TAC TGG GGC CAA GGG ACT CTG GTC ACT GTC TCT GCA
G-- TAC TAT AAT TAC GAC GT CTT GCT TAC TGG GGC CAA GGG ACT CTG GTC ACT GTC TCT GCA
                           |<-N->|-> JH3

 |-> Cγ                     120
 Ala Lys Thr Thr Pro Pro Ser
 GCC AAA ACG ACA CCC CCA TCT GTC TAT CCA CTG GCC CCT GCG
GCC AAA ACG ACA CCC CCA TCT GTC TAT CCA CTG GCC CCT GCG
```

FIG. 2 The nucleotide and deduced amino acid sequence of 845D3 VH and its sterile transcript. The primer sequences are underlined. Dashes indicate identical nucleotides and gaps are inserted (asterisks) to maximize homology. The amino acid numbering and placement of CDRs (overline) are according to E. A. Kabat, T. T. Wu, H. M. Pery, K. S. Gottesman, and C. Foeller, "Sequences of Proteins of Immunological Interest," Fifth Edition, U.S. Dept. Health and Human Services, National Institutes of Health, Bethesda, MD, 1991.

Vα gene usage by rat T cells specific for gp MBP 68–88 has been previously shown by Southern blot analysis to be somewhat restricted as well (5, 6). Using the TCR Vα degenerate primer described in Table I, we were able to amplify Vα regions from the RT1 T-cell line (Fig. 3). Sequencing of gp MBP

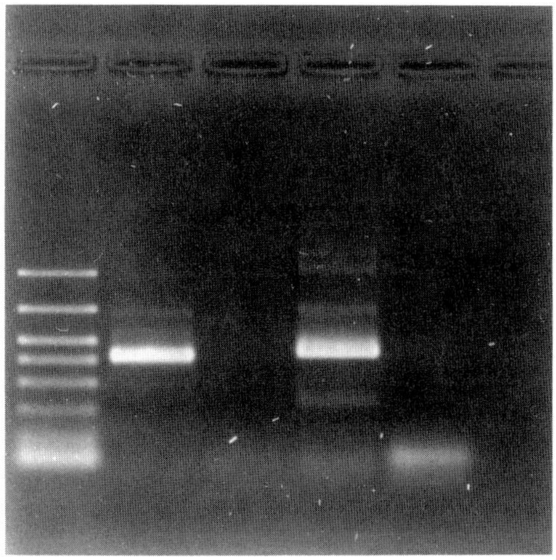

FIG. 3 $V\alpha$ and $V\beta$ PCR products amplified from cDNA of 350 cells of the encephalitogenic rat T-cell line, RT1. Lane 1 is a molecular weight marker with the 400-bp band indicated. Lane 2 shows the 430-bp $V\alpha$ PCR product amplified with the primers rat TCR $V\alpha$ and rat TCR $C\alpha$, while the 450-bp $V\beta$ PCR amplified with primers rat TCR $V\beta$ and rat TCR $C\beta$ is seen in lane 4. No PCR product is produced when amplifying cDNA from 0 cells ($V\alpha$ and $V\beta$ primers, lanes 3 and 5, respectively).

68–88 specific TCR $V\alpha$ elements by ourselves and others (7) reveal several other different $V\alpha$ families are utilized in addition to the predominant $V\alpha$ family (represented by RT1 $V\alpha1$ in Fig.4). Sequences representing three different $V\alpha$ families expressed in the RT1 T-cell line are shown in Fig. 4. The TCR $V\alpha$ primer amplified at least one other family (data not shown) and possibly others; therefore, this primer may be useful in identifying several new families of the poorly studied rat TCR $V\alpha$ structures.

Amplification of Immunoglobulin V Regions of Human Cerebrospinal Fluid Lymphocytes

The power of this technique is exemplified by the ability to amplify Ig V regions from lymphocytes which can only be obtained in small numbers, such as B cells infiltrating the CNS. From one patient 6 ml of CSF was obtained. This contained 2000 lymphocytes/ml, and approximately only 30% of these are expected to be B cells. B cells cannot be cultured, thus to

```
             1
RT1 Vα1      CAGCAGGTGA AGCAGAGACC CATATCTCTT ACAGTCTGGG AAGGAGGACC
RT1 Vα2      ---------- ---------- AGA---A--C -GT----CA- -G----CCAT
RT1 Vα3      ---------- -------C-- AGA---C--C -TT---CCA- -GAAG-CCAT

             48
RT1 Vα1      CACAGTTCTG AACTGCAGTT ATGAGAACAG TGCTTTTGAC TACTTCCCAT
RT1 Vα2      AG-CTC---C -------C-- TCAGCG---- -----C-C-G -C---TTGG-
RT1 Vα3      G--GTC---C -------CA- TCAGTG-TC- -----C-A-- G-----AGG-

             98
RT1 Vα1      GGTATCAGCA GTTCCCTGGG GAAGGCCCTG TACTCCTGAT AGCCATACGA
RT1 Vα2      ----C--A-- ACAT--C--- A-------CA A-A-G----- -T-----TTC
RT1 Vα3      ----CAGA-- GC-TT----- A------T-- AGT-G---G- GT----CTTC

             148
RT1 Vα1      TCAGTGTCCA ATAAAAAGGA AGATGGCCGA TTCACAGTCT TCCTCAGGAA
RT1 Vα2      --CAAT***G GC--C---A- ---A---A-- -------CTC A-----AT-G
RT1 Vα3      --C-AT***G GTG----A-- ---A---A-- -------CTC A-----AT-T

             198
RT1 Vα1      AAGTGAGAAA CAGCTCTCTT TGCACATCGA AGACTCTCAG CCTGGAGACT
RT1 Vα2      -GCCAGCCTG --TG-T--C- --------AC ------G--- --CA-T----
RT1 Vα3      -GCCAGACTG --AG-----C -A-----GAG ----CTGGG- --CA-T----

             248                   → Jα
RT1 Vα1      CAGCCACCTA CTTCTGTGCA GCAGCCCTCA ATAACAACAA TGCC***CCA
RT1 Vα2      -G--AGTT-- -C-------- --GT-AACAT CCTCT----G C***AAG-TG
RT1 Vα3      -T--TGT--- -C-------- -TGAG-AGGC GG--TGCAGG ----AAG-TC

             298                                         → Cα
RT1 Vα1      CGATTTGGAG CAGGAACCAG ACTAACAGTC AAACCAAATG TCACAGACCC
RT1 Vα2      GTG-----GC AG--G--ATC CT--T----- -TT---
RT1 Vα3      ACG------- GG-----A-- GT-G--G--- -----C

             348
Cα           AGAGCCTGCT GTGTACCAGC TGAAAGATCCC CAGTCTGATA ACATCACCCT

             398
Cα           CTGCCTGTTC
```

FIG. 4 The nucleotide sequences of three different Vα elements occurring in the Vα PCR product of the RT1 T-cell line. The primer sequences are underlined and nucleotides numbered starting at the first nucleotide of codon 1. Dashes indicate identical nucleotides, gaps inserted (asterisks) to maximize homology. The 5′ end of the constant region is noted with the arrow.

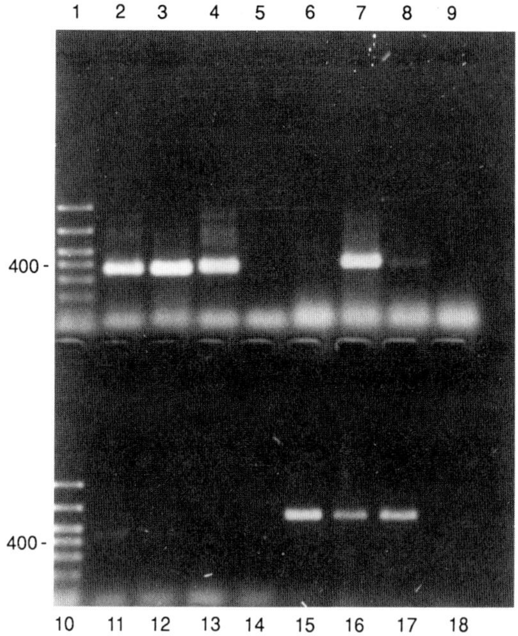

FIG. 5 V regions amplified from human CSF lymphocytes. Lanes 1 and 10 are the molecular weight marker with the 400-bp band indicated. Lanes 2–5 are cDNAs amplified with primers human Ig Vκ and mouse and human Ig Cκ. Lanes 6–9 are cDNAs amplified with primers human Ig VH and human Ig $J_H C\gamma$. Lanes 11–14 are cDNAs amplified with primers human Ig Vλ and human Ig Cλ. Lanes 15–18 are cDNAs amplified with β-actin primers. The order of cDNAs for each primer combination is as follows: CSF of MS patient (12,000 cells; lanes 2, 6, 11, 15), human spleen cDNA (generous gift from D. R. Shaw, UAB, Birmingham, AL; lanes 3, 7, 12, 16), CSF of non-MS patient (6,000 cells; lanes 4, 8, 13, 17), and 0 cells (lanes 5, 9, 14, 18).

determine the repertoire of V regions utilized by B cells infiltrating the CNS, cDNA must be made from a very low number of cells. In the initial attempt to demonstrate that the procedure works on human CSF lymphocytes, degenerate primers listed in Table I were tested for their ability to amplify human Ig V regions. Shown in Fig. 5 are the PCR products generated by the Vκ, VH, and Vλ primer combinations using MS and non-MS CSF lymphocytes (12,000 and 6,000 cells, respectively) and compared to spleen cDNA. β-Actin primers are included as a positive control. The Vκ and VH primers worked well while the degenerate Vλ primer amplified poorly; however, a new degenerate primer has since been designed which should amplify more λ family members. While these degenerate primers obviously do not amplify all Vκ, Vλ, or VH elements, these results support the idea that with well-designed primers, this can be an easy and rapid method for determining the repertoire of V elements utilized by lymphocytes in normal vs autoimmune neurological disorders (see Refs. 8–10 for extensive lists and rationale of V region PCR primer design).

Selection of Thermostable DNA Polymerase

A major difference exists in commercially available thermostable DNA polymerases: The presence or absence of 3′–5′ proofreading activity. The proofreading activity of cloned *Pfu* DNA polymerase results in a 12-fold increase in the fidelity of DNA synthesis when compared to a nonproofreading, thermostable DNA polymerase, such as Amplitaq. Thus, if maintaining the integrity of the template sequence is important, as in cloning projects, then a proofreading DNA polymerase should be used if possible. However, we have found that proofreading polymerases, such as cloned *Pfu* polymerase, will not amplify diverse templates with degenerate primers as efficiently as *Taq* polymerase. For example, in Fig. 6 the Vκ PCR products of CSF lymphocyte and spleen cDNA amplified with Amplitaq and cloned *Pfu* polymerase are compared. Less product is generated with *Pfu* polymerase. Furthermore, some Ig V region cDNAs from hybridomas involved in experimental autoimmune myasthenia gravis amplify nicely with *Taq* polymerase yet will not amplify at all with cloned *Pfu* polymerase when using the same degenerate primers (data not shown). Taken together, this suggests the *Pfu* polymerase is not as tolerant of primer–template mismatches as *Taq* polymerase. Thus repertoire analysis involving degenerate primers should be executed with *Taq* polymerase.

Summary

Presented in this report is a method for the generation of cDNA from a small number of lymphocytes, as few as 10, that might be encountered in the study of human neuroimmune diseases. The method is inexpensive, does not require kits or extraordinary equipment, and is incredibly rapid, making it ideal for analysis of several samples at once. Nonidet P-40 lysis cDNA synthesis has been accomplished in every cell type and disrupted tissue thus far attempted, including hybridomas (11) and B and T lymphocytes, pituitary (2), hypothalamus (2), thymus (2), and liver tissue (unpublished, 1993), and is expected to work on other cell types as well. This technique is therefore

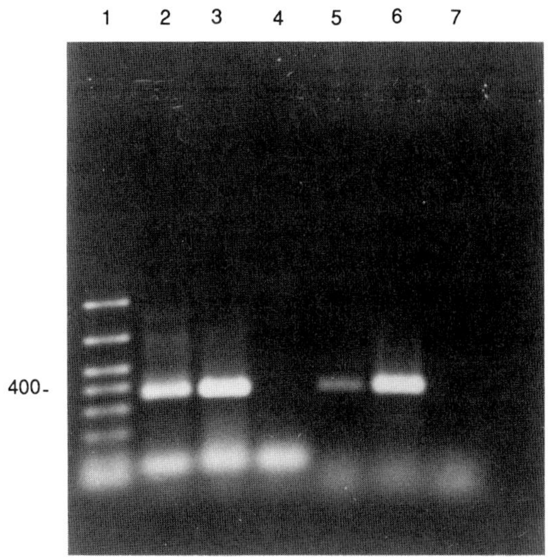

FIG. 6 Comparison of *Taq* DNA polymerase to *Pfu* DNA polymerase when amplifying with Vκ primers. Lane 1, molecular weight marker with the 400-bp band indicated. Lanes 2 and 5 are human CSF lymphocyte cDNA amplified with *Taq* and *Pfu*, respectively. Lanes 3 and 6 are human spleen cDNA amplified with *Taq* and *Pfu*, respectively. Lanes 4 and 7 are cDNA of 0 cells amplified with *Taq* and *Pfu*, respectively.

a legitimate substitute to timely RNA extractions requiring voluminous cells and can be utilized for typical RT-PCR applications.

A possible shortcoming in the method is the ability to convert low abundance or highly unstable mRNAs to cDNA. Because RNases are not immediately denatured with guanidinium and mRNA is not enriched, it is possible the sensitivity to reverse transcribe certain transcripts may be compromised. Parameters for detecting low abundance mRNAs by this methodology have not been analyzed. Furthermore, it is very important to design primers for PCR which flank a noncoding region or intron. Thus if DNA contaminates the first-strand reaction it can be distinguished from cDNA template based on the size of the PCR product.

Acknowledgments

The authors greatly appreciate the helpful discussions with Drs. Robert D. LeBoeuf, John N. Whitaker, and Shan-Ren Zhou. This work was supported by PPG P01 NS29719, NIH DK38021, a Muscular Dystrophy Association grant, and a Multiple

Sclerosis Society pilot grant (PP0317) to JEB. CCM was the recipient of a postdoctoral fellowship from NIH Training Grant T3207335.

References

1. J. O. Price, J. N. Whitaker, R. I. Vasu, and D. W. Metzger, *J. Immunol.* **136,** 2426 (1986).
2. C. C. Maier, B. Marchetti, R. D. LeBoeuf, and J. E. Blalock, *Cell. Mol. Neurobiol.* **12,** 447 (1992).
3. "Promega Protocols and Applications Guide," (D. E. Titus, ed.), 2nd Ed., p. 52. Promega Corporation, U.S.A., 1991.
4. J. Sambrook, E. F. Fritsch, and T. Maniatis, "Molecular Cloning: A Laboratory Manual," 2nd Ed., p. 4.29. Cold Spring Harbor Laboratory Press, Cold Spring Harbor, NY, 1989.
5. E. Heber-Katz and H. Acha-Orbea, *Immunol. Today* **10,** 164 (1989).
6. S. S. Zamvil and L. Steinman, *Annu. Rev. Immunol.* **8,** 579 (1990).
7. A. E. Hinkkanen, J. Määttä, Y.-F. Qin, C. Linington, A. Salmi, and H. Wekerle, *Immunogenetics* **37,** 235 (1993).
8. R. D. LeBoeuf, F. S. Galin, S. K. Hollinger, S. C. Peiper, and J. E. Blalock, *Gene* **82,** 373 (1989).
9. J. D. Marks, M. Tristem, A. Karpas, and G. Winter, *Eur. J. Immunol.* **21,** 985 (1991).
10. M. A. Panzara, E. Gussoni, L. Steinman, and J. R. Oksenberg, *BioTechniques* **12,** 728 (1992).
11. C. C. Maier, R. D. LeBoeuf, S.-R. Zhou, J. N. Whitaker, M. A. Jarpe, and J. E. Blalock, *J. Neuroimmunol.* **46,** 235 (1993).

[23] Modulation of Leukocyte Adhesion, Migration, and Homing by Neurotransmitters and Neuropeptides

Sonia L. Carlson and Joseph P. McGillis

Introduction

The effectiveness of the immune system is largely dependent on the mobile nature of leukocytes and the chance interaction of lymphocytes and antigen. Thus, lymphocytes are constantly recirculating between the blood and tissues as part of immune surveillance. For leukocytes (lymphocytes, monocytes, neutrophils) in the blood to enter a tissue or inflammatory site, the leukocytes must adhere to specialized endothelial cells found in postcapillary venules called high endothelial cells (HEC). These specialized endothelial cells are more cuboidal in shape than other endothelial cells and express specific adhesion molecules that can bind to adhesion molecules expressed on leukocytes. The HEC also can be induced at an inflammatory site by cytokines such as interleukin 1 (IL-1), γ-interferon, and tumor necrosis factor (TNF). One class of adhesion molecules that helps to specify which leukocytes bind to a particular site is the selectins. For example, L-selectins are expressed by lymphocytes, with different L-selectins specifying homing to peripheral lymph nodes or Peyer's patches. Other selectins are specific for other leukocytes such as neutrophils. The selectins bind to counter-receptor adhesion molecules expressed by the HEC and provide the interaction to tether the lymphocyte to the HEC. This interaction is relatively weak and is subsequently strengthened by other adhesion molecules: LFA-1 expressed by lymphocytes and ICAM-1 expressed by endothelial cells. As a result of the signals given to the cells in response to adhesion molecule binding, the lymphocytes migrate between the endothelial cells to enter the tissue. More detailed discussion of the adhesion molecules can be found in recent reviews (1, 2).

Substantial progress has been made in understanding the process of lymphocyte homing. The adhesion molecules have been characterized and antibodies and other reagents have been developed to aid in studying the process of lymphocyte homing. As a result, it is now possible to study in detail the effect of neurotransmitters and neuropeptides on lymphocyte migration and homing to lymphoid tissues or inflammatory sites. Catechol-

Methods in Neurosciences, Volume 24

amines, neuropeptide Y (NPY), substance P, calcitonin gene related peptide (CGRP), and other neurotransmitters are found in nerve terminals in lymphoid tissues and surrounding blood vessels. Thus, these substances are in proximity to the sites where lymphocyte homing occurs and may modulate the number or subsets of cells that home to a particular site. Indeed, we have evidence that catecholamines and CGRP can modulate lymphocyte binding to endothelial cells and homing to lymphoid tissues (3, 4).

Among the techniques that are helpful in studying the effect of the nervous system on lymphocyte homing are methods to examine lymphocyte migration and homing *in vivo* and methods to examine lymphocyte binding to endothelial cells *in vitro*. By correlating the results of these two approaches, we will be able to understand much more about this aspect of neural–immune interactions. The following are methods that we have developed or adapted in our laboratories to examine these questions.

In Vitro Adhesion Assays

Overview

Much of our current understanding of the molecular dynamics of cell migration and homing has been derived from *in vitro* assays using cultured endothelial cells. Several systems have been developed, utilizing endothelial cultures derived from a number of sources including umbilical veins, adipose tissue, neonatal heart tissue, aorta, cerebral blood vessels, and several others. One of the most commonly used systems are cultured endothelial cells derived from human umbilical vein endothelial cells (HUVEC). One concern with HUVECs is that they are a "large vessel" phenotype, and thus may not be the best model for the HEC found in postcapillary venules. This is important in that leukocytes only migrate out of the vascular system in postcapillary venules, and only after attaching to adhesion molecules on HECs. However, the advantages to HUVECs are that it is easy to obtain large quantities of pure endothelial cells, and, in many cases, they have been shown to express adhesion molecules used by HECs for leukocyte binding. The ability of HUVECs to express leukocyte adhesion molecules is probably a reflection of the plasticity of a fetal tissue. Thus, depending on the specific question, HUVECs may be an appropriate model system. However, for many questions, especially regarding site-specific lymphocyte homing, it may be more appropriate to use endothelial cell cultures derived from specific tissues. For these reasons, methods are described for preparing HUVECs as well as mouse lymph node and rat heart microvascular endothelial cells.

Endothelial Cell Culture Methods

Human Umbilical Vein Endothelial Cells

The methods for culturing HUVECs were initially established in the 1970s, and there is an extensive literature describing the use of these cells for studies of angiogenesis, nutrient transport, leukocyte adhesion, etc. The original method for HUVEC culture was described by Gimbrone *et al.* (5). The procedure described here is basically an adaptation of the original method. A key element in the growth and maintenance of HUVECs is the addition of an appropriate endothelial cell growth factor (ECGF). Several growth factors for endothelial cells have been described, some of which are only angiogenic *in vitro* and some of which are only angiogenic *in vivo* (6). One of the most effective for *in vitro* maintenance of HUVECs is basic fibroblast growth factor (bFGF). Some investigators use recombinant bFGF, or "ECGF supplements" which are available commercially. Recombinant bFGF requires the addition of heparin, and the latter ECGF supplements are generally either brain or pituitary extracts. A disadvantage is the cost of the commercial supplements if one is considering extensive use of large numbers of cultured endothelial cells. An alternative to the commercially available ECGFs is a bovine brain extract which is rich in bFGF (7). We have found this extract to be effective with endothelial cells from all of the sources we have cultured to date.

Preparation of Bovine Brain Extract and Human Umbilical Vein Endothelial Cell Medium

A simple bovine brain extract which is very rich in bFGF can be prepared as described by MacCaig *et al.* (7). Briefly, a fresh bovine brain is obtained and the meninges are carefully dissected off. The brain is then cut into 1-cm cubes and added to 1 liter of 0.1 *M* NaCl, pH 7.4. The tissue is then homogenized with a Polytron (9 × 20 sec bursts on medium setting) and stirred for 2 hr at 4°C. The homogenate is then centrifuged at 13,800 *g* for 40 min at 4°C. The supernatant is removed, streptomycin sulfate is added (0.5%, w/v) and the mixture is stirred for 1 hr at 4°C. The mixture is centrifuged 13,800 *g* for 40 min at 4°C. The supernatant is decanted, lyophilized, and stored at −20°C. The efficacy of each batch is tested by titration, with the end point being endothelial cell growth. The optimal concentrations have been in the range of 50 to 100 μg/ml, and typical yields have been 16–17 g of ECGF per bovine brain. Although some investigators have subjected the bovine brain extract ECGF to further purification, we have found the extract described above to be sufficient. Growth and maintenance media for HUVECs is Medium 199 with 10% (v/v) supplemented calf serum (Hyclone),

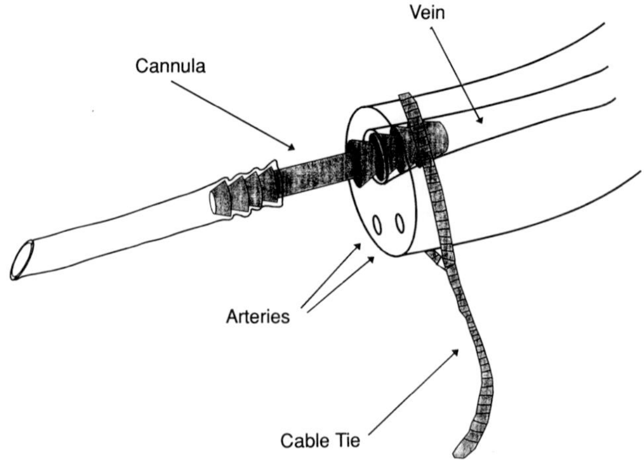

FIG. 1 Schematic of the cannula used in the preparation of endothelial cells from human umbilical vein (HUVECs) as described in the text. Note that the umbilical cord has one vein and two smaller arteries. Drawn by Lorri Ann Morford.

20 m*M* HEPES (Sigma), pH 7.3, 5 U/ml heparin (Elkins-Sinn, Inc., Cherry Hill, NJ), 100 μg/ml ECGF, and 10 μg/ml gentamicin sulfate (GIBCO, Grand Island, NY). For rodent endothelial cells we omit the heparin and use 5% bovine calf serum for rat heart ECs and 10% alpha calf fraction (HyClone) for mouse lymph node ECs.

Preparation of Human Umbilical Vein Endothelial Cell Cultures

Isolation of endothelial cells from the umbilical vein utilizes limited digestion with collagenase to separate the endothelial cells from the basement membrane. Umbilical cords from normal vaginal deliveries are clamped on both ends and are placed in sterile saline. The cords are usually held overnight at 4°C as suggested by van Hinsbergh *et al.* (8) to improve the yield. To remove endothelial cells, the umbilical vein is first cannulated. Several investigators have described the use of glass cannulas with a constriction near the end; however, we have found it preferable to use a barbed polyethylene tubing connector for $\frac{1}{8}$- or $\frac{3}{16}$-inch tubing (Cole Parmer, catalog numbers L-06477-60 or L-06456-10). Silastic tubing, $\frac{1}{8}$ inch inside diameter, is fit over one end of the connector, and the other end can be attached to a syringe (Fig. 1). These cannulas can be autoclave sterilized and reused. Another advantage of these cannulas over the glass cannulas is that they are unbreakable, reducing the potential risk to the personnel working with human tissues.

To cannulate the umbilical cords a fresh cut is made with a sterile scalpel inside the clamps. A cannula is inserted into each end of the vein (there are two smaller arteries and one larger vein). The cannulas are held in place with BAR-LOK cable ties (available in any electrical or hardware store) or heavy thread. Washes and solutions are then added and collected by attaching syringes to the open ends of the cannula tubing. The medium used throughout the preparation is Hanks' balanced salt solution (HBSS) with 20 m*M* HEPES (GIBCO, Gaithersburg, MD). The umbilical vein is flushed with 20 ml of medium to remove blood. A solution of 0.2% collagenase (w/v, Worthington, Freehold, NJ) and 0.2% DNase (w/v, Sigma) in HBSS/HEPES is then perfused into the lumen, and the cord is placed at 37°C for 15 min. DNase is added to degrade DNA (which can be toxic to cultured cells) released from dead cells. After incubation, the contents of the vein are collected into a 50-ml tube, followed by a 20-ml wash to ensure the endothelial cells are washed from the lumen. The cells are then pelleted by centrifugation at 200 *g* for 10 min. The cells are washed three times in HUVEC culture media and resuspended in a final volume of 5 ml. The cells are added to a gelatin-coated 25-cm^2 tissue culture flask and are placed in a humidifed, 5% CO_2 incubator at 37°C. Some investigators have reported the use of trypsin rather than collagenase for removing the endothelial cells. However, in our hands we find that HUVEC cultures prepared with trypsin have contaminating nonendothelial cells at a substantially higher level than do those prepared by collagenase digestion.

Although endothelial cells will grow directly on tissue culture plastic by producing their own substrate layer, they do much better if the tissue culture dishes are precoated with a substrate protein such as collagen or fibronectin. Several commercial sources of highly purified tissue culture grade collagen or fibronectin are available. However, we have found that a relatively inexpensive gelatin solution (gelatin, Type B from bovine skin, 2% solution, Sigma, St. Louis, MO catalog number G-1393) works just as well. Plastic surfaces are coated by incubation with 1% gelatin (diluted 1 : 1, v/v, with HBSS) at room temperature for 30 min. Prior to addition of cells the gelatin is removed and the dish is rinsed with HBSS. Freshly isolated cells from a single umbilical cord are plated in a 25-cm^2 flask and will generally reach confluence within 5–10 days, depending on the initial number of cells plated. Once the HUVECs reach confluence, they are subcultured by digestion with trypsin–EDTA (0.25% and 1 m*M*, respectively, GIBCO) to remove the cells from the plate and are reseeded at a ratio of 1 : 4 or 1 : 5. For adhesion experiments, the cells are generally used in the second to fifth passages.

Characterization of Endothelial Cells

Endothelial cells have a number of unique characteristics that can be used to confirm their identity as endothelial cells and to determine the relative purity of the cultures. The two most common biochemical markers for endo-

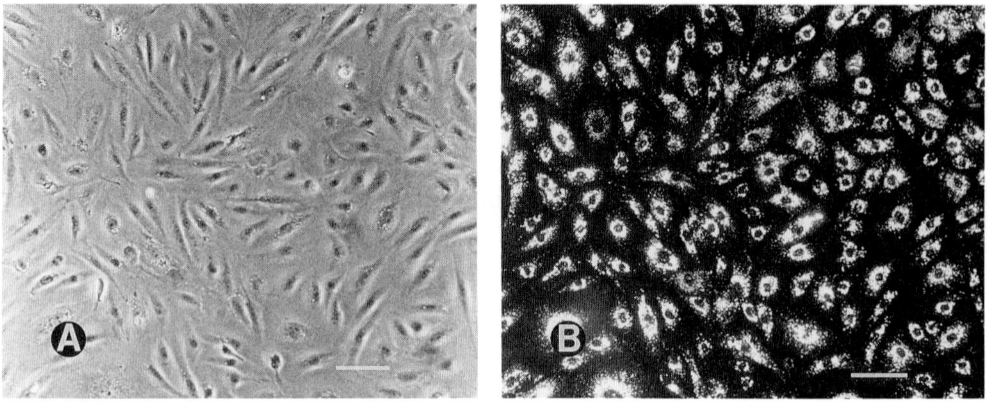

FIG. 2 Microscopy of HUVEC cultures. (A) Phase contrast of near confluent HUVECs showing the characteristic small uniform size of the cells in culture. (B) Fluorescence of the same field of HUVECs showing the uptake of DiI-Ac-LDL used to confirm the cells as endothelial cells. Bar: 100 μm.

thelial cells are the expression of factor VIII, or von Willebrand factor, and the uptake of acetylated low density lipoprotein (ac-LDL). Also, as shown in Fig. 2, HUVECs have a highly characteristic cobblestone morphology in culture. As with any type of primary cell culture system, it is important to establish criteria for the identity of the cultured cells. Factor VIII expression is restricted to endothelial cells and both monoclonal and polyclonal factor VIII antibodies for immunohistochemical staining can be obtained commercially from several sources. A second marker that can be used to identify endothelial cells is their ability to bind and internalize ac-LDL. Acetylated LDL binds to the "scavenger receptor," or the LDL receptor-like protein (LRP), which is expressed only on endothelial cells, macrophages, and astrocytes. Although ac-LDL uptake is not as specific as factor VIII staining, it is much easier, and ac-LDL-positive nonendothelial cells can easily be distinguished by morphology. While there is a potential for monocyte/macrophage contamination, it is not a major concern since monocytes will die out within 10–14 days, especially in HUVEC media. To assess ac-LDL uptake, endothelial cells are cultured at 37°C with DiI-ac-LDL (BTI, Stoughton, MA, 200 μg/ml, or Molecular Probes, Eugene, OR, 100 μg/ml) for 4 hr. After the incubation, the cells are washed with three changes of HBSS or media. Internalized ac-LDL can then be viewed with a fluorescence microsope in live cells or in cells fixed with 4% paraformaldehyde. For HUVECs, we typically find that essentially 100% of the cells are positive for ac-LDL uptake, as shown in Fig. 2B.

Endothelial Cells from Other Sources

While HUVECs are relatively easy to prepare, they may not be the most appropriate model system in all cases. For example, if examining the effect of neural or endocrine mediators on lymphocyte recirculation, it would probably be more appropriate to use endothelial cells derived from lymph nodes. In this section we briefly detail some of the procedures for preparation of endothelial cells from other sources including murine lymph nodes and rat heart microvessels.

Preparation of Mouse Lymphoid Microvascular Endothelial Cells

Lymph node endothelial cells can be cultured from murine peripheral lymph nodes by using an adaptation of the technique described by Ager and Ise *et al.* (9, 10) for rat lymph node ECs. Endothelial cells obtained from lymphoid tissues are likely to be enriched for the HECs that normally interact with migrating lymphocytes and thus should be a more relevant source of ECs for studies of lymphocyte homing. Unfortunately, difficulties in maintaining murine ECs *in vitro* limit the routine use of these cells. The following is the protocol that we have used to isolate mouse peripheral lymph node ECs. Mice are euthanized, and the peripheral lymph nodes collected using sterile technique and placed in sterile washing medium [Dulbecco's modified Eagle's medium (DMEM) with 20 m*M* HEPES and penicillin (100 U/ml)–streptomycin (100 μg/ml)]. The lymph nodes are minced and washed several times by removal of the supernatant after allowing the tissue chunks to settle out. Approximately three to four washes are needed to wash away the lymphocytes. Two milliliters of collagenase (0.5%, w/v, Worthington, Type II collagenase) in washing medium is added and the tissue is incubated for 1 hr, 37°C, with occasional pipetting to break up the tissue chunks. The tissue suspension is filtered through 100 μm nylon mesh into a 15 ml tube, and the collagenase tube is rinsed with medium which is filtered and pooled with the cell suspension. Filtration is greatly facilitated if Swinnex syringe filters (Millipore, Bedford, MA) are used. The cells are pelleted by centrifugation for 7 min at 300*g* at 25°C and washed two additional times. The cell pellet is resuspended in 2 ml endothelial cell growth medium [same as defined above except using DMEM and 10% alpha calf fraction (HyClone)] and added to a gelatin-coated well of a six-well plate. The cells are cultured at 37°C in a humidified 5% CO_2 incubator. The endothelial cells are initially found in small clusters that expand to become dense patches of cobblestone-shaped cells.

Several factors limit the success of culturing murine microvascular endothelial cells. First, it is difficult to obtain pure cultures without contamination by fibroblasts or smooth muscle cells that can rapidly overgrow the endothelial cells. We have used several approaches to enrich the cell population for endothelial cells. First, using alpha calf serum (HyClone) rather than fetal or supplemented bovine calf serum greatly reduces the growth of contaminating cells presumably because of lower levels of growth factors that encourage fibroblast growth. In addition, using medium containing D-valine rather than L-valine in the early stages of the cell culture dramatically reduces the growth of fibroblasts because endothelial cells can convert D-valine to L-valine whereas fibroblasts cannot. We found it necessary to change back to normal growing medium after a few days as the ECs grew slowly in D-valine medium. Another method to enrich for endothelial cells is to change the medium in the culture dish within 2 hr of the initiation of the culture to remove cells that have not adhered. Endothelial cells often adhere to the culture dish more rapidly than other cell types; however, we had limited success with this approach in our culture system. Finally, separating the initial tissue digest on a continuous Percoll gradient (Pharmacia, Piscataway, NJ) can allow selection of cells that have the appropriate density for endothelial cells (1.04–1.05 g/ml), thus eliminating many of the contaminating cells. This approach is limited somewhat if the cell preparation does not yield enough ECs to produce a visible band in the gradient, although a parallel gradient tube containing density marker beads can circumvent this problem. Another limit in the use of murine microvessel ECs is that they do not survive being passaged with trypsin as well as ECs from other sources, which may be due, in part, to using cells derived from adult animals. Thus, murine ECs are best used soon after the initial prep to isolate the cells.

Preparation of Rat Heart Microvessel Endothelial Cells

Fetal rat heart endothelial cultures also have been used to prepare microvessel endothelial cells for adhesion assays. Since over 90% of the blood vessels in the heart are microvessels, it is assumed that the majority of cells in these cultures are derived from microvessels. The following method has been described previously (11, 12). Hearts are dissected aseptically from 10 to 12 four- to five-day old rats and are placed in DMEM. The collected hearts are minced and transferred to a 15-ml tube to which is added 12 ml of DMEM. The fragments are washed by allowing them to settle and then removing the DMEM. This step is repeated until the DMEM remains clear. This step is important in removing free blood elements. The tissue fragments are resuspended in 12 ml of DMEM with 0.2% collagenase (w/v), 0.2% DNase (w/v) and then placed in a shaker bath at 37°C for 15 min. The tissue fragments are then pipetted up and down several times and are allowed to settle. The supernatant cell suspension which contains the endothelial cells is removed and centrifuged at 200*g* for 10 min. The cell pellet is resuspended in culture media and plated in gelatin-coated flasks. The cells are allowed to attach for 1 hr at 37°C and the nonadherent cells are decanted. It is important to keep the initial attachment period brief in that it acts to enrich the cultures for endothelial cells; endothelial cells adhere fairly rapidly whereas smooth muscle cells and other cells require a much longer period to adhere. The flask is washed several times and the cells are cultured and subcultured as described for the HUVECs. Microvascular endothelial cells produced in this manner are generally 80–95% positive for endothelial cell markers (DiI-ac-LDL uptake).

In Vitro Adhesion Assays

In vitro adhesion assays have been used to study both the effects of cytokines on leukocyte adhesion and the regulation of adhesion molecules. The simplest form of these assays measures the percentage of leukocytes which adhere to endothelial cell monolayers following various treatments. The number of leukocytes adhering to the endothelial cell monolayer can be assessed by manual counting after fixation or by using leukocytes labeled with ^{51}Cr or with a fluorescent tag.

Leukocyte Preparation and Labeling

Labeling Leukocytes with ^{51}Cr

The basic procedures for labeling of specific cell types, lymphocytes, neutrophils, monocytes, etc., are essentially the same. A common method for measuring adhesion is to use cells labeled with ^{51}Cr. Leukocytes are prepared as described by Elliott *et al.* (13) and are resuspended in Medium 199 with 20 m*M* HEPES, pH 7.6, 1% BSA at 10^8 cells/ml. An equal volume of $Na^{51}CrO_4$ (1 mCi/ml in sterile PBS) is added and the cells are incubated at 37°C for 1 hr. The cells are then washed by repeated centrifugation and resuspension in media. Radioactivity in the spent media is monitored and washing is continued until the radioactivity is down to background (usually five to seven washes).

Fluorescent Labeling of Leukocytes

In order to avoid the use of radioactivity, lymphocytes can be easily loaded with various fluorescent markers to aid in subsequent data analysis. One effective label is chloromethylfluorescein diacetate (CMFDA, Molecular Probes, Eugene, OR). To load the cells with the CMFDA, the lymphocytes are resuspended at 1×10^7/ml in a 10 μM solution of CMFDA in HBSS, 0.5% BSA, and 20 m*M* HEPES, pH 7.4. The cells are incubated for 15 min at 37°C and then washed two times at 200*g* for 10 min at 25°C. The cells are resuspended in appropriate medium for the subsequent binding assay.

Adhesion Assay Protocols

The effect of biologic mediators on leukocyte–endothelial cell adhesion can be assessed by treatment of the leukocytes and/or the endothelial cell cultures. Extensive studies have been done examining the effect of various cytokines on cell adhesion. Several cytokines, including IL-1 and TNFα, have been identified which upregulate specific adhesion molecules for leukocytes. In a typical experiment, endothelial cells are plated out in gelatin-coated 24-well plates at a concentration of 2×10^4/well and allowed to grow to confluence, usually 2 days. On the day of the binding assay, the endothelial cells are stimulated with 10 U/ml IL-1β for 4 hr, 37°C, to enhance the expression of adhesion molecules. At the end of the incubation, the wells are washed two times, and 500 μl of HUVEC medium is added to each well. Lymphocytes are adjusted to 4×10^6/ml in HUVEC medium, and 500 μl is added to each well to initiate the binding assay. If additional stimulants or reagents are to be added (from 10× stocks) during the binding assay, the volume of medium put in the HUVEC wells after washing away the IL-1 is adjusted such that the final volume per well is 1 ml. The plates are incubated at 37°C for 30–60 min to allow the lymphocytes to adhere. At the end of the incubation, the nonadherent lymphocytes are removed by washing the wells three times with warm (37°C) HBSS supplemented with 0.5% BSA and 20 m*M* HEPES. The number of adherent lymphocytes can be determined by a number of different methods as discussed below.

Analysis Using ^{51}Cr-Labeled Lymphocytes

After the free leukocytes have been removed by washing, the adherent cells are lysed by addition of a minimal volume of 1% Triton X-100 in water. The lysate from each well is then transferred to a tube and the radioactivity measured in a gamma counter. The results from a typical adhesion experiment using ^{51}Cr-labeled human PBLs is shown in Fig. 3. The endothelial cells were pretreated with IL-1 or with CGRP for 4 hr. As expected, treatment with IL-1 caused a dose-dependent increase in the percentage of hPBLs which adhered. In contrast, CGRP by itself had no effect. Interestingly, we have since determined that CGRP can alter the effects of certain cytokines on leukocyte adhesion (4).

Nonisotopic Methods for Analysis

Several methods can be used to avoid the use of radioactivity in lymphocyte–endothelial cell adhesion assays, including flow cytometry, microscopy, or a fluorescence plate reader. For the microscopic method and use of the fluorescence plate reader, the lymphocytes are labeled with the fluorescent tag CMFDA. Unlabeled leukocytes can be used in analysis by flow cytometry.

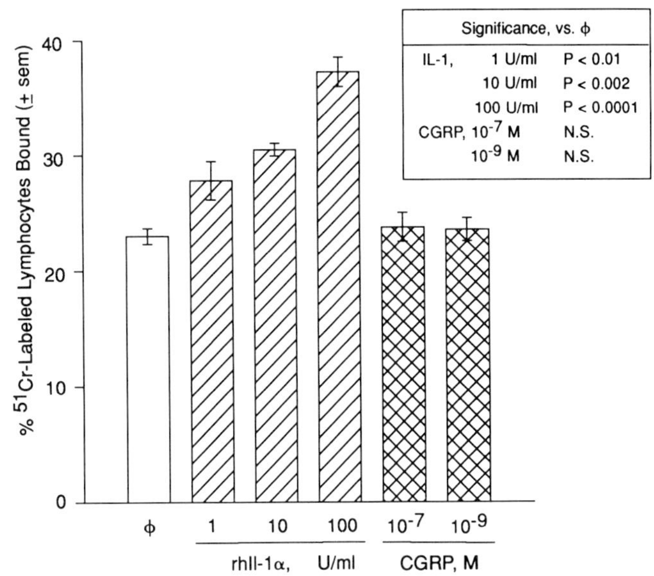

FIG. 3 Adhesion of lymphocytes to IL-1 and CGRP-treated HUVECs. The HUVECs were plated in 24-well gelatin-coated culture plates 24 hr prior to treatment with recombinant human IL-1β or CGRP. The cells were washed and treated with IL-1 at concentrations of 1, 10, and 100 U/ml and concentrations of CGRP of 10^{-7} and 10^{-9} *M* for 4 hr. The cells were then washed three times with HBSS and 3.5×10^6 ^{51}Cr-labeled hPBLs in 0.4 ml were added to each well. After an additional incubation at 37°C for 1 hr nonadherent cells were washed off and 0.4 ml of 1% Triton X-100 was added to lyse the adherent cells. The lysate was transferred to a fresh tube and the radioactivity in the lysate was determined in a gamma counter. The values are the mean ± SE for triplicate samples. The statistical comparison of means was done by Student's *t* test.

Analysis by Flow Cytometry After removal of the nonadherent leukocytes, the adherent lymphocytes and endothelial cells are removed from the plate and analyzed according to the method of Benschop *et al.* (14). Briefly, the endothelial cells are lifted from the plate by adding 250 μl of trypsin–EDTA (GIBCO) and incubating for 1 min. The trypsin activity is stopped by adding 50 μl of serum. Each well is diluted with 1 ml of PBS and the cells from each well are transferred to 12 × 75-mm Falcon snap cap tubes, using an additional 2 × 1 ml of PBS to wash each well. The cells are centrifuged 200*g* for 10 min at 25°C, and the pellet is resuspended in 300 μl 1% paraformaldehyde in PBS. The flow cytometry analysis is based on the distinct forward scatter (cell size) and side scatter (granularity) characteristics

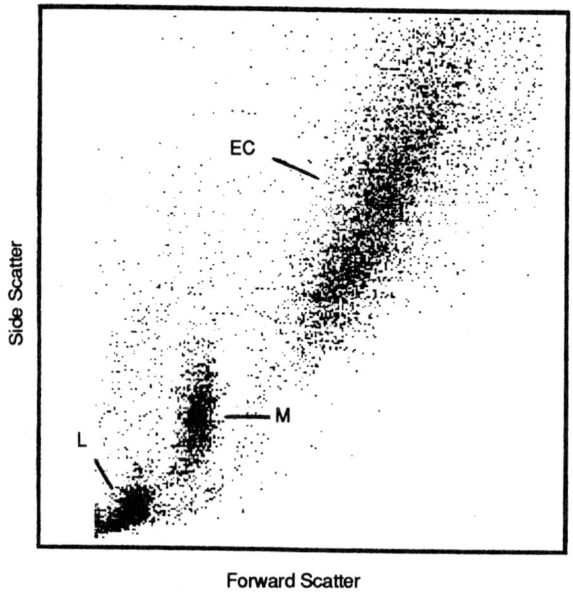

FIG. 4 Cell sorter (FACS) analysis of lymphocyte and monocyte binding to IL-1-activated endothelial cells. Human umbilical vein endothelial cells (HUVECs) were grown to confluence in a 24-well plate and stimulated for 4 hr with 10 U/ml IL-1β. Human peripheral blood lymphocytes (1×10^6/well) were allowed to adhere to the HUVECs for 1 hr, 37°C, and the nonadherent lymphocytes washed away. The adherent cells were lifted from the plate with trypsin as described in the text. Using forward and side scatter with the cell sorter, the lymphocytes (L), monocytes (M), and HUVECs (EC) can be gated on separately to obtain the ratios of lymphocytes or monocytes bound to the HUVECs.

of lymphocytes and endothelial cells (Fig. 4) and the data are expressed as the ratio of lymphocytes to endothelial cells. If macrophages are present in the lymphocyte preparation, they can be gated on separately in the forward and side scatter plot to determine the ratio of macrophages to endothelial cells. In our experience, the ratio of lymphocytes to endothelial cells is doubled if the endothelial cells have been stimulated for 4 hr with IL-1 compared to unstimulated endothelial cells. It is necessary to use wells no smaller than the 24-well format in order to have enough cells to analyze by flow cytometry. It may be possible to phenotypically characterize the adherent leukocytes by using fluorescently tagged antibodies, but in preliminary experiments, we have found that the trypsin treatment decreased antibody staining of T-cell markers.

Microscopic Analysis In microscopic analysis of an adhesion assay, the lymphocytes are prelabeled with CMFDA to aid the analysis. After each well is washed to remove nonadherent lymphocytes, 0.5 ml of 2% glutaraldehyde in PBS is added and incubated for 15 min. The wells are washed twice with PBS and as much of the liquid as possible is removed by aspiration. A drop of Vectashield (Vector Laboratories, Burlingame, CA) or SlowFade (Molecular Probes, Eugene, OR) coverslipping medium is added (to reduce fading of the fluorescence) and a round coverslip placed in each well. The wells are observed using an inverted fluorescence microscope. The endothelial cells and lymphocytes can be seen using phase contrast, but analysis is facilitated by using the fluorescence so that the lymphocytes are readily observed. An eyepiece reticle grid is used to quantify the number of leukocytes bound per reticle field. The area of the reticle field is calibrated using a stage micrometer. To ensure representative data from each well, at least two to three random fields are counted per well, and an average value is obtained. The greatest disadvantage of this technique is the time needed for data collection.

Analysis Using a Fluorescence Plate Reader One of the fastest and most convenient methods of data anlysis utilizes a fluorescence plate reader. The binding assay is carried out as described above using CMFDA-labeled leukocytes. The nonadherent leukocytes are removed and PBS or phenol red-free HBSS is added to each well. The amount of fluorescence per well is rapidly determined by the plate reader. An additional advantage of this method is that it is possible to set up a standard curve of fluorescently labeled cells such that the data can be converted to number of bound cells per well as opposed to fluorescence units (Fig. 5). Using the CytoFluor 2300 (Millipore Corp.) we have been able to detect a minimum of approximately 5000 cells/well in a 48-well plate. Certain plate readers will allow the use of different plate formats from 6- to 96-well, whereas others use only 96-well plates. In preliminary experiments we have found a better HUVEC response to IL-1 using 48-well plates compared to 96-well plates.

In Vivo Assays of Leukocyte Homing to Lymphoid Tissues

The migration and homing of lymphocytes *in vivo* to lymphoid or other tissues can be readily assessed by labeling the lymphocytes with a fluorescent tag prior to iv injection. The mice or rats utilized in these studies must be inbred so that the animals are syngeneic, thus eliminating the generation of immune responses between the host immune system and the newly infused lymphocytes.

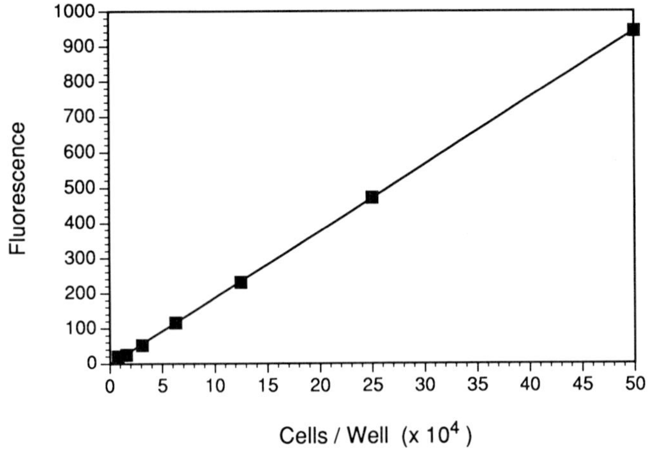

FIG. 5 Standard curve of fluorescently labeled lymphocytes using a fluorescence plate reader. Human T cells were labeled with CMFDA (10 μM) for use in a lymphocyte–endothelial cell binding assay. The standard curve was generated by adding a known number of cells per well of a 48-well plate and represents the average number of fluorescent units per well from duplicate determinations. The data were obtained using a CytoFluor 2300 fluorescence plate reader (Millipore Corp.) with an excitation of 485 nm, emission of 530 nm, and a sensitivity of 4.

In our experiments we have used peripheral lymph node lymphocytes; however, we have found that nylon wool enriched splenic T cells migrate to a similar extent. The lymphoid population from peripheral lymph nodes is 60–70% T cells. The predominant cell type that migrates into the lymphoid tissues in our short-term assays (less than 2 hr) is the T cell. Greater than 95% of the labeled cells that have homed to the spleen or lymph nodes stain positively for CD3, CD4, or CD8 by FACS analysis. Examination of spleen and lymph node sections with a fluorescence microscope shows that the labeled cells are found in T-cell compartments of the tissues (Fig. 6).

The lymphocytes may be labeled with either radioactive or fluorescent tags prior to infusion into recipient mice. The most common radioactive tag is ^{51}Cr. The advantage of chromium is that the total amount of radioactivity per mouse and per lymph node or spleen can be determined; however, there are many disadvantages to working with this substance. The major disadvantages are dealing with radioactive storage and waste disposal as well as the potential for radioactive contamination of laboratory equipment. In addition, it is uncertain how much of the radioactivity measured in a tissue may be the result of ^{51}Cr that has leaked out of labeled lymphocytes. Finally, radioactivity could alter cellular metabolism or function of the la-

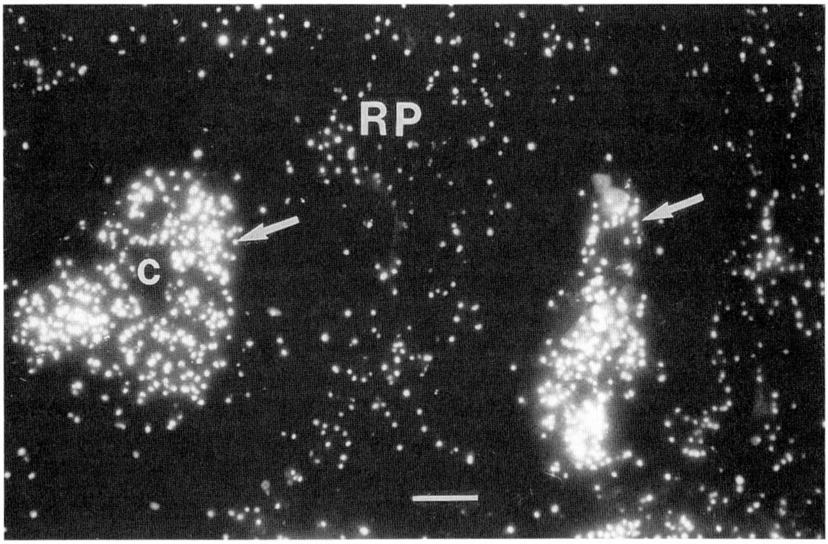

FIG. 6 Fluorescence of CMFDA-labeled lymphocytes that have homed to the spleen. Murine peripheral blood lymphocytes were labeled with CMFDA (10 μM) and injected iv into the tail vein of mice. The mice were sacrificed after 2 hr and the spleen was frozen and cut at 20 μm with a cryostat. The micrograph shows a diffuse distribution of labeled lymphocytes in the red pulp (RP) and the dense collection of cells that have migrated to the T-cell portion of the white pulp (arrows) surrounding the central artery (C). The white bar represents 100 μm.

beled cells. The use of fluorescent tags overcomes many of the problems associated with the use of radioactivity. The biological hazards of the cytosolic fluorescent dyes are much less than that of ^{51}Cr; however, caution should be used with fluorescent tags that bind to the DNA as these pose a significant health hazard. Analysis of the migration of the labeled cells can be done by FACS and by examination of tissue sections microscopically. The FACS samples or tissues sections also can be stained for specific cell-surface markers using fluorescently labeled antibodies in order to phenotypically characterize the lymphocytes which have migrated, thus gaining much more information than is possible with radioactively labeled cells. A disadvantage of the fluorescently labeled cells is that it is difficult to obtain an estimate of the total number of labeled cells that have homed to different tissues without doing extensive cell counts that can be correlated with the FACS data. The basic protocols for labeling and injecting cells are given below, followed by comments on the different dyes that we have used.

TABLE I Fluorescent Dyes Used to Label Lymphocytes for Adhesion and Migration Experiments

Dye	Stock concentration in DMSO[a] (mM)	Final concentration[b] (μM)	Cellular localization and color	Comments
CMFDA	10	10 (M) 0.5 (F)	Cytoplasm, green	For antibody-PE staining, low CMFDA loading concentrations should be used to prevent bleed-through of green fluorescence into red range
CMTMR	10	10–20 (M, F)	Cytoplasm, orange-red	Can be used in combination with CMFDA-labeled cells
CMAC	5	25 (M, F)	Cytoplasm, blue	Decreased mitogen-induced proliferation of splenocytes, thus may have unwanted metabolic effects. May need >30 min loading time to be bright enough for microscopy
H-33342	1	5 (M, F)	Nucleus, blue	Excessive leaching from labeled cells to surrounding cells in tissue. Unsuitable for migration studies.

[a] DMSO, dimethyl sulfoxide.
[b] (M) microscopy; (F) FACS.

Lymphocyte Preparation and Labeling

We have utilized several different fluorescent markers available from Molecular Probes (Eugene, OR) and have found the most satisfactory results with the fluorescein derivatives (Table I). In addition, fewer problems are associated with using cytoplasmic markers compared to markers that bind to the DNA, which could result in altered gene expression and transcription.

The procedure used to label lymphocytes is similar for the different dyes. Lymph node lymphocytes are obtained as described by Elliott *et al.* (13) using density gradient centrifugation to remove dead cells and red blood cells. The cells are resuspended (5–10 × 10^6/ml) in DMEM (supplemented

0.5% BSA and 20 mM HEPES) containing the fluorescent dye (concentrations described below) and incubated for 15 min at 37°C. The cells are washed two times and resuspended at a concentration of 1×10^7 cells per 200 μl. The last wash and resuspension medium is DMEM without BSA or HEPES.

Lymphocyte Injection and Migration

The lymphocytes are taken up into a 1-ml tuberculin syringe and a 26-gauge needle is added. The mice are warmed by placing the cages on heating pads for 20–25 min, thus causing dilation of the tail veins. Each mouse is temporarily placed in a restrainer and the lymphocytes (1×10^7) are infused into a tail vein in a 200-μl volume. Great care must be taken to prevent the cells from settling out in the syringe and to inject exactly the same amount of volume per mouse to limit variability in the data. The cells also should be protected from exposure to light to prevent fading of the dye. We have let cells migrate for 0.5 1, 2, and 24 hr, prior to sacrifice of the mice. After sacrifice, the spleen and various lymphoid tissues are quickly removed and placed in tubes containing washing medium to be prepared for cell sorter analysis or onto a small piece of labeled aluminum foil and immediately frozen on dry ice. Lymph nodes are embedded in a small piece of liver prior to freezing to facilitate later cryostat cutting of these small tissues. For long-term storage, the frozen tissues are kept at −90°C or in a liquid N_2 tank.

In experiments where we have examined the migration of control lymphocytes vs those pretreated with catecholamines, it has been possible to label each of the lymphocyte suspensions with a different color dye and then mix the cells in equal proportions after the washes are completed so that cells from both treatment groups can be infused into the same animal. We have injected 1×10^7 CMFDA-labeled lymphocytes (green, control) plus 1×10^7 CMTMR-labeled lymphocytes (red, catecholamine-treated) in a volume of 200 μl into the same mouse with good results (Fig. 7). The FACS analysis requires, however, a dual-laser cell sorter because CMFDA and CMTMR cannot be excited at the same wavelength. The advantage of this approach is that each mouse can serve as its own control which may eliminate some variability in the data. Some difficulty may be encountered with spleen cell suspensions if the CMTMR is not bright enough because some spleen cells have red autofluorescence that can overlap with weakly labeled CMTMR cells.

Analysis of Tissue-Specific Lymphocyte Migration

FACS Analysis of Lymphocyte Migration

The tissues to be analyzed by FACS must be minced individually. Enough cells (approximately $1–2 \times 10^6$) can be obtained from a single lymph node

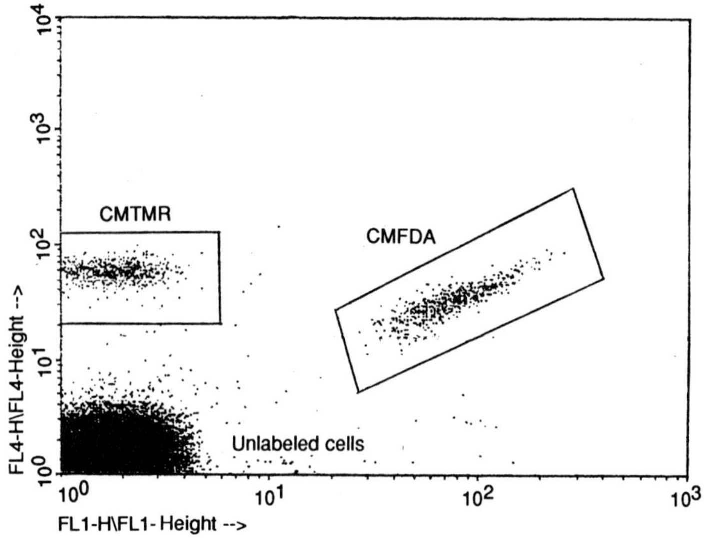

FIG. 7 Analysis of the homing of CMFDA- and CMTMR-labeled lymphocytes to axillary lymph node in mice. Peripheral lymph node lymphocytes were labeled with either CMFDA or CMTMR, washed, and pooled together in equal proportions. The lymphocytes were injected iv into the tail vein and allowed to migrate for 1 hr. The lymphoid tissues were removed and cell suspensions prepared for analysis by dual-laser flow cytometry (FACS). The CMFDA- and CMTMR-labeled cells can be gated on as indicated to determine the percentage of total cells that are labeled, thus giving a measure of the number of cells that have homed to the tissue.

to analyze, but pooling the corresponding nodes from both sides of the body ensures having sufficient cells. Given the large number of cells in a whole spleen, only a portion of this tissue is needed, but a consistent part of the spleen should be used for each sample. The tissues are placed in 0.5 ml of washing medium in 12 × 75-mm Falcon tubes. Lymph nodes or pieces of spleen are removed from the tube and placed on a small piece of 105-μm polypropylene mesh inside a small funnel. We have utilized the base of a 25-mm Swinnex filter holder (Millipore) for this purpose. The funnel is set in the top of the tube and the tissue mashed using the plunger from a 1-ml syringe. The lymphocytes are washed into the tube with 4 ml of medium, and tissue debris remains on the filter. The cell suspensions are washed once, and lymph node samples resuspended in 0.5 ml of 1% paraformaldehyde in PBS. For spleen samples, only a small portion of the original cell suspension is needed for FACS analysis; thus, these cells are resuspended in 1 ml and an aliquot containing approximately 1×10^6 cells is removed to a different tube, spun down, and resuspended in 0.5 ml of 1% paraformaldehyde for FACS analysis.

In order to further characterize the cells that have migrated, the cell suspensions can be stained with fluorescently labeled antibodies against various cell surface markers. Prior to fixation, the cells are resuspended in 100 μl of antibody diluted in PBS with 0.02% azide and 1% fetal calf serum. The cells are incubated with the antibody for 30 min at 4°C, washed twice, then resuspended in 1% paraformaldehyde in PBS. If the lymphocytes for the migration have been labeled with CMFDA (0.5 μM), PE-labeled antibodies work well. The CMFDA-labeled lymphocytes must not be loaded with a high concentration of CMFDA (i.e., 10 μM) as the green fluorescence will be too bright and bleed into the red fluorescence range.

For FACS analysis, 40,000 events are examined because the number of fluorescently labeled lymphocytes that have migrated into the various lymphoid tissues is low. The data are expressed as the percentage of the cells in a tissue that are CMFDA labeled. Typically, 1–3% of the spleen cells and 0.5–1.5% of the lymph node cells have the CMFDA label and thus represent the cells that have homed to the tissue after the iv injection. The CellTracker dyes (CMFDA, CMTMR) become trapped in the cytoplasm of the cells and do not appear to leak out of the cells once they have been loaded.

Microscopic Analysis of Migrated Cells

Frozen tissues are mounted onto a cryostat chuck using TissueTek with care being taken not to thaw the tissue. Tissue sections are cut 10–20 μm thick. Thin sections (10 μm) are preferred for image analysis because the tissue is only one to two cell layers thick. Thicker sections may be preferred for general observation and photography. The sections are thaw-mounted onto gelatin-coated slides and fixed for 15 min in 4% paraformaldehyde in PBS. The slides are rinsed two to three times in PBS, dipped in distilled H_2O, and allowed to drain. The slides are coverslipped using Vectashield (Vector Laboratories, Burlingame, CA). We have found that Vectashield greatly reduces fading of the fluorescence compared to other coverslipping mediums. At all times after the tissues are thaw-mounted onto the slide, they are protected from exposure to room lights as the fluorescence can fade. When observed with a fluorescence microscope and fluorescein filters, the cells labeled with CMFDA are brilliant green compared to the faint autofluorescence of the tissue. In spleen, the cells can be seen to be distributed in red pulp at early time points (30-min migration), but by 2 hr the cells are found tightly clustered in the center of the white pulp (Fig. 6). Thus the cells home to appropriate compartments within the tissue. The CMTMR-labeled cells also can be readily seen using rhodamine filters, but this dye is not as brilliant as the CMFDA. By alternating between fluorescence filters, the distribution of CMTMR- and CMFDA-labeled cells can be compared in the same tissue. If lymphocytes are labeled with high concentrations of CMFDA (10 μM), the fluorescence can bleed through when observing the tissue with rhodamine filters. For slide photography, we use Ektachrome EPL 400 ASA film.

References

1. J. M. Harlan and D. Y. Liu, "Adhesion: Its Role in Inflammatory Disease." Freeman, New York, 1992.
2. Y. Shimizu, W. Newman, Y. Tanaka, and S. Shaw, *Immunol. Today* **13,** 106 (1992).
3. S. L. Carlson, unpublished observations, 1993.
4. J. P. McGillis, unpublished observations, 1993.
5. M. A. Gimbrone, Jr., R. S. Cotran, and J. Folkman, *J. Cell Biol.* **60,** 673–684 (1974).
6. D. Gospodarowicz, *in* "Cell Culture Techniques in Heart and Vessel Research" (H. M. Piper, ed.), pp. 231–244. Springer-Verlag, Berlin, 1990.
7. T. MacCaig, J. Ilsley, P. R. Kelley, and R. Forand, *Proc. Natl. Acad. Sci. U.S.A.* **76,** 5674–5678 (1979).
8. V. W. M. van Hinsbergh, M. A. Scheffer, and E. G. Langeler, *in* "Cell Culture Techniques in Heart and Vessel Research" (H. M. Piper, ed.), pp. 178–204. Springer-Verlag, Berlin, 1990.
9. A. Ager, *J. Cell Sci.* **87,** 133–144 (1987).
10. Y. Ise, K. Yamaguchi, K. Sato, Y. Yamamura, F. Kitamura, T. Tamatani, and M. Miyasaka, *Eur. J. Immunol.* **18,** 1235–1244 (1988).
11. F. H. Kasten, *In Vitro* **8,** 128–149 (1972).
12. P. M. Mattila, Y. A. Nietosvaara, J. Ustinov, R. L. Renkonen, and P. Hayry, *Kidney Int.* **36,** 228–233 (1989).
13. L. H. Elliott, S. L. Carlson, L. A. Morford, and J. P. McGillis, this volume [8].
14. R. J. Benschop, M. B. M. DeSmet, A. C. Bloem, and R. E. Ballieux, *Scand. J. Immunol.* **36,** 793–800 (1992).

[24] Neuropeptides as Immunomodulators: Measurements of Calcitonin Gene-Related Peptide Receptors in the Immune System

Joseph P. McGillis

Introduction

Several hematopoietic cell lineages express high-affinity receptors for calcitonin gene-related peptide (CGRP), and CGRP can modulate the function of several cells, including lymphocytes, monocytes, neutrophils, and eosinophils (1–18). The CGRP receptors in the immune system are linked to cAMP (2, 3, 5, 7, 9, 12), and in general, many of the activities of CGRP which have been reported are inhibitory in nature. This chapter outlines the methods for characterization of CGRP receptors, for studying the effects of CGRP on cAMP production, and for examining the role of CGRP in B-cell differentiation.

Neuropeptides are one of the most logical sets of candidates for the role as molecular mediators of the efferent branch of central nervous system (CNS)–immune system communication. As a group, they have several characteristics which make them ideally suited for a role as immunomodulators. First, they are widely distributed in the peripheral nervous systems (PNS); several have been localized in nerve endings in lymphoid tissues (reviewed in 19). Neuropeptides are relatively stable when compared to amine neurotransmitters, thus when released at a local site they have the potential to influence cells over a period of hours. This is consistent with their role in the brain as neuromodulators, effectors which have long-lasting effects on neuronal function. Finally because of the large number of neuropeptides, there is the potential for different neuropeptides to act on certain processes under highly specific conditions. This would allow the nervous system to fine tune its communication such that it delivers immunomodulatory signals that are meaningful in a temporal and functional context. The functional extent of this efferent arm of CNS–immune system communications is unclear; however, there is evidence that at least four to five PNS neuropeptides act as immunomodulators by specific receptor-mediated mechanisms (reviewed in 20).

Two of the best-studied immunomodulatory neuropeptides are substance

P (SP) and vasoactive intestinal peptide (VIP). Specific high-affinity receptors for both have been identified on lymphocytes and monocytes, and SP can modulate the function of lymphocytes and monocytes *in vitro*. In addition, the role of SP as a major effector in the neurogenic inflammatory response has been well established. Over the past decade it has become clear that SP released antidromically from sensory fibers is playing an integrated role at a local site of inflammation by acting as a vasodilator, by increasing fluid extravasation, by acting as a chemoattractant, and by modulating the function of cells involved in immune and inflammatory responses (reviewed in 21, 22). In the peripheral nervous system, most of the SP-containing C-type sensory fibers also contain CGRP (23).

CGRP was one of the first neuropeptides discovered by molecular cloning. When Amara *et al.* cloned the gene for calcitonin, they discovered an alternatively processed mRNA with the potential to give rise to a novel peptide, CGRP (24). Further studies established that the alternatively spliced CGRP mRNA is expressed *in vivo* and is processed to give rise to the 37 amino acid CGRP. Subsequently, a second gene was identified which encodes a second CGRP (25). This second gene, which appears to have arisen by gene duplication, only encodes CGRP and does not encode calcitonin. The original CGRP is referred to as αCGRP and the second CGRP as βCGRP. The CGRPs are 37 amino acid peptides with an N-terminal disulfide bridge between cysteines at positions 2 and 7 and a C-terminal amide group. As shown in Fig. 1, rat α- and βCGRP differ by 1 amino acid and human α- and βCGRP differ by 3 amino acids. Although rat and human calcitonin also have a disulfide bridge in the N-terminal end, there is very little sequence homology. Salmon calcitonin has some weak sequence homology (Fig. 1) and is thought to be able to bind to certain CGRP receptors in the CNS (26–28).

CGRP is widely distributed in peripheral and central neurons, whereas calcitonin is selectively expressed in thyroid C cells and certain other endocrine cells. In the PNS, CGRP is found in sensory neurons, both independently and colocalized with SP, in enteric neurons, and in a population of motor neurons (23, 29–31). The CGRP containing nerve endings are found around virtually every blood vessel in the body, as well as in lymphoid tissue and in bone marrow (32–36). A major function of CGRP in the PNS is in vascular regulation where CGRP is one of the most potent vasodilators known (37). In addition to its vasodilatory effects, it enhances the vascular permeability induced by various inflammatory mediators including interleukin 1 (IL-1), platelet-activating factor (PAF), histamine, bradykinin, and SP (38–40). The immunomodulatory effects of CGRP include its ability to alter the mitogenic responses of both mouse and human T cells (7, 17, 18) and to inhibit γ-interferon (IFN-γ) induced peroxide production and antigen presentation by macrophages (14). In three of four published studies, CGRP has

	1				5					10					15
Rat αCGRP	Ser	Cys	Asn	Thr	Ala	Thr	Cys	Val	Thr	His	Arg	Leu	Ala	Gly	Leu
Rat βCGRP	-	-	-	-	-	-	-	-	-	-	-	-	-	-	-
Human αCGRP	Ala	-	Asp	-	-	-	-	-	-	-	-	-	-	-	-
Human βCGRP	Ala	-	-	-	-	-	-	-	-	-	-	-	-	-	-
Salmon Calcitonin	Cys	Ser	Asn	Leu	Ser	-	-	-	Leu	Gly	Lys	-	Ser	Gln	Glu

	16				20					25					30
Rat βCGRP	Leu	Ser	Arg	Ser	Gly	Gly	Val	Val	Lys	Asp	Asn	Phe	Val	Pro	Thr
Rat βCGRP	-	-	-	-	-	-	-	-	-	-	-	-	-	-	-
Human αCGRP	-	-	-	-	-	-	-	-	-	Asn	-	-	-	-	-
Human βCGRP	-	-	-	-	-	-	Met	-	-	Ser	-	-	-	-	-
Salmon Calcitonin	-	His	Lys	Leu	Gln	Thr	Tyr	Pro	Arg	Thr	-	Thr	Gly	Ser	Gly

	31				35		
Rat βCGRP	Asn	Val	Gly	Ser	Glu	Ala	Phe-NH_2
Rat βCGRP	-	-	-	-	Lys	-	-
Human αCGRP	-	-	-	-	Lys	-	-
Human βCGRP	-	-	-	-	Lys	-	-
Salmon Calcitonin	Thr	Pro-NH_2					

FIG. 1 Primary structure of human and rat CGRP. The sequences of rat α and β and human α and β CGRP are shown. The entire sequence of rat αCGRP is shown as are the amino acid substitutions in rat β and human α and β CGRP. Salmon calcitonin is also shown.

an inhibitory effect on T-cell proliferation which appears to be mediated by inhibition of IL-2 production (6, 9). *In vivo,* CGRP can enhance neutrophil infiltration following injection of IL-1 and can enhance neutrophil binding to cultured endothelial cells *in vitro* (40, 41). Neutral endopeptidase (CD10) can generate a fragment of CGRP which acts as chemotactic factor for eosinophils (15). CD10 is expressed in several tissues, including lymphoid progenitor cells and a subpopulation of mature B cells where it may play a coregulatory role by regulating the effect of neuropeptides.

The CGRP receptors have been identified and characterized in several tissues, including brain, pituitary, pancreas, endothelium, smooth muscle, and cardiovascular tissue (5, 28, 33, 42–46). The first indication of CGRP receptors in lymphoid tissue came from studies by several laboratories which identified CGRP binding sites in spleen (47–49). It was interesting to note that spleen contained relatively high levels of CGRP binding relative to other tissues. However, since these studies were done with cell membranes prepared from unfractionated spleens, they provided no information on the specific cell types in spleen which express CGRP receptors. More recent studies have characterized CGRP binding sites on purified and cultured lymphocytes and macrophages (1, 3–5, 10, Table II), thus confirming that the CGRP binding in earlier studies with spleen membranes was due in part to binding to CGRP receptors on immune cells. However, this does not rule out the possibility that CGRP is also binding to erythrocytes and stromal tissue in the spleen. Functional studies have found that lymphocyte and monocyte CGRP receptors are linked to adenylyl cyclase (2, 3, 5–7, 9, 10). Further characterization of immune system CGRP receptors and of the functional consequences of CGRP receptor activation will be necessary to define further the role of CGRP in modulation of immune and inflammatory responses.

Characterization of Lymphocyte Calcitonin Gene-Related Peptide Receptor

Characterization of a neuropeptide receptor in the immune system should satisfy the same criteria used to establish authenticity of receptors in other tissues. This includes demonstration that the binding site is dependent on receptor concentration, that binding is reversible, that it is saturable, and that it is specific. Further evidence for the authenticity of a receptor should include identification of the receptor protein and demonstration of a dose-dependent second-messenger response. One of the major pitfalls to receptor characterization in the immune system is that simple studies measuring only displaceable binding (binding of hot ligand vs. binding in the presence of a high concentration of cold ligand) can be misleading. This is in part due to the nature of cells in the immune system: they have evolved to bind, internalize, and process protein antigens. While one can detect displaceable binding with many iodinated peptides and proteins, especially with B cells and macrophages, subsequent studies may find that the binding is not due to a specific high-affinity receptor. In fact some premature reports on putative lymphocyte neuropeptide receptors have not held up to further scrutiny.

The binding characteristics of neuropeptide receptors in the immune system can be studied using membrane binding assays or whole-cell binding assays. In most other tissues, receptor binding studies have been done using cell membrane preparations. An advantage to studying neuropeptide receptors in the immune system is that it is relatively easy to do binding studies with live cells. Advantages to using live cells are that (i) it eliminates the need to prepare cell membranes in which receptor loss may be significant and variable, (ii) receptor densities are measured in terms of binding sites per cell, and (iii) changes in receptor affinity and density can be measured following experimental manipulation of the cells. A disadvantage to whole-cell binding assays is that it is more difficult or impossible to examine the role of receptor-associated proteins such as GTP binding proteins. Many of the drugs necessary for these studies are quite toxic to cells. The methods described here are for the production of ^{125}I-[His^{10}]-CGRP and for the characterization of lymphocyte CGRP receptors. However, they can easily be adapted for characterization of other receptors by substitution of the appropriate ligand, or for CGRP receptors on other cell types. These protocols are similar to those which have been successfully used for characterization of the lymphocyte SP (50, 51).

Iodination and Purification of Calcitonin Gene-Related Peptide

Several methods have been described for the iodination of peptides and hormones (52–54). The major goal for ligand binding studies is to introduce a radioactive atom into the peptide without altering its intrinsic ability to bind to its receptor. A convenient approach for peptides and proteins has been the use of oxidizing agents to link ^{125}I covalently to tyrosines or histidines. The major difficulty that has been encountered is the damaging effects of the oxidizing agent on other reactive amino acids, particularly on methionines. In many neuropeptides such as corticotropin-releasing hormone or SP, oxidation of the methionines to the sulfoxide will destroy the ability of the peptide to bind to its receptor. However, oxidation does not usually affect the ability of an iodinated peptide to be recognized by antibodies. Thus, many methods for iodination of peptides which are suitable for producing labeled peptides for use in radioimmunoassays (RIA) are not suitable for producing ligands for radioreceptor assays. In particular, use of a strong oxidizer such as chloramine-T can significantly damage the intrinsic binding of peptides by oxidizing methionines. A further complication with iodination procedures is that they may yield several iodinated species, only one or two of which may be suitable for use in radioreceptor assays. Compounding factors include mono- vs diiodination of tyrosines, multiple tyrosines, and variable oxidative damage to the peptide. For these reasons it is recommended (and usually necessary) that radiolabeled neuropeptides for binding assays be purified by high-performance liquid chromatography (HPLC).

Experience has shown that CGRP is very easy to label. Although it has no tyrosines, the histidine at position 10 can be labeled using Na^{125}I and chloramine-T. Purification with HPLC yields two major peaks (Fig. 2), both of which have binding activity. Only human βCGRP contains methionine (Fig. 1), although there is currently no information on whether oxidation of the methionine alters its ability to bind to the receptor. The method described here works equally well with rat α- or βCGRP or human αCGRP. [Tyr^0]CGRP analogs are available; however, we have found that ^{125}I-[Tyr^0]CGRP has a significantly lower binding affinity than does ^{125}I-[His^{10}]-CGRP. Following

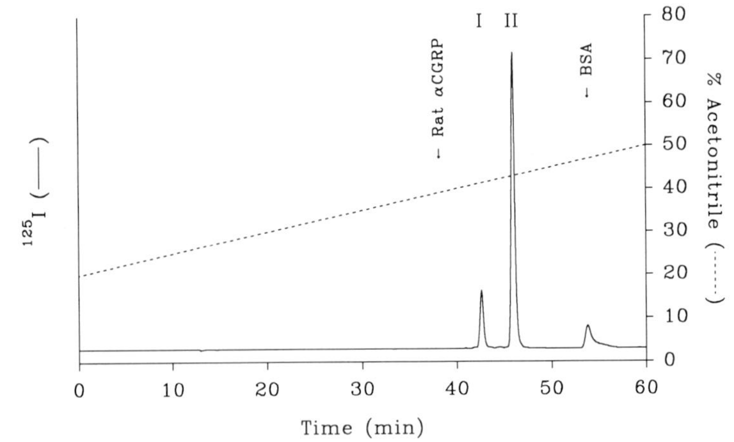

FIG. 2 High-performance liquid chromatography purification of rat α ^{125}I-[His^{10}]-CGRP. Rat αCGRP is iodinated with chloramine-T and Na^{125}I as described in the text. The ^{125}I-[His^{10}]-CGRP is injected onto a Vydac 4.6 × 200-mm C18 column and is eluted with a linear gradient form 0.1% TFA/20% acetonitrile/H_2O to 0.1% TFA/50% acetonitrile/H_2O over 60 min at a flow rate of 0.5 ml/min. ^{125}I is monitored with an on-line isotope detector (solid line). Two ^{125}I-[His^{10}]-CGRP peaks, I and II, elute at 42.6 and 45.9 min. ^{125}I-labeled BSA elutes at 53.8 min. The elution time of unleveled rat αCGRP is also shown (38.1 min).

removal of unreacted ^{125}I, ^{125}I-[His^{10}]-CGRP can be separated into two reactive species by reversed-phase HPLC as shown in Fig. 2. The second peak is routinely used for binding assays, although both species have binding activity. The difference between the two species is unknown; however, we suspect that the early peak is CGRP in which the N-terminal disulfide bridge is reduced. This is because reduction of the disulfide bridge will decrease the retention time of noniodinated CGRP. Commercial sources of [^{125}I]CGRP are available; however, we have found them to be prohibitively expensive if extensive binding studies are planned and have found that the quality is variable from batch to batch. The procedure described here is relatively simple, but does require the use of an HPLC.

The iodination procedure can be divided into three steps: (i) the iodination reaction, (ii) removal of unreacted ^{125}I, and (iii) HPLC purification. The major hazards to personnel are from volatile I_2 and from the high levels ^{125}I present in the initial reaction mixtures. The initial iodination procedures should be done in a chemical fume hood that is properly vented. All ^{125}I solutions should be handled behind lead shielding. A suitable shield can be constructed from $\frac{3}{16}$-inch lead sheets. Additional protection is afforded by protective breathing masks fitted with activated charcoal filters (Fisher Scientific). Three pairs of polyvinyl chloride (PVC) gloves are worn when handling ^{125}I solutions during the first two steps, especially when opening the Na^{125}I vial. A survey meter with a sodium iodide detector (LUDLUM Instruments, Sweetwater, TX) is kept nearby and gloves and pipettors are checked frequently for contamination. All pipetting is done with positive displacement pipettors (Gilson Microman, Models R-25, R-50, and R-250, Rainin Instrument Co. Inc., Woburn, MA). Because the plunger and the pipette tip are an integral unit that is ejected simultaneously, these pipettors are much less prone to contamination than are the air displacement pipettors (Pipetman, Eppendorf, etc.) used in most laboratories.

Synthetic CGRP peptides for iodination are obtained from Peninsula Laboratories, Inc. (Belmont, CA) or BACHEM California (Torrance, CA). The neuropeptides are dissolved in 0.01 *N* acetic acid and 20-μl aliquots are stored at -70°C. Once thawed, unused peptide is discarded and is not refrozen. The protocol described here is for 2 μg although it may be scaled up proportionately. We routinely iodinate up to 8 μg if necessary; however, we find that efficiency drops off above this level. If more ^{125}I-[His^{10}]-CGRP is desired, it is better to do multiple iodinations and pool them prior to HPLC purification.

For the iodination reaction, 8 μl of sodium phosphate buffer (0.5 *M*, pH 8.0) is added to 2 μg of CGRP, followed by 1 mCi of Na^{125}I (high concentration, Cat. No. 63035, ICN Biomedicals Inc., Irvine, CA). Two microliters of chloramine-T (1 mg/ml in water) is added and the mixture is gently agitated for 30 sec. The reaction is quenched by the addition of 25 μl of 1% bovine serum albumin (BSA, Sigma, RIA grade) followed by 0.5 ml of 0.5 *N* acetic acid. Although many iodination protocols use reducing agents such as sodium metabisulfite or 2-mercaptoethanol to quench the reaction, these agents will also reduce the disulfide bridge in the N terminus of CGRP. Free ^{125}I is removed using a Waters C_{18} Sep-Pak (Millipore Corporation, Millford, MA). A C_{18} Sep-Pak is prepared ahead of time by washing once with 10 ml of methanol, twice with 10 ml of water, and twice with 10 ml of HPLC buffer A [0.1% trifluoroacetic acid (TFA)/H_2O*]. The iodination mixture is drawn up into a syringe containing 3 ml of buffer A and is cycled through the Sep-Pak five times by washing it back and forth with syringes attached to both sides of the Sep-Pak. The ^{125}I-[His^{10}]-CGRP will stick to the Sep-Pak and

* Trifluoroacetic acid (TFA), Sequenal Grade (Pierce Chemical Company, Rockford, IL) is diluted to 1% TFA in HPLC H_2O (Burdick and Jackson, Baxter, CO). High-performance liquid chromatography A buffer is prepared by diluting the 1% TFA to 0.1% TFA with HPLC H_2O and buffer B is prepared by diluting the 1% TFA to 0.1% TFA with HPLC grade acetonitrile (Burdick and Jackson, Baxter).

the free ^{125}I is removed by washing the Sep-Pak twice with 10 ml of buffer A. The washes are collected into a 50-ml tube containing an absorbent such as cat box litter or vermiculite. If allowed by local regulations, the tube can be sealed and disposed of as solid waste. The ^{125}I-[His^{10}]-CGRP is eluted with five 1-ml washes of HPLC buffer B (0.1% TFA/9.9% H_2O/90% acetonitrile). Each fraction is collected into a 12 × 75-mm polypropylene tube containing 0.1 ml of 1% BSA in water. The first 1 ml of buffer B is pushed onto the Sep-Pak and allowed to sit for 1 min before continuing. Air is pushed through the Sep-Pak between elutions. The radioactivity is measured in each fraction. The first tube usually contains greater than 90% of the radioactivity. If the first tube contains less than 90%, then the first two tubes can be combined. The tubes are then concentrated to dryness in a Speed-Vac (SAVANT Instruments, Inc., Farmingdale, NY) prior to purification by HPLC.†

^{125}I-[His^{10}]-CGRP is purified by reversed-phase HPLC using a Vydac C_{18} column (The Separations Group, Hesperia, CA). We use a Hewlett–Packard 1090 HPLC equipped with a Hewlett–Packard 1050 UV/VIS spectrophotometer and a Beckman Model 170 isotope detector. The system is set up with separate Rheodyne injectors for radioactive and nonradioactive samples that can be selected by a Rheodyne switching valve. The dried ^{125}I-[His^{10}]-CGRP is redissolved in 200 μl of A buffer and 50 μl of B buffer. The sample is injected onto the column and eluted with a gradient of 20 to 50% B over 60 min at a flow rate of 0.5 ml/min. As shown in Fig. 2 there are two major radioactive peaks which elute at 42.6 and 45.9 min and are referred to as peaks I and II. The smaller broad peak at 53.8 min is ^{125}I-labeled BSA. The arrow shows the elution time for unlabeled rat αCGRP, 38.1, which is completely separated from ^{125}I-[His^{10}]-CGRP. The eluates are collected into tubes containing 100 μl of 1% BSA. The isotope detector has a built-in integrator which controls the fraction collector. The fraction time is set for 4 min. When the isotope detector senses a peak start or end it automatically switches tubes. A printout indicates which tubes contain the peaks. The advantage to this system is that it minimizes handling of the radioactive samples. If an isotope detector is not available, 1-min fractions should be collected. To determine the location of the ^{125}I-[His^{10}]-CGRP peaks, 1 μl from each fraction is transferred to a 12 × 75-mm tube and is counted in a gamma counter. If peaks I and II are not as well separated by the system being used, it may be necessary to decrease the fraction size to 0.5 min. Once the general elution times have been determined for a given column, it may be necessary to measure the radioactivity in the tubes around where the peaks elute (± 10 min). We have found that over a period of 3 years,

† To prevent ^{125}I contamination of the Speed-Vac condensor and the vacuum pump a chemical trap is placed between the Speed-VaC head and the condensor.

there was less than ± 0.2 min variation in the elution times. However, it should be noted that there can be a significant variation between identical columns from the same manufacturer. With the Vydac columns, we have observed differences up to 1 to 2 min between individual columns.

The second peak is aliquoted into several screw-cap microcentrifuge tubes and is stored at −20°C for up to 2 months. Since both peaks I and II are completely separated from unlabeled CGRP, the specific activity of the ^{125}I-[His^{10}]-CGRP is that of ^{125}I. If carrier free Na^{125}I is used, then the specific activity of the ^{125}I-[His^{10}]-CGRP is 2125 Ci/mmol on the batch date of the Na^{125}I. The ^{125}I-[His^{10}]-CGRP is very stable and several cycles of repeated freezing and thawing seem to have no effect on its intrinsic binding activity. Peak I can be saved and can be used for RIA. For saturation binding assays and for competition binding studies it is best to use label which is no older than 2 to 3 weeks. The reason for this is that as the specific activity decreases due to decay it becomes more difficult to accurately estimate parameters for binding sites which have a very high affinity (< 0.2 n*M*). For this reason we generally do not use labels of less than 1700 Ci/mmol for saturation or competition binding assays. The specific activity of the ^{125}I-[His^{10}]-CGRP on a given day is determined by multiplying the initial specific activity by the decay factor for the number of days since the label was prepared. An ^{125}I decay table is usually provided with the Na^{125}I by the supplier.

Radioligand Binding Studies

The characterization of a binding site requires a systematic series of experiments which will satisfy the criteria binding site and which will provide estimates of receptor affinity and density. Studies on the lymphocyte CGRP receptor have found that it reaches equilibrium binding fairly rapidly and that it binds with high affinity (K_d range from 0.35 to 48 n*M*, Table I). The examples shown here are from studies on ^{125}I-[His^{10}]-CGRP binding to rat lymphocytes, to murine 70Z/3 cells, and to mouse bone marrow cells (1, 3, 4). However, the same methods of analysis could be used for CGRP receptor characterization on other leukocytes as well. The basic method for the radioligand binding assay using whole cells is outlined in Fig. 3. The lymphocytes (or other leukocytes) are prepared as described by Elliott *et al.* (55) and resuspended in binding buffer‡ at an appropriate concentration. Total binding is determined by incubating cells with ^{125}I-[His^{10}]-CGRP and nonspecific

‡ Hanks' balanced salt solution (HBSS, GIBCO, Grand Island, NY) with 20 m*M* HEPES, pH 7.3, with 0.5% BSA (Sigma, RIA Grade).

TABLE I CGRP Receptor Affinity and Density on Cells of the Immune System

Cells	K_d[a] (nM)	B_{max}	Ref.
Rat spleen T	0.873 ± 0.019	774 ± 387 sites/cell	(3)
Mouse lymph node T	0.35 ± 0.1 (K_1)	265 ± 96 sites/cell	(5)
	48 ± 6 (K_2)	13,000 ± 321 sites/cell	(5)
Rat spleen B	0.387 ± 0.072	747 ± 244 sites/cell	(3)
Mouse bone marrow	3.92 ± 1.24	2796 ± 365 sites/cell	(4)
Murine 70Z/3 pre-B[b]			
Undifferentiated	0.166 ± 0.064 (K_1)	105 ± 21	(1)
	3.16 ± 0.49 (K_2)	18,962 ± 1784	(1)
Differentiated	0.206 ± 0.040 (K_1)	401 ± 138	(1)
	3.46 ± 0.85 (K_2)	20,716 ±2805	(1)
Murine P388 D1 macrophages[c]	1.76	85.48 fmol/mg protein	(10)

[a] K_d values are expressed as nM ± SEM. In studies where both high- and low-affinity binding sites were detected, the affinities and densities of both sites, K_1 and K_2, are shown.

[b] 70Z/3 pre-B cells are a mouse cell line which can be induced to differentiate by treatment with LPS.

[c] P388 D1 macrophages are a mouse cell line which constituitively produces IL-6 and IL-1.

binding (NSB) is determined by including unlabeled CGRP at a final concentration of 1 μM. Specific ^{125}I-[His^{10}]-CGRP binding is defined as the displaceable binding—the difference between the total binding and NSB. After the incubation period, the incubation mixture is layered over a mixture of phthalate oils in 0.4-ml microcentrifuge tubes. ^{125}I-[His^{10}]-CGRP bound to cells is separated from free ^{125}I-[His^{10}]-CGRP in the supernatant by centrifugation; the cells will pass through the oil interface whereas the supernatant will remain above the interface. The tube is then sliced through the oil interface and the portions containing the pellet and the supernatant are placed in tubes and counted in a gamma counter. A major advantage to this method of separating bound and free ligand is that the NSB due to ligand binding to the tube is very low. This is due to the fact that the reaction mixture never comes in contact with the portion of the tube which contains the pellet. Thus, the NSB that is actually measured is only that which is due to binding to the cells. Although bound ^{125}I-[His^{10}]-CGRP can also be separated from free ligand by filtration methods, we find that the NSB is much higher when using filtration.

The specific method described here has been used to characterize CGRP binding sites on rat T and B lymphocytes, murine 70Z/3 B cells, and mouse bone marrow cells (1, 3, 23). The incubation reaction can be set up in 12 × 75-mm polystyrene tubes or in 96-well flat-bottomed microtiter plates. We have found that polystyrene plastic adsorbs less ^{125}I-[His^{10}]-CGRP than does polypropylene. An advantage to using microtiter plates is that multichannel

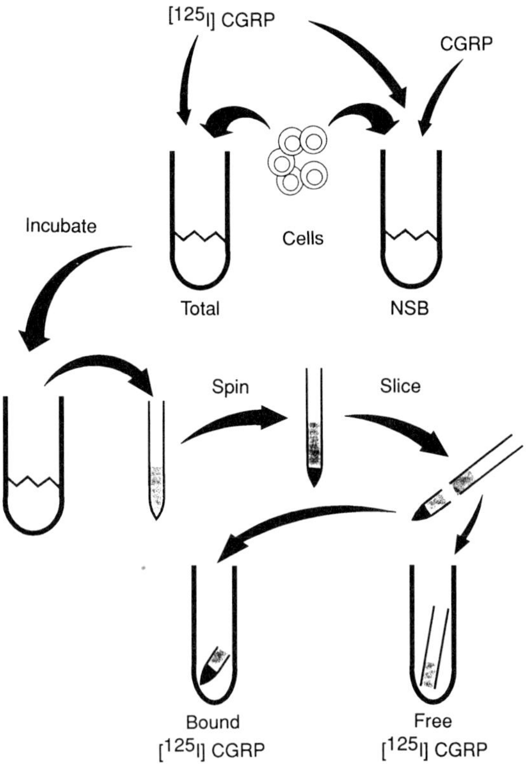

FIG. 3 Radioreceptor binding assay with live cells. Lymphocytes or other cell suspensions are incubated with ^{125}I-[His^{10}]CGRP in polystyrene tubes or in 96-well microtiter plates. The NSB tubes include cold CGRP at a final concentration of 0.5 to 1 μM. Following the incubation, the binding reaction is transferred to a 0.4-ml polyethylene tube containing 0.1 ml of phthalate oil and is centrifuged at 5500g for 4 min. The cells pellet through the oil interface and the supernatant is retained above the oil interface. The tube is sliced through the oil interface and the bound ^{125}I-[His^{10}]-CGRP in the pellet and the free ^{125}I-[His^{10}]-CGRP in the supernatant-containing fractions are placed in 12 $\times$ 75-mm tubes. The radioactivity in each fraction is determined by counting in a gamma scintillation counter.

pipettors can be used to set up the assay. The first series of experiments should demonstrate that ligand binding has a linear dependence on cell concentration and should examine the time course of binding. Figures 4 and 5 show examples of the dependence of ^{125}I-[His^{10}]-CGRP on cell concentration and a time course of ^{125}I-[His^{10}]-CGRP binding by 70Z/3 cells. The incubation reaction, which has a final volume of 0.2 ml is set up by adding the components (shown in the tabulation) in order.

Component	Volume (μl) for binding	
	Total	Nonspecific
1. Binding buffer	60	40
2. Unlabeled CGRP (0.5 μ*M* final)	—	20
3. ^{125}I-[His^{10}]-CGRP	20	20
4. Bacitracin, 20 mg/ml	20	20
5. Cells	100	100

Triplicate or quadruplicate total and NSB tubes are set up for each time point or cell concentration. A 10× stock of unlabeled CGRP is prepared by diluting a 20-μl aliquot of 10^{-4} *M* CGRP to 400 μl with binding buffer. ^{125}I-[His^{10}]-CGRP is diluted to give approximately 150,000 to 200,000 counts per minute (cpm)/20 μl. Following the incubation period the binding mixtures are transferred to a 0.4-ml polyethylene microcentrifuge tube containing 100 μl of a phthalate oil mixture (77% dibutyl phthalate/23% dinonyl phthalate) and are centrifuged at 5500 *g* for 4 min (56). Following centrifugation, the tubes are sliced with a scalpel or a razor blade through the middle of the oil interface. The portions containing the pellet and the supernatant are placed in 12 × 75-mm tubes and are counted in a gamma scintillation counter. To examine the dependence of binding on cell concentration, we have used concentrations ranging from 10,000 cells per well up to 10^8 cells per well. The concentration of cells which fall on the linear portion of the curve will vary depending on the actual receptor density in a given population of cells. With rat lymphocytes, 70Z/3 cells, and mouse bone marrow cells significant levels of binding can be detected with cell concentrations as low as 500,000, 40,000, and 100,000 cells/0.2 ml, respectively (1, 3, 4). For subsequent binding studies, a concentration of cells should be selected at which specific binding is somewhere between 5,000 and 20,000 cpm. If competition binding studies are done with fewer counts, the differences between adjacent concentrations of competing ligand may overlap, making parameter estimation less precise. To determine the time course of binding, assays are done in which binding is measured at several time points. In our studies, we find that CGRP binding at room temperature is fairly rapid, with equilibrium binding being reached by 1 hr, and being stable for 2 to 4 hr, as shown in Fig. 5. In our earlier study on rat lymphocytes we observed a peak in binding at about 30 to 40

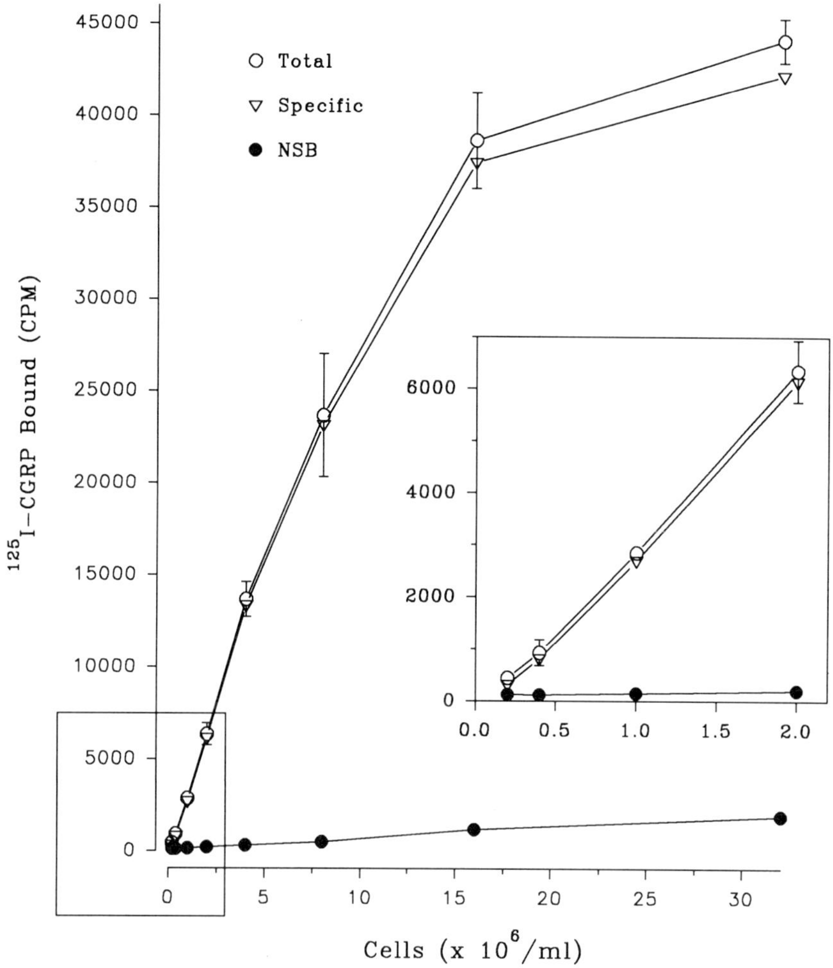

FIG. 4 ^{125}I-[His^{10}]-CGRP binding to 70Z/3 is dependent on cell concentration. 70Z/3 cells at concentrations ranging from 2×10^5 to 3.2×10^7 cells/ml were incubated for 1 hr at room temperature with approximately 250,000 cpm ^{125}I-[His^{10}]-CGRP in the absence (total binding, ○) or presence of 0.5 μM unlabeled CGRP (NSB, ●). Total and NSB are the mean ± SE for quadruplicate samples. Specific binding (∇) is plotted as the subtracted difference between total binding and NSB. The inset shows the lower cell concentrations with an expanded scale. Significant binding was observed at all concentrations tested. Reprinted with permission from J. P. McGillis, S. Humphreys, V. Rangnekar, and J. Ciallella, *Cell. Immunol.* **150,** 391 (1993).

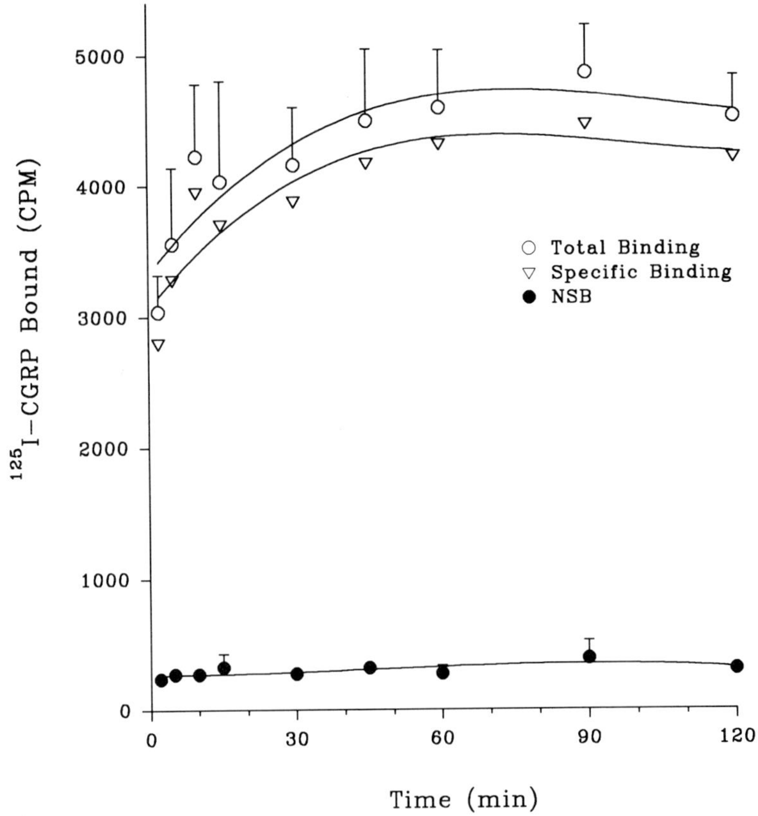

FIG. 5 Time course of binding of ^{125}I-[His^{10}]-CGRP to 70Z/3 cells. 70Z/3 cells at a concentration of 10^7 cells/ml in 0.25 ml were incubated with approximately 150,000 cpm ^{125}I-[His^{10}]-CGRP for periods ranging from 2 to 60 min. The NSB was determined by including rat CGRP at a final concentration of 0.5 μM. Each total binding (○) point represents the mean ± SE for triplicate samples and each NSB (●) point represents the mean for triplicate samples. The SE is shown for NSB where the %SE was greater than 2%. Specific binding (∇) is the subtracted difference between total binding and NSB. Reprinted with permission from J. P. McGillis, S. Humphreys, V. Rangnekar, and J. Ciallella, *Cell. Immunol.* **150,** 391 (1993).

min which decreased over the next 2 to 4 hr (3). In subsequent studies with 70Z/3 cells we examined the effect of several protease inhibitors on CGRP binding (1). Either bacitracin or chymostatin enhanced the binding of CGRP to 70Z/3 cells and prevented the decline in binding seen at later times (1 to 4 hr). Thus, the decline in binding observed in the earlier study was probably due to degradation of the ligand. While bacitracin is a broad spectrum protease inhibitor, the activity of chymostatin suggests that ^{125}I-[His^{10}]-CGRP can be degraded by cysteine proteases. The studies shown here have all been done at room temperature. ^{125}I-[His^{10}]-CGRP binding can also be examined at other temperatures. We find that binding at 4°C is quantitatively similar, although slower. Binding at 37°C is very rapid, reaching equilibrium within 5 to 10 min, after which it declines significantly. Because the decreased binding at later time points at 37°C cannot be inhibited by bacitracin or chymostatin, it could be due to degradation by some other protease or by desensitization of the CGRP receptor.

Estimation of Receptor Affinity and Density

A preliminary estimate of the affinity and demonstration of the reversibility can be determined by allowing the cells to reach equilibrium binding and then adding cold CGRP (0.5 μM final). Binding is then measured at several time points after the addition of cold CGRP. Affinity is described by the dissociation constant, K_d, which is equal to the dissociation rate divided by the association rate ($K_d = k_{off}/k_{on}$). A more definitive estimation of the affinity is determined by saturation binding studies which can also detect the presence of multiple binding sites (high- and low-affinity sites or states). For this analysis a series of incubations are set up in which replicate total and NSB tubes are incubated with a range of concentrations of ^{125}I-[His^{10}]-CGRP. For the lymphoid populations we have examined so far, we have used concentrations of ^{125}I-[His^{10}]-CGRP ranging from approximately 0.01 nM up to 8 nM. Saturation assays should include a minimum of 10 to 12 concentrations of hot ligand. A saturation binding assay with 12 concentrations of hot ligand and quadruplicate total and NSBs can be set up on a 96-well plate using a multichannel pipettor. The hot ligand is first diluted directly on the plate by a series of twofold serial dilutions. A 5× stock of the highest concentration of ^{125}I-[His^{10}]-CGRP is prepared (approximately 50 nM). Forty microliters of binding buffer is first added to columns 2 through 12 on the plate, and 40 μl of the 5× ^{125}I-[His^{10}]-CGRP is added to the first 2 columns. Starting with the second column a twofold serial dilution is done by transferring 40 μl to the third column. At each step, the dilutions are mixed by pipetting up and down three times and 40 μl is then transferred to the next column. After the last column, 40 μl is removed and discarded. Twenty microliters of binding buffer is then added to the total binding wells and 20 μl of unlabeled CGRP (0.5 μM final) is added to the NSB wells. Forty microliters of bacitracin (10 mg/ml in binding buffer) is added to all wells followed by 100 μl of cells. After the binding assay has incubated for a sufficient time to reach equilib-

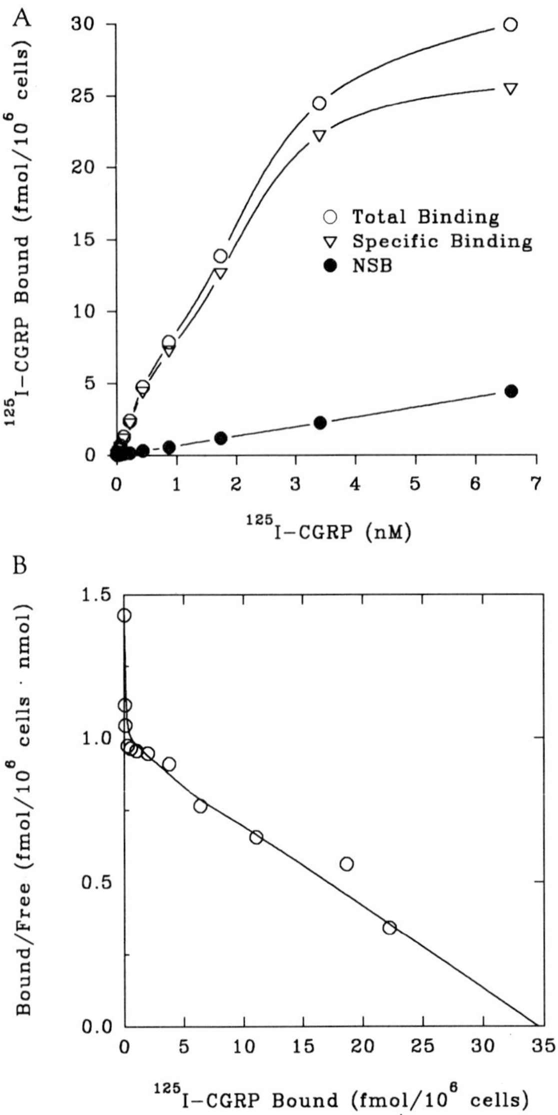

FIG. 6 Saturation isotherm analysis of ^{125}I-[His^{10}]-CGRP binding to 70Z/3 cells. 70Z/3 cells at a concentration of 10^7 cells/0.2 ml were incubated with ^{125}I-[His^{10}]-CGRP at concentrations ranging from 0.01 to 8 n*M*. (A) Saturation plot of ^{125}I-CGRP bound vs the concentration of ^{125}I-[His^{10}]-CGRP. Total binding (○) and NSB (●) are the mean of quadruplicate samples, and specific binding (∇) is the subtracted difference between total and NSB. (B) Scatchard–Rosenthal plot of bound/free

rium, bound ligand is separated from free by centrifugation over oil. The 0.4-ml tubes with oil can be placed in an empty pipette tip rack and the reaction mixtures can be transferred using an eight-channel pipettor. The total ligand for each concentration of hot is estimated by adding the average counts in the pellets and the supernatants. Although this is slightly less than the total amount of hot ligand actually added—some ^{125}I-[His^{10}]-CGRP remains stuck to the plate—it is assumed that the ^{125}I-[His^{10}]-CGRP stuck to the plate was not available for binding to cells and that the total of the pellet and supernatant represents the actual concentration that was available for binding. Figure 6 shows a typical saturation curve and a Scatchard–Rosenthal plot of ^{125}I-[His^{10}]-CGRP binding to 70Z/3 cells. K_d and B_{max} (binding site density) can be estimated by nonlinear regression analysis using various programs. We routinely use Lundon-1 and Lundon-2 (Lundon Software, Inc., Cleveland, OH), but have also found the analysis with LIGAND (BioSoft, Milltown, NJ) gives essentially the same results. LIGAND will provide estimates for one- and two-site models and Lundon-1 will provide estimates for one-, two-, and three-site models and will do a statistical analysis to predict the best fit. On freshly isolated lymphocytes and bone marrow, we only detected a single site (3, 4), whereas on 70Z/3 cells we are able to detect both low- and high-affinity sites (1). Table I provides a comparison of the CGRP binding affinity and receptor densities reported for several lymphoid tissues. For lymphocytes, we only included those studies which used whole cell binding assays and not those which used cell membrane preparations (17). The K_d values were in a similar range in these studies, but it is not possible to compare the actual receptor densities.

Specificity of ^{125}I-[His^{10}]-CGRP Binding

Characterization of the specificity of receptor binding serves two purposes. First it establishes that the binding site being studied is specific. Many neuropeptides are known to bind to other receptors at higher concentrations. Second, if there are multiple receptors, and if specific analogs are available, it is possible to determine which receptor a ligand is binding to. For certain neuropeptides such as the tachykinins and opiates there are a number of

^{125}I-[His^{10}]-CGRP (B/F) vs bound ^{125}I-[His^{10}]-CGRP. Analysis of the data with the Lundon-1 program determined that ^{125}I-[His^{10}]-CGRP binding by 70Z/3 cells is best described by a two-site model, which is shown by the line. Reprinted with permission from J. P. McGillis, S. Humphreys, V. Rangnekar, and J. Ciallella, *Cell. Immunol.* **150,** 391 (1993).

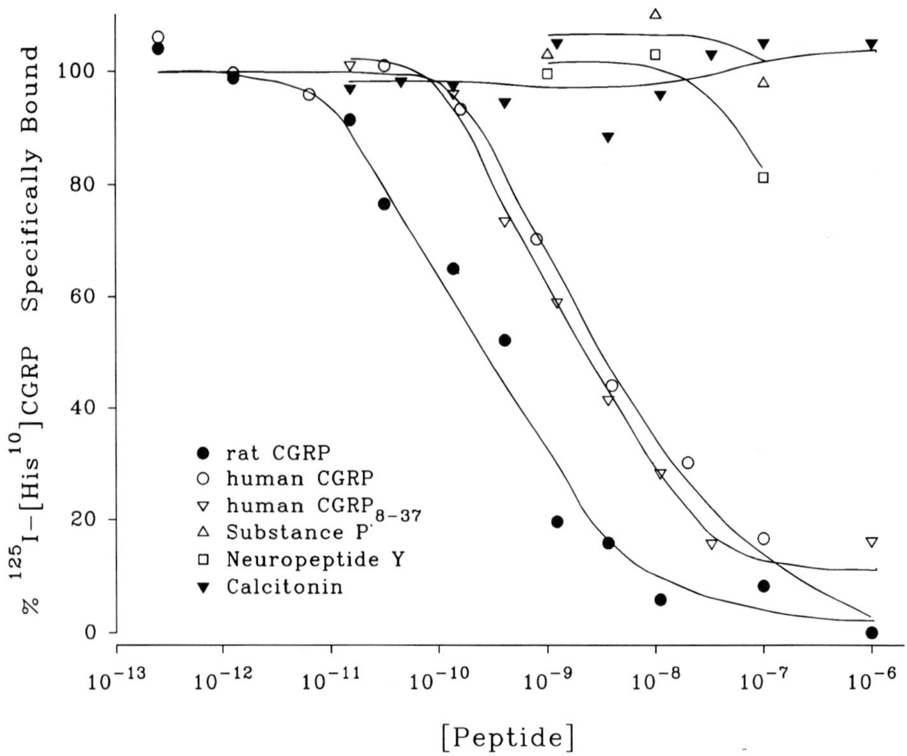

FIG. 7 Specificity of ^{125}I-[His^{10}]-CGRP binding to rat spleen lymphocytes. Rat lymphocytes, 2.5×10^6 cells/0.25 ml, were incubated for 1 hr at 22°C with 200,000 cpm ^{125}I-[His^{10}]-CGRP and unleveled neuropeptides at concentrations ranging from 10^{-13} to 10^{-6} *M*. The percent of specific ^{125}I-[His^{10}]-CGRP binding is plotted vs unleveled peptide concentration. Specific binding is defined as the difference between total binding (no unlabeled peptide) and NSB (0.5 μM rat CGRP). Ech point and line represent the averages from three to six separate experiments. Rat CGRP (●) inhibited ^{125}I-[His^{10}]-CGRP binding at the lowest concentrations, followed by human CGRP (○), and CGRP (8–37) (▽). Substance P (△), neuropeptide Y (□), and calcitonin (▼) had no effect of ^{125}I-[His^{10}]-CGRP binding at concentrations up to 10^{-7} and 10^{-6} *M*. Reprinted with permission from J. P. McGillis, S. Humphreys, and S. Reid, *J. Immunol.* **147,** 3482 (1991). Copyright 1991, The Journal of Immunology.

receptor subtype-specific agonists and antagonists that can be used to differentiate binding to specific classes of receptors. However, for many neuropeptides, there are few if any site-specific analogs available. Based on *in vitro* and *in vivo* binding asays, as well as binding studies, there is evidence for up to three different CGRP binding sites. Two of these, the CGRP1 and

CGRP2 sites, have been proposed by Quirion and co-workers and the prototype tissues are rat or guinea pig atria and rat vas deferens, respectively (42, 48, 57). They differ primarily in their agonist sensitivity to a reduced and methylated linearized form of CGRP and in the antagonist potency of C-terminal analogs. A third site which has been described in nucleus accumbens is sensitive to salmon calcitonin, but not to human calcitonin (26, 58). The CGRP receptor in the immune system does not bind salmon calcitonin; however, it is unclear at present whether it fits into the proposed CGRP1 or CGRP2 categories.

Competition binding studies can be set up on 96-well plates as described for saturation binding assays, except that a constant amount of ^{125}I-[His^{10}]-CGRP is added and the concentration of the unlabeled ligand is varied. For these assays, we set up the total binding and NSB are set up in quadruplicate. The competition curves are generally set up by doing a threefold serial dilution of unlabeled peptide in quadruplicate, at concentrations ranging from 10^{-6} *M* to 10^{-13} to 10^{-15} *M*. The results are usually expressed as the percentage of ^{125}I-[His^{10}]-CGRP specifically bound ([CPM bound at a given peptide concentration − NSB]/[total binding − NSB] × 100). Figure 7 shows a typical series of competition displacement curves for the inhibition of ^{125}I-[His^{10}]-CGRP binding to rat lymphocytes. The concentration which inhibits 50% of the binding (IC_{50}) and the inhibitory constant (K_i) can be estimated using the Lundon-2 or LIGAND software programs. For many neuropeptides such as the tachykinins and opiates, the rank order of potency of various analogs can be used to distinguish between receptor subtypes. Such analogs for CGRP have yet to be developed or identified. Table II summarizes the K_i values we have estimated for various CGRPs on different lymphocyte preparations. The rank order of potencies are as follows

Rat lymphocytes:	rat α CGRP ≫ human αCGRP human αCGRP(8–37)
Mouse bone marrow cells:	rat αCGRP, rat βCGRP ≫ human αCGRP ≫ human αCGRP(8–37)
70Z/3 Pre B cells	rat αCGRP ≫ human αCGRP ≫ human αCGRP(8–37)

The greater potency of human αCGRP(8–37) on rat lymphocytes may be due to species differences between rat and mouse CGRP receptors. As more specific CGRP receptor analogs become available, it should be possible to better distinguish CGRP receptors on the basis of radioligand binding assays and *in vivo* bioassays.

TABLE II Specificity of Murine Lymphocyte CGRP Receptors: K_i Values[a] for CGRP Peptides

Peptide	Rat spleen lymphocytes (3)	Mouse bone marrow cells (4)	70Z/3 pre-B cells (1)
Rat αCGRP	0.192 ± 0.073	0.899 ± 0.186	44.1 p*M* (K_{i1}) 0.60 n*M* (K_{i2})
Rat βCGRP	ND[b]	0.771 ± 0.287	ND
Human αCGRP	2.06 ± 0.97	2.97 ± 0.54	3.92 n*M*
Human αCGRP (8–37)	2.59 ± 0.52	18.0 ± 3.86	6.50 n*M*
Salmon calcitonin	NI[c]	NI	NI
Human calcitonin	NI	NI	NI
SP, NPY, CRH[d]	NI	NI	NI

[a] K_i, Inhibitory constant. Both high and low affinity inhibitory constants (K_{i1} and K_{i2}) are shown for 70Z/3 cells.
[b] Not determined.
[c] No inhibition (NI) seen at concentrations up to 1 μ*M*.
[d] SP, substance P; NPY, neuropeptide Y; CRH, corticotropin-releasing hormone.

Affinity Labeling

One of the standard methods for demonstrating that a binding site is a protein receptor is to identify the protein by affinity labeling. This approach has been used extensively in the characterization of many receptors in the brain and other tissues and has been useful in the characterization of the SP receptor on lymphocytes (59–61). In addition to demonstrating that binding is mediated by a receptor protein, affinity labeling can be a useful tool in the biochemical characterization of receptor proteins. Two general approaches have been used for affinity labeling of neuropeptide and protein hormone receptors. The method described here is very simple in design and uses a homobifunctional cross-linking reagent to covalently link the ligand to the receptor protein. An alternative approach not described here is the derivatization of the ligand with photoactivatable cross-linking reagents. The advantage to the latter procedure is that it is less prone to nonspecific cross-linking artifacts. The preparation of biologically active photoactivatable radiolabeled ligand can be a fairly complex procedure. We have successfully used two different cross-linking reagents for the identification of lymphocyte CGRP receptors, disuccinimidyl suberate (DSS, Pierce Chemical Co., Rockford, IL) and a membrane-impermeable analog of DSS, bis(sulfosuccinimidyl) suberate (BS^3, Pierce Chemical Co.). The reactive groups on both DSS and BS^3 are *N*-hydroxysuccinimide esters which react with primary amino groups to form stable covalent bonds. Thus, the amino group on a lysine or on the amino terminus is cross-linked to an adjacent primary amino group on the receptor protein. In addition to DSS and BS^3, there are several other cross-linking reagents available. Many of these agents use similar reactive groups, but have different length spacers between the reactive groups. Thus, depending on the distances between the reactive groups on the receptor and the ligand, some cross-linking reagents may work better than others. There are currently no empirical rules for selecting the appropriate cross-linking reagent, other than trial and error. However, DSS is one of the most commonly used and has worked well with a number of receptor ligand pairs.

The cross-linking reaction is set up similar to a binding assay. Cells (10^7) in 0.4 ml of binding buffer are incubated with 500,000 cpm of ^{125}I-[His^{10}]-CGRP at room temperature for 1 hr. The specificity of labeling is demonstrated by performing a parallel incubation with 1 μM unlabeled CGRP (nonspecific labeling). Following the incubation, the cells are pelleted by centrifugation at 200*g* for 10 min at 4°C. The supernatant is removed and the cells are resuspended in 0.36 ml of prechilled (4°C) HBSS/HEPES without BSA. A 10× stock of DSS or BS^3 (10 m*M*) is prepared by resuspending the cross-linking reagent in dimethyl sulfoxide (DMSO) immediately before it is used. Forty microliters is added and the reaction is incubated on ice for 15 min. The cross-linking reaction is then quenched by the addition of 100 μl of 25 m*M* Tris in saline (0.9% NaCl). The cells are pelleted by centrifugation at 200*g* for 10 min at 4°C and the pellet is vigorously resuspended in 100 μl of SDS–PAGE sample buffer (62.5 m*M* Tris–HCl, pH 6.8, 10% glycerol, 2% SDS, 5% 2-mercaptoethanol, 0.01% bromophenol blue) and heated at 95°C for 10 min. After being chilled on ice, DNA is sheared by drawing the sample in and out of a syringe with a 22-gauge needle. The lysate is then centrifuged at 19,000*g* at 4°C for 15 min to remove debris. Fifty to 200 μl of the total and nonspecific affinity-labeled supernatants containing the solubilized cell membrane proteins are then resolved on a standard SDS–polyacrylamide gel (7.5 to 10% acrylamide) as described by Laemmli (62). After the gel has been run it is exposed to Kodak X-Omat film (Rochester, NY) for 7 to 14 days. A representative autoradiograph is shown in Fig. 8.

The major protein bands which are affinity-labeled on rat lymphocytes and mouse 70Z/3 cells have molecular weights of 74,500 and 103,000, respectively (1, 3). The CGRP receptor-like binding proteins have also been affinity-labeled in other tissues including cerebellum, placenta, and SK-N-MC neuroblastoma cells, with reported molecular weights ranging from 13,700 to 240,000 (63–65). The differences in molecular weights could be due to a number of factors including species differences in the receptor protein, differences in glycosylation, and the existence of multiple CGRP receptors. Tissue-specific differences in glycosylation of the same receptor have been found to produce receptor proteins with widely varying sizes. Another possibility is differential splicing of the mRNA for the receptor. However, this possibility

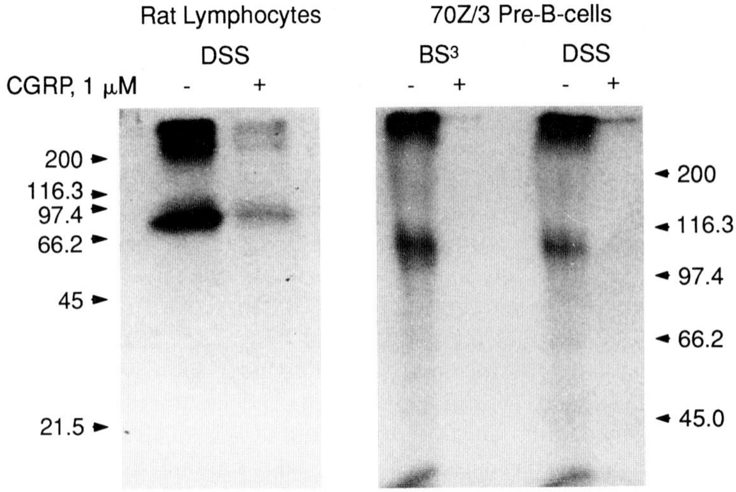

FIG. 8 Affinity labeling of the CGRP receptor protein on lymphocytes. ^{125}I-[His^{10}]-CGRP was covalently cross-linked to its cell membrane receptor on rat lymphocytes and/or on 70Z/3 cells with DSS or BS^3 as described in the text. Nonspecific labeling was delineated from specific labeling by including 1 *μM* CGRP in a parallel reaction. Following cross-linking, detergent-solubilized cellular proteins were analyzed by SDS–polyacrylamide gel electrophoresis. The dried gels were exposed to Kodak X-Omat film. Affinity labeling of rat lymphocytes identified three major protein bands on rat lymphocytes, one at the origin of the gel, and bands with molecular weights of 220,000 and 74,500. Densitometric analysis on a BioImage Analyzer revealed that nonspecific labeling accounted for 14 to 24% of specific labeling. Affinity labeling of 70Z/3 cells identified two protein bands, one at the origin and one with a molecular weight of 103,000. The bands at the origin and at 220,000 (rat lymphocytes) are probably aggregated and incompletely solubilized receptor proteins. The bands at 74,500 and 103,000 are probably monomeric CGRP receptor proteins. Reprinted with permission from J. P. McGillis, S. Humphreys, and S. Reid, *J. Immunol.* **147,** 3482 (1991) and J. P. McGillis, S. Humphreys, V. Rangnekar, and J. Ciallella, *Cell. Immunol.* **150,** 391 (1993). Copyright 1991, The Journal of Immunology.

is not as likely. Although the gene for the CGRP receptor has yet to be cloned, it is highly probable that it belongs to the 7-transmembrane domain family of G-protein-linked receptors. Of the 70-some members of this family that have been cloned, few have introns, and some investigators suggest that intronless genes are a characteristic of this family of receptors. Once the CGRP receptor has been cloned, receptor cDNA probes will be a useful tool for further study of the expression and function of the CGRP receptor in the immune system.

Characterization of Calcitonin Gene-Related Peptide Signal Transduction in Lymphocytes

The functionality of receptor in a given cell or tissue can be demonstrated by showing that it is linked to a specific second-messenger response. The nature of the second-messenger response also can provide information on the functional consequences of a neuropeptide receptor activation. Signal transduction following CGRP binding is linked to activation of adenylyl cyclase in lymphocytes as well as in other tissues (2, 3, 5, 10, 43, 44, 66). In the older literature, any agent which stimulated cAMP in lymphocytes was considered to be inhibitory. This was based on the observations that mitogen responses were inhibited by agents which elevated or mimicked cAMP. However, it is now known that cAMP is required in certain stages of lymphocyte expansion and development. Thus, the inhibitory effect of cAMP could be due to blocking the cells from entering the cell cycle, or could be due to its driving them out of the cell cycle. For many cells, differentiation includes moving proliferating cells out of the cell cycle concomitantly with the acquisition of a mature functional phenotype. To complicate a simple interpretation of a second-messenger response further, it is now clear that different agents which elevate cAMP in the same cells can have different effects (67). In addition, there have been contradictory reports on the effects of CGRP on T cells. Wang *et al.* (9) reported that CGRP inhibits T-cell proliferation by inhibiting IL-2 production, whereas Boudard and Bastide (6) reported in an earlier study that CGRP has no effect on IL-2 production.

Changes in intracellular cAMP in lymphocytes can be measured by RIA. We have used an anti-cAMP antibody provided by Dr. Brian Jackson (University of Kentucky) and [^{125}I]cAMP purchased from Dupont NEN Research Products (Boston, MA) or BTI (Stoughton, MA). cAMP antibodies are available commercially from a number of vendors, as are cAMP RIA kits. We have examined the cAMP response to CGRP in rat lymphocytes and in mouse 70Z/3 cells. These studies were performed essentially as described by Elliott *et al.* (55). Briefly, the cells are first preincubated with IBMX for 10 min at 37°C. We used rat lymphocytes or 70Z/3 cells at a concentration of 1.25×10^6 cells/0.25 ml. Following incubation with CGRP or other peptides, cAMP was extracted and acetylated as described. As shown in Fig. 9, CGRP induces a rapid prolonged elevation of cAMP in rat lymphocytes. A similar

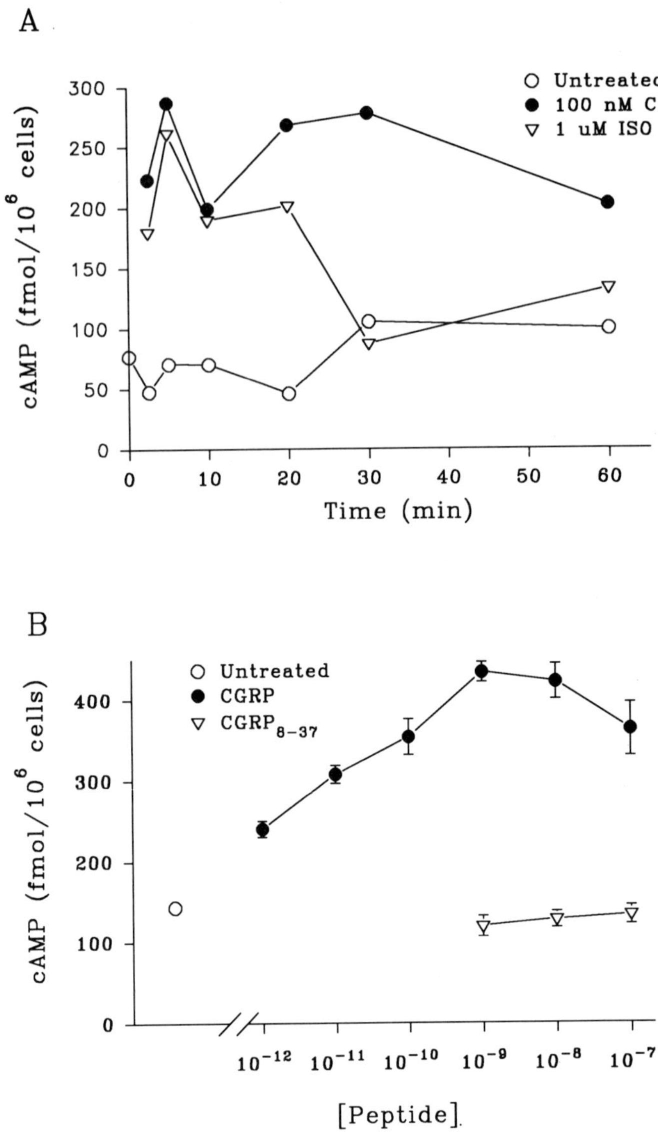

FIG. 9 Stimulation of cAMP production in rat spleen lymphocytes by CGRP. Rat spleen lymphocytes were stimulated for times ranging from 2 to 60 min (A), or 20 min (B) at 37°C. cAMP in acetylated cell extracts was measured by RIA as described in the text. (○) Untreated. (A) CGRP (●), 100 n*M*] stimulated a rapid sustained elevation in cAMP which was still significantly elevated at 60 min ($p < 0.05$ for all time points) relative to untreated cells. In contrast, cAMP levels had returned to

response was seen in 70Z/3 cells and in bone marrow (2). One of the interesting aspects of the cAMP response to CGRP in lymphocytes is its duration. When lymphocytes are stimulated through the β-adrenergic receptor with isoproterenol, there is a rapid elevation in cAMP that peaks within 5 to 10 min and then returns to baseline by 30 min. In contrast, when the same cells are treated with CGRP, cAMP is still elevated after 1 hr (2, 3).

At present, the reasons for the sustained elevation in cAMP following CGRP treatment are not known. However, there are two possible consequences which merit further consideration. The first is the functional consideration. The sustained elevation following CGRP treatment suggests that the effects of CGRP might be more sustained than those resulting from adrenergic stimulation. One consequence is that in two- and three-signal models, CGRP stimulation affords a larger temporal window through which potential immunomodulatory effects of CGRP can be elicited. The second consideration is the cellular mechanism of the sustained response. Two possibilities are that the CGRP receptor is not desensitized or that phosphodiesterase activity is inhibited. The first possibility can be better examined once the lymphocyte CGRP receptor is cloned. One possibility is that the CGRP receptor might be lacking phosphorylation sites through which similar cAMP-linked receptors are desensitized.

The dose–response shown in Fig. 9B shows that the cAMP response is fairly potent, with an optimal effect at 10^{-9} *M* and a significant effect being seen at 10^{-12} *M*. In 70Z/3 cells which have a higher receptor density, the optimal response is seen at 10^{-11} *M* and a significant response can be seen at concentrations as low as 10^{-16} *M* (2). The higher sensitivity of 70Z/3 cells is predicted in part by the higher receptor density in these cells (Table I). When examining the effect of CGRP on cAMP, controls should include unrelated peptides such as calcitonin and groups which are coincubated with the CGRP antagonist CGRP(8–37). The calcitonin control is important in that it has been reported that CGRP can bind to the calcitonin receptor. In lymphocytes, we have found that calcitonin has no effect of cAMP and that CGRP(8–37) is a weak antagonist (inhibition

baseline by 30 min following isoproterenol [(∇), 1 μM) treatment. (B) CGRP stimulated a dose-dependent increase in cAMP in lymphocytes. Cells were incubated with CGRP [($\bullet$) 10^{-12} to 10^{-7} *M*] or CGRP (8–37) [(∇) 10^{-9} to 10^{-7} *M*]. CGRP treatment caused in a dose-dependent increase in cAMP with an ED_{50} of approximately 8 p*M*. The CGRP receptor antagonist CGRP (8–37) had no effect of cAMP levels. Reprinted with permission from J. P. McGillis, S. Humphreys, and S. Reid, *J. Immunol.* **147,** 3482 (1991). Copyright 1991, The Journal of Immunology.

requires a 10- to 100-fold higher concentration). The high sensitivity of this response is important since CGRP levels in tissue are likely to be very low. Levels of CGRP in human serum have been reported to range from approximately 0.5 to 32 p*M* (49, 68). The ability of lymphocytes to respond to very low concentrations of CGRP supports a physiological role for CGRP in modulating lymphocyte function.

Inhibition of B-Cell Differentiation by CGRP

As reviewed in the introduction, CGRP has a number of effects of T lymphocytes, macrophages, and granulocytes. We have examined the effect of CGRP on early B-cell differentiation (2, 4). An effect of CGRP on B cells is suggested by the presence of CGRP receptors on mouse 70Z/3 cells and by the presence of CGRP-containing nerve endings in bone marrow (34–36). 70Z/3 cells have been used extensively as a model system to study early B-cell differentiation (69). These cells have rearranged μ and κ genes, and express cytoplasmic μ protein. Following exposure to LPS or lymphokines, 70Z/3 cells transcribe the κ gene and assemble and express surface immunoglobulin (sIg) protein. Thus, they represent a defined step in early B-cell differentiation—the transition from a pre B cell to an immature B cell. The expression of sIg can be assessed by fluorescence-activated cell sorter (FACS) analysis and the expression of the μ and κ genes can be assessed by Northern blot analysis. Although CGRP by itself has no effect on sIg expression in 70Z/3 cells, it inhibits the effect of LPS on sIg expression.

Analysis of sIg Expression by FACS

The expression of sIg can be examined by FACS analysis using anti-sIg antibodies. The general procedures for FACS analysis are discussed elsewhere in this volume (55). For the analysis of sIg on 70Z/3 cells we use an antibody directed against the mouse κ chain. An antibody to the light chain is used rather than to the μ heavy chain since undifferentiated 70Z/3 cells express cytoplasmic μ heavy-chain protein. For these experiments 70Z/3 cells are cultured at a density of 2×10^5 cells/ml with the various treatments for 48 hr. To stain sIg-positive cells the treated cells are first washed two times with buffer (HBSS/20 m*M* HEPES, pH 7.3/0.1% BSA). The cells are then resuspended at a concentration of 10^6 cells/0.1 ml and are incubated with a 1 : 100 dilution of anti-κ (goat anti-mouse κ, Caltag, South San Francisco, CA) on ice for 1 hr. After incubation with the primary antibody, the cells are diluted to 1 ml with buffer and are pelleted by centrifugation at 200g for 10 min. The cells are then resuspended in 100 μl of buffer containing a 1 : 100 dilution of the second antibody, donkey anti-goat fluorescein isothiocyanate (DAG-FITC, Jackson Immunoresearch, West Grove, PA) and are incubated on ice for an additional hour. The cells are again diluted to 1 ml with buffer and are pelleted. The supernatant containing the unbound DAG-FITC is removed and the cells are resuspended in 1 ml of buffer for FACS analysis. Control groups should include unstained, unstimulated 70Z/3 cells and cells incubated with only the second antibody (DAG-FITC). Ideally there should be no difference between the profiles of unstained cells (autofluorescence control) and the cells stained with only the second antibody. Five to 10% of untreated 70Z/3 cells will normally be positive for sIg, thus comparison of the second antibody control and untreated cells stained with both the primary and secondary antibodies should reveal a small population of cells (5 to 10%) which are clearly positive. The window for positive sIg expression is set such that it contains this population. This window should contain no more than 1 to 2% of the cells in the secondary antibody control.

An example of the results from this type of analysis is shown in Fig. 10. Treatment of 70Z/3 cells with CGRP will reduce the percentage of sIg-positive cells by up to 40 to 50%. When doing any type of functional study using neuropeptides, it is important to demonstrate that the response is dependent on peptide concentration and to include controls for specificity. Ideally, the magnitude of the response should have a dependence on peptide concentration over a concentration range that is likely to be found *in vivo*. Typically, the ED_{50} will be within 1 to 2 orders of magnitude of the K_d or K_i for the peptide. Controls for specificity should include both related and unrelated peptides. In the case of CGRP, one could use both the α and β forms, as well as forms from different species. Unrelated peptides should include peptides of similar size and charge. For CGRP, rat or human calcitonin is an ideal negative control. If available, an antagonist should be used to block the effect of the peptide. Table III shows that high concentrations of CGRP(8–37) can block the inhibitory effects of cGRP on LPS-induced sIg expression. Antagonism by CGRP(8–37) only at higher concentrations is consistent with its lower affinity as determined by competition binding studies (1; Table II).

Experiments can also be done to examine the cellular mechanisms by which CGRP inhibits sIg expression. As shown in Table III, dibutyryl-cAMP can also block the effect of LPS-induced sIg expression. This suggests that the effects of CGRP on sIg expression are induced by its induction of cAMP. Using this system, it should be possible to do more extensive studies on the cellular mechanisms by which CGRP inhibits sIg expression.

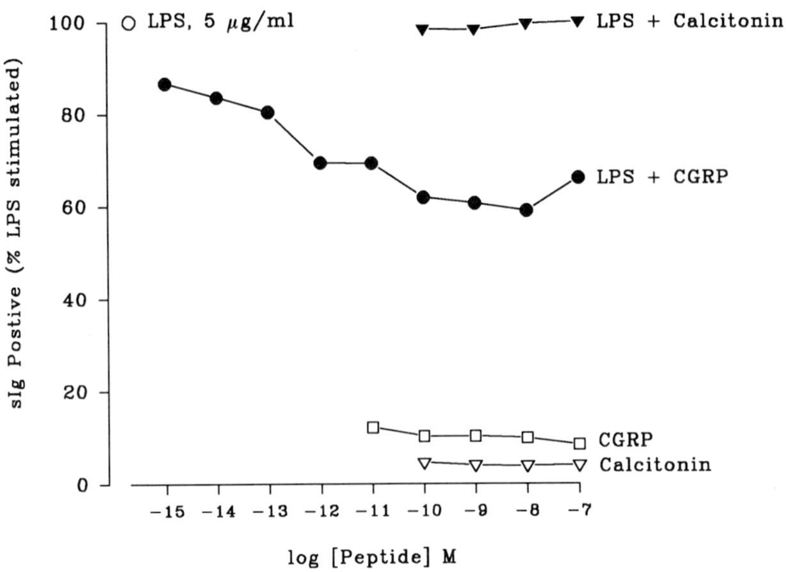

FIG. 10 CGRP inhibits LPS induction of sIg in 70Z/3 pre-B cells. 70Z/3 cells were treated for 48 hr with LPS (1 μg/ml), CGRP (10^{-11} to 10^{-7} *M*), calcitonin (10^{-10} to 10^{-7} *M*), LPS + CGRP (10^{-15} to 10^{-7} *M*), or LPS + calcitonin (10^{-10} to 10^{-7} *M*), CGRP, or calcitonin, or with combinations of LPS and CGRP or calcitonin. The percentage of cells expressing sIg was determined by FACS analysis of cells with an anti-κ antibody. The data are expressed as the percentage of LPS-stimulated controls. Each data point represents the mean from three to five separate experiments. The percentage SE for each point was less than 8%. CGRP, but not calcitonin, inhibited LPS induction of sIg in a dose-dependent manner. Reprinted with permission from J. P. McGillis, S. Humphreys, V. Rangnekar, and J. Ciallella, *Cell. Immunol.* **150,** 405 (1993).

Analysis of Immunoglobulin Gene Expression

The major regulatory point for immunoglobulin gene expression is the transcription of the heavy and light chain genes. Once both chains are transcribed, Ig protein is synthesized and is expressed on the surface of the cell or is secreted. Depending on the developmental and activational stage of the B cell, different heavy-chain isotypes can be expressed following class switching. Post-transcriptional splicing can give rise to either membrane-bound or secreted forms. All of these points, transcription, class switching, splice site selection, are points at which neuropeptides could have regulatory effects. Immunoglobulin mRNA is an abundant mRNA in B cells, thus differences

TABLE III CGRP Inhibition of sIg Expression Reversed by CGRP (8–37) and Mimicked by Dibutyryl-cAMP

Treatment	CGRP (8–37) (*M*)	Dibutyryl-cAMP (*M*)	sIg expression[a] (%)
Untreated	—	—	9.8
LPS, 1 μg/ml	—	—	100
LPS, 1 μg/ml + CGRP, 10 n*M*	—	—	55.0
+ CGRP (8–37)	10^{-9}	—	41.5
	10^{-8}	—	52.3
	10^{-7}	—	46.8
	10^{-6}	—	91.9
LPS + dibutyryl-cAMP	—	10^{-3}	50.0
	—	10^{-4}	55.4
	—	10^{-5}	75.7
	—	10^{-6}	98.7
	—	10^{-7}	108.1
	—	10^{-8}	101.4

[a] 70Z/3 cells were treated for 48 hr and sIg expression was analyzed by FACS. The results are expressed as the % of LPS stimulated controls. Each point represents the mean from two separate experiments. [These data are reprinted with permission from J. P. McGillis, S. Humphreys, V. Rangnekar, and J. Ciallella, *Cell. Immunol.* **150,** 405 (1993)].

in expression of specific isotypes and differentially spliced forms can easily be examined by Northern blot. We have found this approach useful for studying the effects of CGRP on Ig gene expression in 70Z cells. Using Northern blot analysis, we find that CGRP reduces the steady-state levels of both μ and κ mRNA in LPS-treated 70Z/3 cells by about 50%, a level similar to the reduction of sIg protein expression (Fig. 11).

To examine the effect of LPS, CGRP, calcitonin, LPS and CGRP, or LPS and calcitonin on μ and κ mRNA expression, 70Z/3 cells are treated for 48 hr and cellular RNA is prepared by the method of Chomczynski and Sacchi (70). Ten micrograms of each RNA sample is resolved on a 1.2% agarose formaldehyde gel (71) and RNA is transferred to DURALON membranes (Stratagene, San Diego, CA) by capillary blotting (71). Following transfer, RNA is cross-linked to the membrane by exposure to 1200 μJ (microjoules) of UV light. The blots are probed with a 483-bp fragment of κ derived from spCκ or a 787-bp fragment of μ derived from pGEMCμ. These probes recognize the constant regions of κ and μ, respectively. The probes are labeled with [α-^{32}P]dCTP (ICN, Irvine, CA) using a random hexamer labeling kit (Amersham, Arlington Heights, IL). Following a 3- to 5-hr prehybridization, the blots are hybridized overnight with 5×10^5 cpm/ml of the probe in hybridization buffer (5× Denhardt's, 5× SSC, 50 m*M* sodium phosphate,

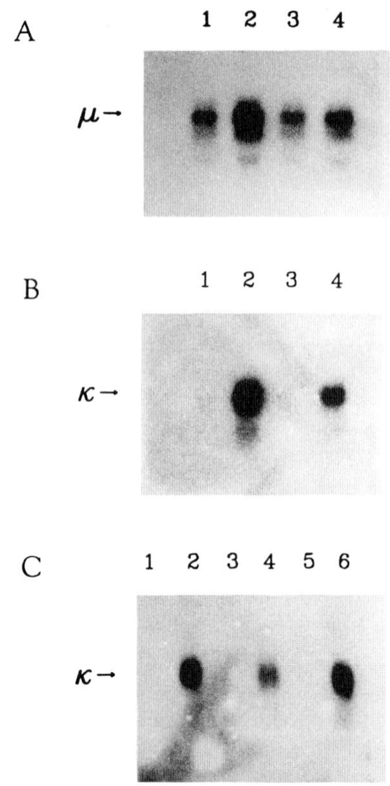

FIG. 11 Downregulation of LPS induced μ and κ mRNA by CGRP. 70Z/3 cells were treated for 48 hr with LPS at 1 μg/ml, with CGRP or calcitonin at 1 n*M*, or with LPS + CGRP or calcitonin. Northern blots were prepared as described in the text and probed with μ or κ constant region probes. (A and B) Cells were untreated (lane 1), treated with LPS (lane 2) or CGRP (lane 3), or with LPS and CGRP (lane 4). The location of the μ (A) and κ (B) bands is shown by the arrows. (C) Lanes 1–4 are the same as in (A) and (B). Lane 5 is from 70Z/3 cells treated with calcitonin, and lane 6 is from cells treated with LPS and calcitonin. The blot was probed with κ and the position of the κ band is shown by the arrow. CGRP treatment by itself had no effect on μ or κ expression, but inhibited LPS induction of both μ and κ by about 50%. Calcitonin had no effect by itself or when given with LPS. Reprinted with permission from J. P. McGillis, S. Humphreys, V. Rangnekar, and J. Ciallella, *Cell. Immunol.* **150,** 405 (1993).

pH 7.5, 0.1% SDS, 50% formamide, 250 μg/ml salmon sperm DNA) at 42°C. The blots are then washed twice with 2× SSC[¶]/0.1% SDS for 30 min at room

[¶] SSC (saline sodium citrate) washes are prepared by diluting 20× SSC (3 *M* NaCl, 0.3 *M* sodium citrate, pH 7.0) and 10% SDS in distilled H_2O.

temperature, twice with 0.1× SSC/0.1% SDS for 60 min at 65°C, and twice with 1× SSC/0.1% SDS at room temperature and then rinsed briefly with water. Autoradiographs are prepared by exposing the blots to Kodak X-Omat film. In the representative studies shown in Fig. 11, untreated 70Z/3 cells only expressed μ. Following treatment with LPS, μ expression is upregulated about fourfold and κ expression is induced. The CGRP has no effect by itself, but reduces the levels of μ and κ expression induced by LPS.

Conclusion

Using the protocols described here, we have found that a number of different lymphocyte populations express CGRP receptors, that the receptors are functional, and that CGRP may have an inhibitory role in early B-cell differentiation. The presence of CGRP receptors on specific cells in the immune system has been reported by other investigators, as have effects on other cells in the immune system. However, several major questions remain to be answered concerning the expression and function of CGRP receptors in the immune system. With respect to receptor expression, it is not clear whether CGRP receptors are expressed on all T and B cells, or whether CGRP receptors are expressed on distinct subpopulations. In earlier studies using a fluorescent analog of SP and two-color FACS analysis, Payan *et al.* found that the SP receptor is expressed on distinct subpopulations of both CD4 and CD8 human T cells (51). We have attempted to use similar methods to produce a biologically active fluorescent CGRP analog but have been unsuccessful so far. An alternative approach would be to try to characterize the CGRP receptor on purified subpopulations by radioligand binding. The limitation to this approach is that it would be prohibitively expensive to purify sufficient numbers of cells for a complete series of binding studies. Moreover, even if purified cells were used for binding studies, one could still not be certain whether all the cells in the purified subpopulation expressed the receptor. A more definitive approach would be to use a receptor cDNA probe to analyze expression of CGRP receptor mRNA by *in situ* hybridization histochemistry. This approach will be invaluable in analyzing CGRP receptor expression in bone marrow cells. Although our studies have found high levels of CGRP receptors in bone marrow (4), there is no information on which cell lineages express the CGRP receptor. Although we have some preliminary functional data that pre B cells in bone marrow express the CGRP receptor, it is probable that other lineages also have CGRP receptors. This is based on the presence of CGRP receptors on the mature cells. Further studies on which cell lineages express CGRP receptors, and at what stage in their development, will be necessary to understand fully the potential role of CGRP in hematopoiesis.

More information on the immunomodulatory effects of CGRP is needed to fully understand its role in immune and inflammatory responses. The number of different cells which it can influence suggests that its role is pleiotropic. With respect to a role in B-cell differentiation, the studies on 70Z/3 cells suggest that it has an inhibitory role. In studies with sIg^+-depleted bone marrow we have found that CGRP has a similar inhibitory effect on B-cell differentiation (72). Based on this and the other reported activities of CGRP, its overall role seems to be inhibitory, suggesting that its general role may be to act as an endogenous "anti-inflammatory agent." With respect to its inhibitory effect on B-cell differentiation, it is possible that CGRP acts as a negative feedback inhibitor to downregulate B-cell differentiation which has been upregulated in response to an inflammatory or immune response. Further studies will be needed to substantiate this and other roles of CGRP in the immune and inflammatory systems.

References

1. J. P.McGillis, S. Humphreys, V. Rangnekar, and J. Ciallella, *Cell. Immunol.* **150,** 391 (1993).
2. J. P. McGillis, S. Humphreys, V. Rangnekar, and J. Ciallella, *Cell. Immunol.* **150,** 405 (1993).
3. J. P. McGillis, S. Humphreys, and S. Reid, *J. Immunol.* **147,** 3482 (1991).
4. M. S. Mullins, J. Ciallella, V. Rangnekar, and J. P. McGillis, *Reg. Pept.,* **49,** 65 (1993).
5. Y. Umeda and M. Arisawa, *Neuropeptides* **14,** 237 (1990).
6. F. Boudard and M. Bastide, *J. Neurosci. Res.* **29,** 29 (1991).
7. Y. Umeda, M. Takamiya, H. Yoshizaki, and M. Arisawa, *Biochem. Biophys. Res. Commun.* **154,** 227 (1988).
8. J. Richter, R. Andersson, L. Edvinsson, and U. Gullberg, *Immunology* **77,** 416 (1992).
9. F. Wang, I. Millet, K. Bottomly, and A. Vignery, *J. Biol. Chem.* **267,** 21,052 (1992).
10. J. Abello, D. Kaiserlian, J. C. Cuber, J. P. Rèvillard, and J. A. Chayvialle, *Neuropeptides* **19,** 43 (1991).
11. C. Singaram, A. Sengupta, C. Stevens, S. J. Spechler, and R. K. Goyal, *Gastroenterology* **100,** 560 (1991).
12. A. Vignery, F. Wang, and M. B. Ganz, *J. Cell. Physiol.* **149,** 301 (1991).
13. J. Hosoi, G. F. Murphy, C. L. Egan, E. A. Lerner, S. Grabbe, A. Asahina, and R. D. Granstein, *Nature (London)* **363,** 159 (1993).

14. Y. H. Nong, R. G. Titus, J. M. C. Ribeiro, and H. G. Remold, *J. Immunol.* **143,** 45 (1989).
15. D. Davies, M. S. Medeiros, J. Keen, A. J. Truner, and L. W. Haynes, *Biochem. Pharmacol.* **43,** 1753 (1992).
16. H. C. Manley and L. W. Haynes, *Neuropeptides* **13,** 29 (1989).
17. K. Bulloch, T. Radojcic, R. Yu, J. Hausman, L. Lenhard, and S. Baird, *Prog. Neuroendocrinimmunol.* **4,** 186 (1991).
18. A. Casini, P. Geppetti, C. A. Maggi, and C. Surrenti, *Naunyn Schmiedebergs Arch. Pharmacol.* **339,** 354 (1989).
19. D. L. Bellinger, D. Lorton, T. D. Romano, J. A. Olschowka, S. Y. Felten, and D. L. Felten, *Ann. N.Y. Acad. Sci.* **594,** 17 (1990).
20. M. S. O'Dorisio and A. Paneria (eds.), "Neuropeptides and Immunopeptides: Messengers in a Neuroimmune Axis." The New York Academy of Sciences, New York, 1990.
21. J. P. McGillis, M. Mitsuhashi, and D. G. Payan, *Ann. N.Y. Acad. Sci.* **594,** 85 (1990).
22. J. P. McGillis, M. Mitsuhashi and D. G. Payan, *in* "Psychoneuroimmunology" (R. Ader, D. L. Felten, and N. Cohen eds.), p. 209. Academic Press, Orlando, FL, 1991.
23. Y. Lee, K. Takami, Y. Kawai, S. Girgis, C. J. Hillyard, I. MacIntyre, P. C. Emson, and M. Tohyama, *Neuroscience* **15,** 1227 (1985).
24. S. G. Amara, V. Jones, M. G. Rosenfeld, E. S. Ong, and R. M. Evans, *Nature (London)* **298,** 240 (1982).
25. S. G. Amara, J. L. Arriza, S. E. Leff, L. W. Swanson, R. M. Evans, and M. G. Rosenfeld, *Science* **229,** 1094 (1985).
26. P. M. Sexton, J. S. McKenzie, and F. A. O. Mendelsohn, *Neurochem. Int.* **12,** 323 (1988).
27. H. Henke, S. Sigrist, W. Lang, J. Schneider, and J. A. Fischer, *Brain Res.* **410,** 404 (1987).
28. F. A. Tschopp, H. Henke, J. B. Petermann, P. H. Tobler, R. Janzer, T. Hokfelt, J. M. Lundberg, C. Cuello, and J. A. Fisher, *Proc. Natl. Acad. Sci. U.S.A.* **82,** 248 (1985).
29. J. Rodrigo, J. M. Polak, L. Fernandez, M. A. Ghatei, P. Mulderry, and S. R. Bloom, *Gastroenterology* **88,** 444 (1985).
30. L. Kruger, J. D. Silverman, P. W. Mantyh, C. Sternini, and N. C. Brecha, *J. Comp. Neurol.* **280,** 291 (1991).
31. P. Popper and P. E. Micevych, *Brain Res.* **496,** 180 (1989).
32. E. Weihe, S. Muller, T. Fink, and H. J. Zentel, *Neurosci. Lett.* **100,** 77 (1989).
33. P. Popper, C. R. Mantyh, S. R. Vigna, J. E. Maggio, and P. W. Mantyh, *Peptides* **9,** 257 (1988).
34. A. Bjurholm, *Int. Orthod.* **15,** 325 (1991).
35. C. L. Kimberly and M. R. Byers, *Anat. Rec.* **222,** 289 (1988).
36. M. Hukkanen, Y. Konttinin, R. G. Rees, S. J. Gibson, S. Santavirta, and J. M. Polak, *J. Rheumatol.* **19,** 1252 (1992).
37. S. D. Brain, T. J. Williams, J. R. Tippins, H. R. Morris, and I. MacIntyre, *Nature (London)* **313,** 54 (1985).

38. S. M. Louis, A. Jamieson, N. J. W. Russel, and G. J. Dockray, *Neuroscience* **32,** 581 (1989).
39. G. G. Wong, J. S. Witek, P. A. Temple, K. M. Wilkens, A. C. Leary, D. P. Luxenberg, S. S. Jones, E. L. Brown, R. M. Kay, E. C. Orr, C. Shoemaker, D. W. Golde, R. J. Kaufman, R. M. Hewick, E. A. Wang, and S. C. Clark, *Science* **228,** 810 (1985).
40. T. L. Buckley, S. D. Brain, P. D. Collins, and T. J. Williams, *J. Immunol.* **146,** 3424 (1991).
41. C. P. Sung, A. J. Arleth, N. Aiyar, P. K. Bhatnagar, P. G. Lysko, and G. Feuerstein, *Peptides* **13,** 429 (1992).
42. T. Dennis, A. Fournier, S. St. Pierre, and R. Quirion, *J. Pharmacol. Exp. Ther.* **251,** 718 (1989).
43. A. Haegerstrand, C.-J. Dalsgaard, B. Jonzon, O. Larsson, and J. Nilsson, *Proc. Natl. Acad. Sci. U.S.A.* **87,** 3299 (1990).
44. Y. Hirata, Y. Takagi, S. Takata, Y. Fukuda, H. Yoshimi, and T. Fujita, *Biochem. Biophys. Res. Commun.* **151,** 1113 (1988).
45. H. Seifert, P. Sawchenko, J. Chesnut, J. Rivier, W. Vale, and S. J. Pandol, *Am. J. Physiol.* **249,** G147 (1985).
46. S. Sigrist, A. Franco-Cereceda, R. Muff, H. Henke, J. M. Lundberg, and J. A. Fischer, *Endocrinology* (*Baltimore*) **119,** 381 (1986).
47. H. Nakamuta, Y. Fukuda, M. Koida, N. Fufii, A. Otaka, S. Funakoshi, N. Mitsuyasu, and R. C. Orlowski, *Jpn. J. Pharmacol.* **42,** 175 (1986).
48. T. Dennis, A. Fournier, A. Cadieux, F. Pomerleau, F. B. Jolicoeur, S. St. Pierre, and R. Quirion, *J. Pharmacol. Exp. Ther.* **254,** 123 (1990).
49. S. J. Wimalawansa, *Ann. N.Y. Acad. Sci.* **657,** 70 (1992).
50. D. G. Payan, D. R. Brewster, and E. J. Goetzl, *J. Immunol.* **133,** 3260 (1984).
51. D. G. Payan, D. R. Brewster, A. Nissirian-Bastian, and E. J. Goetzl, *J. Clin. Invest.* **74,** 1532 (1984).
52. F. C. Greenwood, W. M. Hunter, and J. S. Glover, *Biochem. J.* **89,** 114 (1963).
53. M. A. K. Markwell, *Anal. Biochem.* **125,** 427 (1982).
54. A. E. Booton and W. M. Hunter, *Biochem. J.* **133,** 529 (1973).
55. L. E. Elliott, S. L. Carlson, L. A. Morford, and J. P. McGillis, this volume (8).
56. D. W. Goldman and E. J. Goetzl, *J. Immunol.* **82,** 1600 (1982).
57. R. Quirion, D. Van Rossum, Y. Dumont, S. St-Pierre, and A. Fournier, *Ann. N.Y. Acad. Sci.* **657,** 88 (1992).
58. T. Dennis, A. Fournier, S. St-Pierre, and R. Quirion, *Brain Res.* **539,** 59 (1991).
59. J. P. McGillis, M. L. Organist, and D. G. Payan, *Anal. Biochem.* **164,** 502 (1987).
60. J. P. McGillis, M. L. Organist, K. H. Scriven, and D. G. Payan, *J. Neurosci. Res.* **18,** 190 (1987).
61. D. G. Payan, J. P. McGillis, and M. L. Organist, *J. Biol. Chem.* **261,** 14,321 (1986).
62. U. K. Laemmli *Nature* (*London*) **259,** 680 (1970).
63. S. Dotti-Sigrist, W. Born, and J. A. Fisher, *Biochem. Biophys. Res. Commun.* **151,** 1081 (1988).
64. S. M. Foord and R. K. Craig, *Eur. J. Biochem.* **170,** 373 (1987).
65. R. Muff, D. Stangl, W. Born, and J. A. Fischer, *Ann. N.Y. Acad. Sci.* **657,** 106 (1992).

66. T. Chiba, A. Yamaguchi, T. Yamatani, A. Nakamura, T. Morishita, T. Inui, M. Fukase, T. Noda, and T. Fujita, *Am. J. Physiol.* **256,** E331 (1989).
67. M. M. Bartik, W. H. Brooks, and T. L. Roszman, *Cell. Immunol.* **148,** 408 (1993).
68. C. D. Joyce, R. R. Fiscus, X. Wang, D. J. Dries, R. C. Morris, and R. A. Prinz, *Surgery* **108,** 1097 (1990).
69. C. J. Paige, P. W. Kincade, and P. Ralph, *J. Immunol.* **121,** 641 (1978).
70. P. Chomczynski and N. Sacchi, *Anal. Biochem.* **162,** 156 (1987).
71. J. Sambrook, E. F. Fritsch, and T. Maniatis, "Molecular Cloning, A Laboratory Manual." Cold Spring Harbor Laboratory Press, Cold Spring Harbor, NY, 1990.
72. J. P. McGillis, M. W. Mullins, and J. R. Ciallella, unpublished observation, 1993.

[25] Effects of Cocaine on the Immune Response

Ian R. Tebbett and Janet Karlix

Introduction

Cocaine is a major drug of abuse which has increased in popularity over the past few years (1). Its use throughout the United States has reached epidemic proportions, with an estimated 20 million users, and has become a major concern of recent government administrations. Cocaine hydrochloride is readily absorbed from mucous membranes including the nasal mucosa. After administration by this route (snorting), maximum euphoria is experienced after 15–20 min, with peak plasma levels of 10–500 ng/ml approximately 30 min after ingestion (2–5). Cocaine is also absorbed orally with peak plasma levels being attained 20–60 min after ingestion (1). Intravenous administration (iv), produces an immediate intense rush with corresponding high plasma concentrations. The freebase form of the drug, known as "crack," provides an active drug for smoking, since it is not destroyed at the temperatures required for pyrolysis (6).

Metabolism

Cocaine is metabolized by plasma and liver cholinesterases to water-soluble metabolites that are excreted in the urine. The two major metabolites are benzoylecgonine and ecgonine methyl ester. Smaller amounts of ecgonine, norcocaine, and various hydroxylated products are also found in the urine after cocaine administration [7].

Cocaine is rapidly eliminated from the body with a biological half-life of 45–90 min. Because plasma cholinesterase activity is lower in the elderly, in patients with various states of liver disease, in pregnant women, and in fetuses, cocaine toxicity may be exacerbated in these groups (8). Studies have indicated that premature infants have a reduced capacity to metabolize cocaine to the major adult metabolite benzoylecgonine, indicating immature liver esterase function (9–11). Instead, relatively high concentrations of unchanged cocaine and the *N*-demethyl metabolite, norcocaine, were identified. The reduced cocaine metabolism in the fetus prolongs the half-life of cocaine and central nervous system (CNS)-active metabolites such as norcocaine thereby prolonging the exposure of the fetus to toxic effects of the drug.

Methods in Neurosciences, Volume 24

Toxicology

The effects of cocaine on the CNS are well-characterized and demonstrate a biphasic pattern of intense stimulation followed by depression. Cortical stimulation is manifested by euphoria, restlessness, and excitability. However, none of the known neurochemical actions of cocaine singly provide a full explanation of how the drug produces euphoria. It has been demonstrated that cocaine blocks dopamine uptake causing increased dopamine concentrations in the synaptic cleft. This, in turn, increases neurotransmission in the reward systems (12). In addition, cocaine has multiple actions on several neurotransmitters, affecting noradrenergic, dopaminergic, serotonergic, and cholinergic systems (12). Blockage of catecholamine uptake at adrenergic nerve endings potentiates sympathetically mediated vasoconstriction and hypertension (5, 8). This action is associated with many of the toxic effects of cocaine which include pyrexia (5), respiratory collapse, seizures, and cerebrovascular infarction. In addition, the accumulation of catecholamines predisposes the myocardium to arrhythmias which may compromise cardiac output, in some cases resulting in myocardial infarction and ischemia. Cocaine toxicity has also been implicated in sudden arrhythmic death, contraction band necrosis, fibrosis, and myocarditis. Intestinal ischemia may result from cocaine-induced catecholamine stimulation of α receptors in mesenteric vasculature, causing intense vasoconstriction and reduced blood flow (5). Additionally, women who use cocaine during pregnancy are noted to have more sexually transmitted diseases than those who are drug-free. This is thought to be due to a more sexually promiscuous lifestyle. Complications which may occur due to intravenous use of any drug include endocarditis, hepatitis, human immunodeficiency virus (HIV) infection, and abscesses. Freebase users may complain of cough or sore throat. Cocaine insufflation is associated with upper airway lesions, nasal and septal defects, sinusitis, and an inability to smell or taste (8). Other severe problems of crack abuse include nervous agitation, cardiac arrhythmia, hypertension, paranoia, and heart failure. Anorectic effects associated with nutritional deficiencies of drug users may affect the immune system (13). Malnutrition may be an indirect effect of cocaine resulting in altered disease and tumor resistance (13).

Effects of Cocaine on the Newborn

Of considerable concern is the increasing cocaine use among young women and the high incidence of the highly addictive form of the drug crack. A number of case reports have linked such medical problems in the newborn as perinatal cerebral infarction, ophthalmic abnormalities, chromosome abnormalities, necrotizing enterocolitis, ventricular tachycardia, and aortic thrombosis and hypertension to maternal cocaine use during pregnancy. Studies have documented an increase in such perinatal problems as spontaneous abortion, abruptic placentae, preterm labor and delivery, precipitous labor, stillbirth, premature rupture of the membranes, and meconium-stained amniotic fluid. Clinical studies have also documented a series of problems in neonates who are prenatally exposed to cocaine. These problems have included lower gestational age; lower birth weight, length, or head circumference; a higher rate of congenital malformations; a higher incidence of intrauterine growth retardation and/or small for gestational age infants; and lower Apgar scores with poorer general outcome. Prenatal cocaine exposure has also been shown to decrease thymus/body weight ratios but increase spleen/body weight ratios. Although these ratios are not functional measures of immunity they may reflect a long-term alteration in components of the immune system (14).

Only sparse data are available which relate outcome to the type of cocaine used or the point in time during gestation that the drug was used. A study published by Graham *et al.* (15) reported the pregnancy outcome of 25 women who were social cocaine users during the first trimester of pregnancy only. Although no control group was available for comparison, the pregnancy outcomes of these 25 women were not different from that of the general population. Chasnoff *et al.* reported the outcomes of 23 women who used cocaine during the first trimester, 52 women who used cocaine throughout pregnancy, and 40 women who were drug-free. The first trimester users were similar to the drug-free group for rate of preterm delivery, low birth rate, intrauterine growth retardation, and infant birth weight, length, and head circumference. The group who used cocaine throughout pregnancy had worse outcomes on all of the above measures than the drug-free group. Surveys of primarily inner city populations have indicated that 10–15% of women entering their hospitals for delivery used cocaine during pregnancy. Those figures are in line with the overall incidence of 11% (range 0.4–27%) found in a survey of 36 hospitals representing different geographical areas across the country. Undoubtedly these prevalence figures are underestimates, as urine screening performed at delivery only identifies infants of mothers who used cocaine within a few days prior to delivery and maternal histories obtained at a single interview can be misleading (16).

Central Nervous System

Cocaine has sympathomimetic activity which involves at least two mechanisms: the release of catecholamines from the adrenal medulla and inhibition of reuptake of norepinephrine and other catecholamines by the sympathetic nervous system (17). It has also been reported that acute and chronic treatment with D-amphetamine and cocaine increased the number of β receptors in the brain at doses of 10 ng/kg. Animal studies have shown that cocaine causes β- and α-adrenergic receptor supersensitization and increased norepinephrine and dopamine turnover (18). Catecholamines have direct and indirect inhibitory effects on various immune phenomena. Lymphocytes, macrophages, granulocytes, and mast cells all possess B catecholamine receptors (19). Stimulation of these receptors decreases the lymphocyte response to mitogen and antigens as well as the response of mast cells and skin reaction to antigen histamine. Catecholamines also inhibit macrophage and neutrophil activation (19). Sympathetic innervation of lymphoid organs is documented, as well as innervation of thymus gland, bone marrow, spleen, and lymph nodes. Disruption of this innervation has been shown to result in enhanced immune responses (20, 21).

Dopamine has important stimulatory roles in hypothalamus–pituitary–adrenal (HPA) regulation and dopamine and serotonin produce adrenocortical stimulation via D1 and D2 receptors. Dopamine tonically inhibits prolactin release and both dopamine and norepinephrine stimulate growth hormone release from the pituitary gland (18). Neurophysiological alterations in dopaminergic and noradrenergic systems have been observed in chronic cocaine abusers (18). Chronic cocaine administration blocks dopamine and norepinephrine reuptake in various brain regions which in turn depletes endogenous neuronal neurotransmitter stores. It has been demonstrated that chronic cocaine exposure in rats also results in reduced endogenous levels of norepinephrine in the spleen and heart (22). These depleted cardiac levels may indicate the etiology of cardiac-related traumas reported in cocaine abusers (22).

Cocaine stimulates the HPA axis, and modifies the activity of acetylcholine, serotonin, norephinephrine, and dopamine. All of these neurotransmitters are stimulants of CRH as an effect of the local anesthetic effect of cocaine and in opposition to increasing the actual levels of these neurotransmitters (23). In addition to the potentiating effects of cocaine on neurotransmitters, and the consequent direct and indirect effects on neurohormone secretion, it is important to consider second-messenger effects. Epinephrine, glucocorticoids, histamine (H2), prostaglandin A, and prostaglandin E can all increase cyclic AMP levels. Elevated levels of cyclic AMP have been shown to have immunosuppressive effects, by inhibiting mature, differentiated lymphocyte functions. Cyclic GMP concentrations generally oppose the effects of cAMP and are increased by acetylcholine, interleukin 1, serotonin, and thymic hormones (24). Stimulation of acetylcholine and muscarinic and nicotinic receptors, present on lymphoid cells, generally enhances immune responses including T-lymphocyte reactions and complement synthesis (19).

Neuroendocrine Effects of Cocaine

Evidence supports the possibility that neurophysiological adaptations occur after prolonged cocaine administration and that neuroendocrine measures might reflect such changes (17). It is recognized that a reciprocal transmission of information exists between the neuroendocrine and immune system. These two systems share a common set of hormones and receptors (25). The hypothalamus plays a central role in neuroendocrine function through the regulation of endocrine and neurotransmitter processes. Both of these systems are thought to participate in the modulation of cellular and humoral mediated immunity and both systems have been shown to be affected by cocaine (26). Both human and animal studies have shown that acute cocaine administration induces the secretion of adrenocorticotropic hormone (ACTH), β-endorphin, and corticosterone (13, 26, 27). Although these hormones are released from the pituitary, cocaine had no effect on the ACTH production of cultured pituitary cells *in vitro,* suggesting the effects of cocaine are mediated via the hypothalamus (26). The administration of other dopamine, norepinephrine (NE), and serotonin uptake blockers also stimulated HPA axis activity (28). It is possible then that cocaine stimulates the hypothalamus to increase the secretion of CRF and to decrease the secretion of prolactin inhibition factor. The result of the elevated CRF level in the pituitary is a potentiated secretion of β-endorphin and ACTH (13). Chronic cocaine administration to rats has also been shown to produce adrenocortical hypertrophy. This may occur following an increase in plasma ACTH, followed by an increase in corticosterone production in the adrenal cortex (13). β-Endorphin, ACTH, and corticosterone have multiple effects on the immune response. *In vitro* studies have shown that very high concentrations of cocaine inhibit numerous immune responses indirectly mediated via ACTH, β-endorphine, and corticosterone (19, 21). The ACTH increases the circulating levels of norepinephrine and glucocorticoids which also have modulatory effects on the immune system (19, 21). Glucocorticoid receptors are present on all leukocytes and largely influence leukocyte recirculation. Increased levels of glucocorticoids cause atrophy of the lymphoid organs, profound suppression of humoral and cell-mediated immune mechanisms, and the inhibition of mononuclear and polymorphonuclear phagocytosis (19). An increase in plasma norepinephrine levels following ACTH stimulation could potentially increase natural killer (NK) cell activity (29). The ACTH also inhibits γ-interferon production of murine spleen cells and the antibody response to sheep red blood cells (SRBC) (13). In addition, ACTH has been shown to bind to receptors on lymphocyte membranes probably mediating suppressive effects of cocaine on γ-interferon production (13).

Acute administration of CNS stimulants has been shown to result in a decrease in serum prolactin concentrations and an increase in growth hormone (GH) (17, 30). Chronic administration of cocaine may therefore result in prolonged increases in GH or decreases in prolactin (17, 18, 27).

GH is needed for maintenance of lymphatic tissue, and decreases lead to atrophy of the thymus and secondary lymphatic tissue (20). Prolactin receptors are present on T and B cells and monocytes. The hormone regulates γ-interferon production by T lymphocytes and can reverse lowered antibody responses in hypophysectomized rat PRL also induces interleukin 2 (IL-2) receptor expression (31).

Cocaine causes a decrease in plasma prolactin concentrations. This may be due to cocaine induced changes in norepinephrine and dopamine levels in the hypothalamus which modulate LH and PRL release from the pituitary (18, 32), to decreased functional dopamine tone, or to cocaine activation of the serotonin neurotransmitter (27, 33). Thyroid-stimulating hormone is blunted in cocaine patients due to chronically elevated TRH levels as a result of the potentiation of dopamine receptors (18, 27). TRH inhibits monocyte activities and results in decreased immunoglobulin G (IgG) activity by peripheral mononuclear blood cells (PBMC).

Acute cocaine administration has been observed to increase luteinizing hormone concentration, while higher cocaine concentrations cause a decrease (18, 32). Also observed is an acute increase in the amount of testosterone which then rapidly decreases (18, 27). Cocaine has been shown to stimulate the endogenous opiate system. Endogenous opiates appear to facilitate the immune responses *in vitro*, but *in vivo* studies show that opiates inhibit immune responses and impair tumor rejection (27). β-Endorphin is a potent stimulator of NK cell activity and γ-interferon secretion. It was also found to trigger the release of prostaglandin E_2 from PBMC (14). Prostaglandin E_2 (PGE_2) is a potent inhibitor of some monocyte and lymphocyte functions (14). β-Endorphins can blind to opioid receptors on monocytes and lymphocytes and exert multiple stimulating effects on these cells including the release of immunomodulatory cytokines (13). β-Endorphin suppresses responses of primary IgG plaque-forming, rat spleen cells to antigenic stimulation (34) and has been shown to enhance the proliferative response of spleen cells to T-cell mitogens. This effect of β-endorphin was dose-dependent and occurred at physiological concentrations of the peptide in rat plasma (35). T lymphocytes possess surface receptors for met enkephalin, and studies have shown natural killer cell activity and interleukin 2 production are enhanced by this compound *in vitro*.

Immunomodulatory Effects

In addition to the toxic effects of cocaine outlined above, evidence exists to suggest that cocaine may have a marked effect on the immune system. Although several studies have investigated the effects of cocaine and metabolites on human and animal immune functions, the data are often contradictory.

Effects on Cellular Immune Function

Human T-Lymphocyte Studies

Cocaine has been reported to affect the immune system in animal models; however, recently, more reports have appeared demonstrating an effect of cocaine on human T lymphocytes. Klein *et al.* (36) initially investigated the effect of cocaine on mitogen-stimulated human and mouse T lymphocytes in concentrations of 0–400 μg/ml and discovered immunosuppression at the higher cocaine concentrations. Klein *et al.* (37) also evaluated the effect of lower cocaine concentrations on suboptimally phytohemagglutinin (PHA)-stimulated T lymphocytes from healthy volunteers. In this experiment, the PBMCs were purified to increase the T-lymphocyte population in the tissue culture wells by a well-described adherent procedure. Low concentrations of cocaine (0.09–12 μM) were unable to suppress the proliferation of suboptimum (0.2 μg/ml) PHA-stimulated PBMCs. However, cocaine-induced suppression was seen in the PHA stimulated T-cell-enriched peripheral blood lymphocytes (PBL) suggesting that cocaine may not have as great an effect on inhibiting antigen-presenting cells. The immunosuppressive effect of cocaine could be decreased by increasing the amount of mitogen; however, this effect could be reversed by incubating the cells with cocaine for 24 hr prior to the assay. Calcium mobilization was also investigated and it was found that cocaine suppressed the cytosolic free calcium mobilization in suboptimally stimulated T cells. These results suggest the immunosuppressive effects of cocaine may not appear in low concentrations of mitogen stimulation or when accessory cells such as antigen-presenting cells are present.

Another report investigates the effects of cocaine through T lymphocytes stimulated through the T-cell receptor pathway (37, 38). In this study, human PBMCs were cultured with OKT3, a mitogen which stimulates proliferation through the CD3 pathway. A dose-dependent response was observed with cocaine achieving a plateau of immunosuppression at 0.75 μM. Cocaine was found to inhibit the nonspecific IL-2 and calcium-dependent pathways of stimulation by concanavalin A (Con A) in human PBMCs in a dose-dependent fashion. This study also suggested that cocaine may not be stable in tissue culture environments which may skew results (39). Cocaine has also been shown to stimulate the immune system by reversing the heroin-mediated suppression of rosette formation *in vitro* (40). Mononuclear cells were stimulated with mitogen *in vitro* in the presence and absence of various concentrations of cocaine. In doses which altered behavior, cocaine did not suppress responses to antigenic challenge, nor did it affect tumor growth or susceptibility to infection (41).

Human cells exposed *in vitro* to a range of cocaine concentrations showed no modulation of T- or B-cell subsets. However, after a single dose of cocaine, nonhabitual users showed a significant stimulation of natural killer cell activity. Levels of some T-cell subsets were elevated while levels of T-helper cells, suppressor cells, B cells, and monocytes were unchanged (42). In humans, NK activity is increased by exercise or by the administration of adrenergic agents. This suggests that NK cells may be partially regulated by the adrenergic system and therefore susceptible to the effects of cocaine.

We have been investigating the effects of cocaine and its metabolites on lymphocytes from normal volunteers (Fig. 1). We found phytohemagglutinin (PHA)-stimulated T lymphocytes were inhibited by cocaine from 0.039 to 300 μg/ml as has been previously described in both human and mouse lymphocytes. Cocaine exerted a much greater effect on inhibiting lymphocyte proliferation in Con A, phorbol 12-myristate 13-acetate (PMA), and mixed lymphocyte reaction (MLR) experiments. IC_{50} values for Con A, PMA, and MLR were 90 μg/ml, 70 mg/ml, and 30 μg/ml, respectively. As compared to cocaine, benzoylecgonine was much less potent in inhibiting any of the T-lymphocyte responses. Benzoylecgonine exerted a much greater effect on inhibiting lymphocyte proliferation in the MLR and PMA systems; however, neither effect was as great as the cocaine inhibitory effect. IC_{50} values for Con A, PHA, PMA, and MLR were 300, 300, 25, and 50 μg/ml, respectively (Fig. 2). Norcocaine exerted a much greater effect on inhibiting PHA- and PMA-stimulated lymphocytes in these experiments as compared to cocaine and benzoylecgonine. IC_{50} values for PHA and PMA were 90 μg/ml and 70 mg/ml, respectively (Fig. 3).

The cocaine concentrations employed covered a much wider range than previously investigated. Despite this, we found the dose-dependent range to be similar to that of previous reports (42). The inhibitory effects of cocaine, benzoylecgonine, and norcocaine in the PMA-stimulated T-lymphocyte assays suggest that cocaine and these two metabolites may inhibit T lymphocytes through the protein kinase C pathway and may bypass the antigen presentation step in T-cell activation. Interestingly, norcocaine appears to be much more potent in inhibiting the PMA-stimulated lymphocytes. Because of the increased immunosuppressive activity of norcocaine as compared to

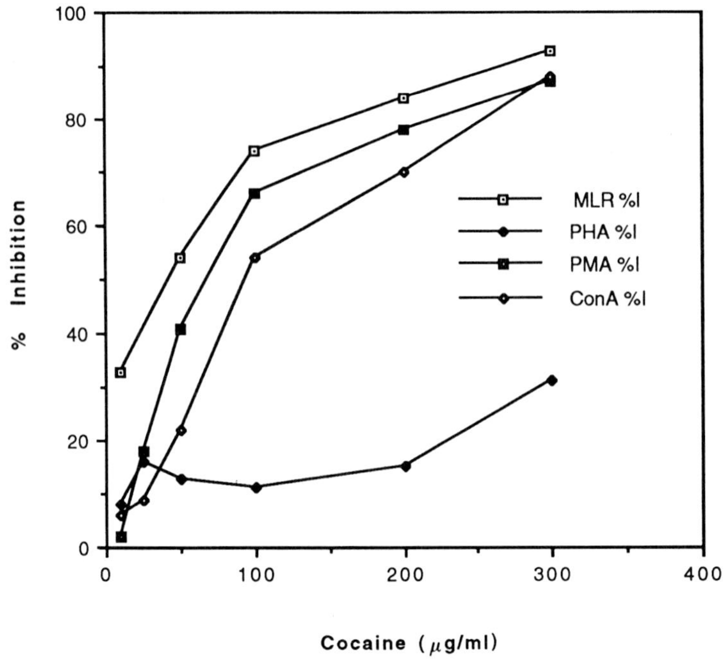

FIG. 1 Inhibition of lymphocytes by cocaine. (⊡) MLR, (◆) PHA, (■) PMA, (◇) Con A.

either cocaine and benzoylecgonine in inhibiting PMA-stimulated T lymphocytes, there is increased need to evaluate the role of this metabolite in influencing the immune system in the patient population which may have elevated concentrations of norcocaine such as newborns exposed to cocaine *in utero*. By inhibiting Con A and to a lesser degree PHA, cocaine and norcocaine appear to possess nonspecific inhibitory capacities through calcium and interleukin 2-dependent pathways. Benzoylecgonine also had an effect in inhibiting PHA- and Con A-stimulated lymphocytes but was less potent than cocaine. The inhibition of the MLR by cocaine validates that cocaine can inhibit allogeneic immune responses in the *in vitro* model that may correlate to *in vivo* findings in patients.

Because there may be differences of metabolism in various populations and therefore differences in concentrations of cocaine and its metabolites in individual subjects, it would be interesting to test for immunosuppressive synergy of cocaine and some of its metabolites by adding varying concentrations of the compounds in the tissue culture cell well. Because of the effect of cocaine, benzoylecgonine, and norcocaine on PMA-stimulated lymphocytes,

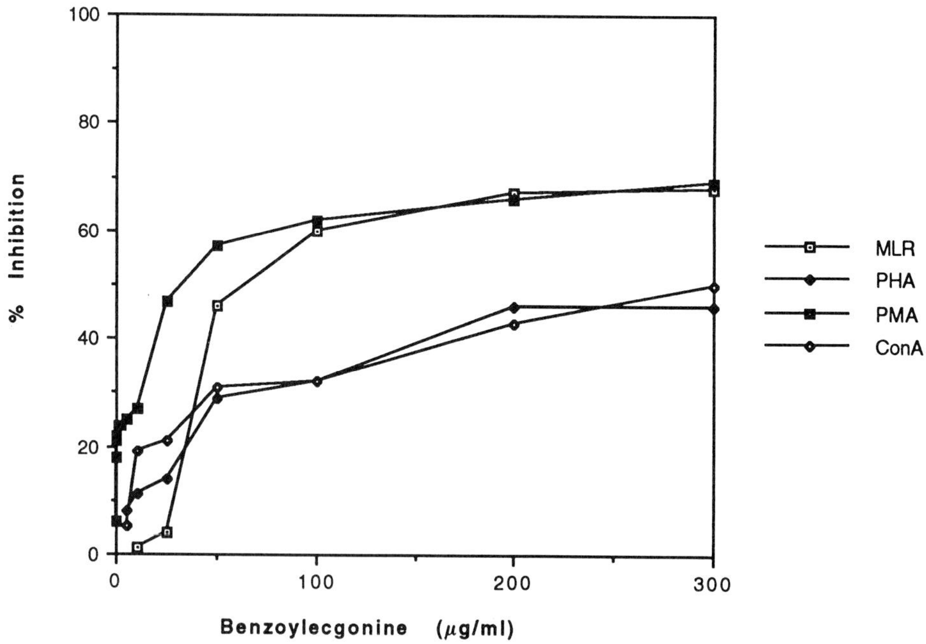

FIG. 2 Inhibition of lymphocytes by benzoylecgonine. (□) MLR, (◆) PHA, (■) PMA, (◇) Con A.

additional information on the influence of these agents on second signal transduction pathways such as CD28 would further complement our knowledge of the immune modulating properties of cocaine and its metabolites.

Techniques

Isolation of Peripheral Blood Mononuclear Cells Peripheral blood mononuclear cells are isolated from healthy volunteers from heparinized blood by Ficoll–Hypaque density gradient centrifugation. Blood is collected in sterile vacuum tubes that contain 500 U heparin. If separation of lymphocytes will not be completed within 10 hr of collection, blood should be diluted in RPMI medium with an anticoagulant (heparin, 500 U) and be stored between 4 and 20°C. Ficoll–Hypaque is available as a commercial product and can be purchased from most tissue culture companies. To increase the yield of leukocytes, all materials used should be at approximately room temperature (22°C). Under sterile conditions, blood is diluted with RPMI in equal ratios. Twenty milliliters of blood is placed in a 50-ml conical tube and diluted with 20 ml of RPMI. Ten milliliters of Ficoll–Hypaque is drawn into a 10-ml

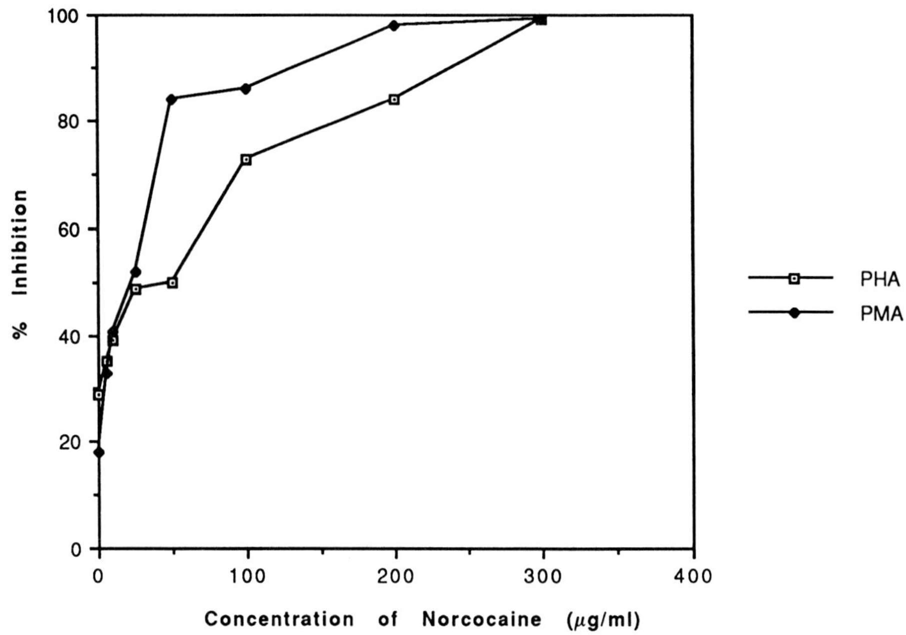

FIG. 3 Inhibition of lymphocytes by norcocaine. (⊡) PHA, (◆) PMA.

pipette. The pipette containing the Ficoll–Hypaque is plunged into the blood–RPMI mixture. The Ficoll–Hypaque is released slowly into the blood mixture forming a layer on the bottom of the 50-ml conical tube. The tube is centrifuged for 30 min at 1200 rpm. Erythrocytes and polymorphonuclear leukocytes from a pellet at the bottom of the tube and the platelets remain in the plasma. The mononuclear leukocytes are suspended at the interface of the plasma and the Ficoll–Hypaque. Using a Pasteur pipette, PBMCs are removed (approximately 10–15 ml) from the 50-ml conical tube and placed in another tube. The cell suspension is immediately diluted with four times its volume of 5% human albumin RPMI. In most instances, if the cell suspension is placed in a 50-ml conical tube, the tube can be filled up to the 50-ml mark with 5% human albumin RPMI. The cell suspension is then washed by centrifuging for 10 min at 1200 rpm. The PBMCs will form a pellet at the bottom of the conical tube. The RPMI is removed and the cells are resuspended in a small, known volume to count and assess cell viability. Trypan blue is used to stain the lymphocytes and determine visual contrast between live and dead cells. If an excess of red blood cells is found on the phase-contrast microscopy analysis of the cell suspension, the cells can be washed again with 5% human albumin RPMI and recounted.

Mixed Lymphocyte Reaction The MLR measures the cellular immune response of responder cells against mismatched HLA antigens from stimulator cells. The primary HLA antigens responsible for the reaction are the class II, HLA-DR antigens. The MLR provides an excellent *in vitro* model with which to measure immunosuppressive activity of drugs.

Mononuclear cells are isolated under sterile conditions as described earlier. The cells that are to be used as stimulator cells are irradiated at 3000 rads with a cesium gamma source. Cells are counted and suspended with 5% human albumin RPMI. The cell suspensions should be adjusted to a concentration of 1×10^5 cells/100 μl. One hundred microliters of each cell suspension (1×10^5 cells/100 μl) is dispensed into a round-bottom well of a 96 U-bottom microtiter plate. All data points should be done in triplicate. If the MLR is performed to assess drug activity, the cell suspensions should be 1×10^5 cells/50 μl. The volume of drug added to the cell well is 100 μl. Therefore, drug concentration desired should be doubled in the working solution because of the 1 : 1 dilution in the cell well. If drug solutions are to be used, the drug solution should be added to the cell wells before the cell suspensions. The microtiter plates are placed in a 37°C incubator with a 5% CO_2 atmosphere. On Day 5, each cell well is pulsed with 1 μCi of tritiated thymidine that has been diluted in RPMI and delivered in 10-μl aliquots. On Day 6, the cells are harvested on nylon paper with an automatic cell harvester. After the paper is dry, the individual disks are placed into vials containing liquid scintillation fluid and counted on a scintillation counter. The counts per minute are reported for each cell well. If drug activity is to be assessed using an MLR, there should be adequate controls in the microtiter plate including stimulated cells in wells with no drug added (100% control), wells with RPMI only, and stimulated cells in wells exposed to the drug diluent. Most studies reporting the effects of drugs on the MLR will calculate the percent inhibition of proliferation as follows: 1-[(cells without drug cpm − cells with drug cpm)/cells without drug cpm] × 100.

Mitogen Stimulation

Mitogens are used to stimulate lymphocytes through different pathways. When assessing drug activity, mitogen-stimulated assays are useful in determining mechanism of action. Phorbol 12-myristate 13-acetate is known to stimulate T lymphocytes through protein kinase C pathways within the cytosol of the lymphocyte and thought to work independently of antigen-presenting cells.

In contrast to the MLR, the mitogen assay is completed within 72 hr. The optimum mitogen concentration for each mitogen should be assessed by the individual laboratory and for each lot of mitogen. Mitogens, PHA, PMA, and Con A are available from most tissue culture companies including Sigma Chemical Co. (St. Louis, MO).

In our laboratories we have found the optimum final cell concentrations for individual mitogens to be in range of the following: Con A, 10 μg/ml; PMA, 50 ng/ml; and PHA, 5 μg/ml. After lymphocyte preparation as described earlier, the cell suspensions should contain 1×10^5 cells/200 μl. The mitogen is added before dispensing the cell aliquots into the microtiter plate to the desired final concentration. We have found in our laboratory that 0.5×10^5 cells/200 μl for the PHA experiments can produce adequate lymphocyte stimulation. If the mitogen assays will be measuring drug effect on the stimulated lymphocytes, the cells should be diluted to an appropriate concentration for 100-μl aliquots. As described in the MLR, the working stock solution of drug concentration should be double that of the desired concentration in the cell well to allow for the 1 : 1 dilution within the well. If the experiments include evaluating the drug effect, the 100 μl of drug solution should be dispensed into the microtiter plate prior to the cells. After 48 hr, each cell well is pulsed with 1 μCi of tritiated thymidine that has been diluted in RPMI and delivered in 10-μl aliquots. Twenty-four hours after the thymidine pulse, the cells are harvested on nylon paper with an automatic cell harvester. After the paper is dry, the individual disks are placed into vials containing liquid scintillation fluid and counted on a scintillation counter. The counts per minute are reported for each cell well. If the mitogen experiments are designed to assess drug activity, there should be adequate controls in the microtiter plate including wells containing stimulated cells with no drug added (100% control), wells with RPMI only, and wells containing stimulated cells exposed to the drug diluent. Most studies reporting the effects of drugs on mitogen assays will calculate the percent inhibition of proliferation: 1-[(cells without drug cpm − cells with drug cpm)/cells without drug cpm] × 100. All experimental data points should be done in triplicate.

Animal T-Lymphocyte Studies

In vitro work has shown that increasing concentrations of cocaine suppress mouse T-lymphocyte proliferation in response to mitogen stimulation. Short-term exposure of mice to cocaine showed reduced body, spleen, and thymus weight and an increased responsiveness of lymphocytes to mitogens (41). Administration of cocaine to mice has been shown to enhance tumor growth, decrease both primary cellular and humoral responses, and inhibit peritoneal macrophage phagocytosis. T-suppressor cell function in rats may also be diminished following cocaine injection (39). T-cell subsets were seen to malfunction after cocaine exposure. These are considered direct effects, not on mature T-cell subset functions but on cellular differentiation (39). In murine cells, cocaine was found to inhibit the cellular response of delayed-type hypersensitivity (43).

Since intravenous drug users are at significant risk for HIV and other infections, there has been some speculation that cocaine use may contribute to decreased immune function in drug abusers. Malnourished mice exposed to cocaine were studied and found to have a significant decrease of $CD4^+$ and $CD8^+$ cells independent of the malnourished controls suggesting that cocaine *in vivo* may alter T-lymphocyte populations (44). These researchers also reported increases in B cells from the spleen in both groups.

The immunologic effects of cocaine *in utero* in humans are unknown. Sobrian *et al.* reported that rats exposed to cocaine prenatally decreased thymus/body weight ratio and increased spleen/body ratios, suggesting that cellular function may be diminished while humoral response may be enhanced by *in utero* cocaine exposure (14).

Effects on Humoral Immune Function

The exact effect of cocaine on humoral function is unclear. To date, there have been conflicting reports demonstrating both stimulatory and suppressive effects of cocaine on the humoral arm of the immune system.

Human B-Lymphocyte Studies

Antibody responses to T-dependent antigens were increased at lower concentrations and were suppressed at higher concentrations. *In vitro* studies did not show stimulation of B-cell populations indicating that a metabolite of cocaine or release of other host factors may be responsible for this immunomodulation (45). Splenocytes stimulated by B-cell mitogen were not affected, and a range of concentrations of cocaine had no effect on the cytotoxicity of murine natural killer cells (13, 14). The responsiveness of B lymphocytes to mitogens was suppressed and phagocytic activity was also shown to be decreased in a dose-related response.

Animal B-Lymphocyte Studies

The humoral response in mice was reported by Havas *et al.* to be enhanced in mice exposed to varying concentrations of cocaine. Even at lethal doses of cocaine, these investigators found that the B-cell response was elevated. The enhanced effect was more evident in female mice than in the male mice (41). Similar responses were reported when the humoral response was evaluated in female mice which included a nutritionally depleted group to simulate the malnourished state of drug abusers. Mice were given ip doses of cocaine beginning with 5 mg/kg/day to 40 mg/kg/day by Week 4. The malnourished rats had reduced B-cell numbers, but the well-nourished rats showed an increase in B cells. This could be due to the handling of the rats; however, the control rats did not show an increase in B cells. It was also suggested that the stress of the ip injection could account for the elevated B cells, but the saline controls did not have the same elevation as the cocaine-treated rats (46). Rats treated with cocaine had increased numbers of plaque-forming cells and increased antibody responses to specific antigens. The magnitude of elevation was related to the dose of cocaine administered. In converse, the humoral effect of cocaine and its metabolites were found to be suppressed in mice by using the Jerne hemolytic plaque assay (PFC). It was found that cocaine, norcocaine, ecgonine, and benzoylecgonine suppressed the PFC spleen cell response. However, when any of these agents were used in combination with alcohol the inhibitory effects were antagonized by approximately 50% (43).

We have also been investigating the influence of cocaine on the humoral arm of the immune system in rats.

Techniques

Cocaine hydrochloride is obtained from Sigma Chemical Co. (St. Louis, MO). Radialimmunodiffusion kits for immunoglobulin analyses are obtained from ICN, (Irvine, CA). Male Sprague–Dawley rats, 2.5 months old, are purchased from Harlan Sprague–Dawley (Indianapolis, IN). Rats are housed two per cage in a temperature- and humidity-controlled laboratory with a 12-hour light/dark cycle. The animals have free access to food and water. The rats are allowed to acclimate for 3 days before cannulation.

The jugular vein of each rat is cannulated using aseptic technique while the rat is under ethyl ether anesthesia. The cannula is inserted so that the tip stays in the inferior vena cava rather than the external jugular vein. The rats are allowed to recover for 7 days after surgery. Twenty rats (10 controls and 10 cocaine-exposed) are closed, via the cannula, with either 300 μl normal saline and 30 units of heparin or the same solution containing 1 mg/kg of cocaine hydrochloride. The infusions are given over a period of 30 sec. The dose is repeated every 12 hr for 12 days after which time the animals are sacrificed.

Blood samples (300 μl) are collected 1 hr before the first dose and 24 hr after the last administration. These are collected into borosilicate sample tubes and allowed to stand at 4°C for 1 hr to coagulate. The clotted blood samples are then centrifuged at 1500*g* for 10 min at room temperature and the sera are transferred to 500-μl plastic tubes. The levels of IgA, IgG, and IgM are measured using a radial immunodiffusion (RID) technique. Five microliters of sample is used for each immunoglobulin determination. Systems are allowed to diffuse for 144 hr before the results are read. At the end of the diffusion the ring edges of the diffused rat immunoglobulin formed by immunoprecipitation are marked and the diameters of these rings are measured using a low-power microscope. Calibration curves are constructed for all three immunoglobulins using linear regression of reference standards. Each measurement is made in triplicate.

An alternative method for the determination of immunoglobulins in rat serum uses an enzyme-linked immunosorbent assay (ELISA) as follows.

All chemicals can be purchased through Sigma Chemicals (St. Louis, MO), Fisher Chemicals (Itasca, IL), and Zymed (San Francisco, CA). A 0.1 *M* bicarbonate coating buffer should be prepared by mixing 4.24 g Na_2CO_3 (0.04 *M*) with 5.04 g $NaHCO_3$ (0.06 *M*) into 1 liter distilled H_2O and adjusting to pH 9.6. Excess solution can be stored at 4°C. Goat anti-rat IgA polyclonal antibody (Sigma R-9630) is diluted to a concentration of 100 μg/ml in bicarbonate buffer. Goat anti-rat IgG polyclonal antibody (Fisher OB1320-UNL) is diluted to a concentration of 5 μg/ml in bicarbonate buffer. For either assay, 100 μl of the desired solution is placed into each well of a pretreated microtiter plate and incubated overnight at 4°C. Wash buffer consisting of 0.01% Tween in PBS is used to wash the plate three times. Then 100 μl of PBS 5% BSA is added to each well to block the plate which is then incubated at room temperature for 1 hr. The plate is then washed again three times, before diluted samples, standards, and controls are added. The plate is then incubated at room temperature for 2 hr. Standard curves consist of the following: purified rat IgA (Zymed 02-9400), 100–1.9 μg/ml and purified rat IgG (Sigma I-4131), 1000–3.9 ng/ml. For each batch of assays, the best serum dilutions are determined by evaluating the following serum dilutions in PBS: 1 : 100, 1 : 1,000, 1 : 10,000. Controls consist of PBS with 1% BSA, blank serum. Fresh labeled antibody is prepared from biotinylated mouse anti-rat monoclonal antibody (Zymed 03-9440), concentration 1 : 100 in PBS and rabbit anti-rat IgG (whole molecule) (Sigma A-5795) horseradish peroxidase conjugate, concentration 1 : 100,000. The labeled antibody (100 μl) is dispensed into each well of the plate, covered and incubated at room temperature for 2 hr. Then the plate is washed three times. When using the biotinylated antibody for the anti-rat IgG, an extra step must be performed following labeled antibody incubation and washing. Streptavidin peroxidase (100 μl) at a concentration of 1 μg/ml is added to each well. The plate is then incubated at 37°C for 40 min and then washed three times. OPD Peroxidase Substrate (Sigma P-9187) is prepared by dissolving two tablets into 20 ml distilled water, and 100 μl placed into each well. The substrate should be prepared no more than 10 min before use since it is light sensitive and unstable. The plate is incubated at room temperature while protected from light for

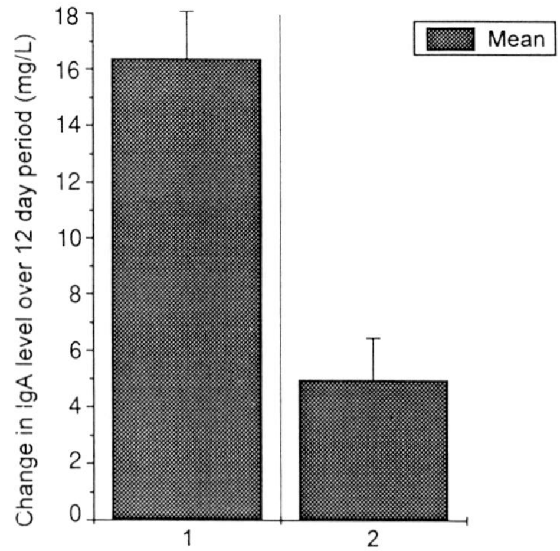

FIG. 4 Change in IgA levels after chronic exposure of mice to cocaine. 1, Controls; 2, cocaine exposed.

approximately 10 min or until a deep yellow color develops. At this point 2 *N* sulfuric acid (50 μl) is added to each well to stop the reaction. The plate is read by measuring the absorbance from the color reaction using an ELISA reader at 492 nm.

Results

The total serum immunoglobulin levels for 10 control and 10 cocaine-exposed rats were determined. The changes occurring in serum IgA levels after 12 days of infusion were significantly lower ($p < 0.001$) in the cocaine-exposed group (4.95 ± 4.79 mg/liter) than in the control animals (16.36 ± 5.41 mg/liter). Conversely, IgG levels of the cocaine-treated rats significantly increased ($p < 0.05$) compared to the control group, with mean serum concentrations of 28.6 ± 1.76 and 687.0 ± 7.89 mg/liter, respectively. Immunoglobulin M levels showed a decrease over the 12-day treatment period with no significant difference being detected between the two groups ($p > 0.05$). (Figs. 4 and 5).

Intraperitoneal or subcutaneous injection of cocaine is frequently reported as the route of administration for studying the immunological effects of the drug. These routes of administration, however, introduce an adsorption phase that may result in significant variations in pharmacokinetic and pharmacodynamic effects, particularly when a vasoconstrictor such as cocaine is administered. We, therefore, chose to use the intravenous route for this study.

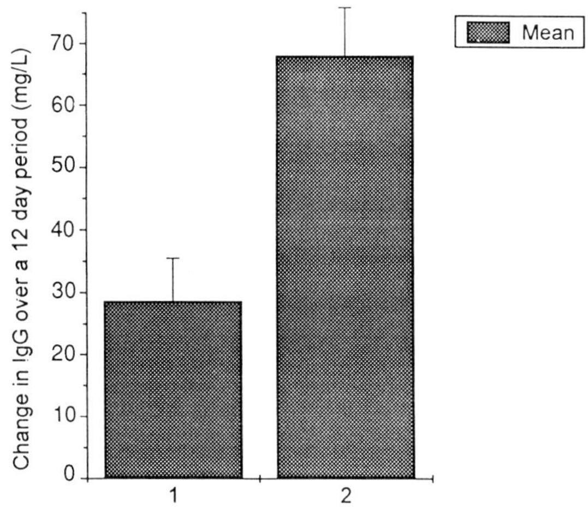

FIG. 5 Change in IgG levels after chronic exposure to cocaine. 1, Controls; 2, cocaine exposed.

We found significant changes in immunoglobulin levels in the control animals which could be explained as being associated with the stress of handling during the course of the study. Despite this, there were significant differences observed in the IgA and IgG levels of the control and cocaine-exposed groups: IgA levels being significantly lower and IgG levels being significantly higher in cocaine-treated animals. Although both cocaine-exposed and control animals showed a decline in IgM levels over the course of the study, there were no significant differences between the two groups.

Conclusion

Cocaine continues to be a major drug of abuse, prompting the further exploration of multiple biological activities. One of the most startling effects of cocaine which has only recently come to light is its immunomodulatory activity. Cocaine and its metabolites have been shown to suppress the cellular immune response, while reported effects of cocaine on the humoral arm of the immune system are presently contradictory. The exact immunotoxicological outcome of the immunosuppressive activity of cocaine in humans is unknown but will become clearer with further investigation of the effects of cocaine in immunosuppressed patients such as HIV-positive patients. Since cocaine metabolites also demonstrate immunomodulatory effects, patient populations with altered cocaine metabolism, such as the fetus, pregnant women, or those with esterase deficiencies, may be exposed to a different, perhaps more pronounced, immunomodulatory effect of this drug. The impact of cocaine on the integrity of the immune system may have a significant effect in the development of the fetal immune system and the contraction and progression of various diseases.

References

1. C. Van Dyke, P. Jatlow, J. Ungerer, P. G. Barash, and R. Byck, *Science,* **200,** 211–213 (19780.
2. M. W. Fischman, *J. Clin. Psychiatry* **49(2 Suppl.),** 7–10 (1988).
3. J. Javaid, M. W. Fischman, G. R. Schuster, H. Dekirmenjian, and J. M. Davis, *Science* **202,** 227–228 (1987).
4. C. E. Johanson, and M. W. Fischman, *Pharmacol. Rev.* **41(1),** 3–24 (1989).
5. C. Van Dyke, P. G. Barash, P. Jatlow, and R. Byck, *Science* **191,** 859–860 (1976).
6. S. O. Isaacs, P. Martin, and J. Hamil-Willoughby, *Oral Surg. Oral Med. Oral Pathol.* **63,** 12–16 (1987).
7. P. Jatlow, *Yale J. Biol. Med.* **61,** 105–113 (1988).
8. K. A. Loper, *Med. Toxicol. Adv. Drug. Exp.* **4,** 174–185 (1989).
9. S. Roberts, Center for Environmental and Human Toxicology, University of Florida. Personal communication, 1993.
10. H. C. Walls, "Valid and Reliable Drug Testing Techniques," presented at the 2nd National Conference on Drug Abuse, NIDA, Washington DC, July 1993.
11. A. M. Dusick, R. D. Covert, M. D. Schreiber, G. T. Yee, S. P. Browne, C. M. Moore, and I. R. Tebbett, *J. Pediatr.* **122,** 438–445 (1993).
12. F. H. Gawin, *J. Clin. Psychiatry* **49,2(Suppl.),** 11–16 (1988).
13. B. Watzl, and R. R. Watson, *Life Sci.* **46,** 1319–1329 (1990).
14. S. K. Sobrian, L. E. Burton, N. L. Robinson, W. K. Ashe, H. James, D. L. Stokes, and L. M. Turner, *Immunol. Biochem. Behav.* **35,** 617–629 (1990).
15. K. Graham, D. Dimitrakoudis, E. Pellegrini, and G. Koren, *Vet. Hum. Toxicol.* **31,** 143–148 (1989).
16. I. J. Chasnoff, M. E. Bussey, R. Savich, and C. M. Stoack, *J. Pediatr.* **108(3),** 456–459 (1986).
17. F. H. Gawin, and H. D. Kleber, *Br. J. Psychiatry* **147,** 569–573 (1985).
18. T. Di Paolo, C. Rouillard, M. Morissette, and D. Levesque, *Can. J. Physiol. Pharmacol.* **67,** 1177–1181 (1989).
19. I. Berczi, *Rev. Comp. Immunol.* **13,** 329–341 (1989).
20. E. J. Blalock, *J. Immunol.* **132(3),** 1067–1070 (1984).
21. H. O. Besedovsky, A. E. Del Rey, and E. Sorkin, *J. Immunol.* **135(2),** 750s–754s (1985).
22. K. St. John-Allan, P. R. Vulliet, and E. V. Avakian, *Proc. West. Pharmacol. Soc.* **32,** 61–63 (1989).
23. A. E. Calogero, W. T. Gallucci, M. A. Kling, G. P. Chrousos, and P. W. Gold, *Brain Res.* **505,** 7–11 (1989).

24. R. G. Coffey, and J. W. Hadden, *Fed. Proc.* **44**(1/1), 112–116 (1988).
25. J. Wybran, L. Schandene, J. P. Van Vooren, G. Vandermoten, D. Latinne, J. Sonnet, M. De Bruyere, H. Taelman, and N. P. Plotnikoff, *Ann. N. Y. Acad. Sci.* **496,** 108–114 (1987).
26. R. L. Moldow, and A. J. Fischman, *Peptides* **8,** 819–822 (1987).
27. L. J. Forman, and S. Estilow, *Life Sci.* **43,** 309–315 (1988).
28. B. Borowsky, and C. M. Kuhn, *J. Pharmacol. Exp. Ther.* **256**(1), 204–210 (1989).
29. C. Van Dyke, A. Stesin, R. Jones, A. Chuntharapai, and W. Seaman, *J. Clin. Invest.* **77,** 1387–1390 (1986).
30. R. Hart, F. Wagner, W. Steffens, C. Lersch, H. Dancygier, L. Duntas, and M. Classen, *Regul. Pept.* **27,** 335–342 (1990).
31. Pinku Mukherjee, A. M. Mastro, and W. C. Hymer, *Endocrinology* **126**(1), 88–94, 1990.
32. J. H. Mendelson, S. K. Teoh, U. Lange, N. K. Mello, R. Weiss, A. Skupny, and J. Ellingboe, *Am. J. Psychiatry* **145**(9), 1094–1098 (1988).
33. J. H. Mendelson, N. K. Mello, S. K. Teoh, J. Ellingboe, and J. Cochin, *J. Clin. Endocrinol. Metab.* **69(6),** 1256–1260 (1989).
34. F. Martinez, and R. R. Watson, *Life Sci.* **47,** PL59–PL64 (1990).
35. S. G. Gilman, J. M. Schwartz, R. J. Milner, F. E. Bloom, and J. D. Feldman, *Proc. Natl. Acad. Sci. U.S.A.* **79,** 4226–4230 (1982).
36. T. W. Klein, C. A. Newton, and H. Friedman, *in* "Psychological, Neuropsychiatric and Substance Abuse Aspects of AIDS" (T. P. Bridge et al., eds.), pp. 139–143. Raven Press, New York, 1988.
37. T. W. Klein, K. Matsuri, and C. A. Newton, *et al. Int. J. Immunopharm.* **15,** 77–86 (1993).
38. K. Matsuri, H. Friedman, and T. W. Klein, *Int. J. Immunopharm.* **14,** 1213–1220 (1992).
39. J. C. Delafuente, and C. L. DeVane, *Immunopharmacol. Immunotoxicol.* **13,** 11–23 (1991).
40. R. M. Donohoe, J. K. Nicholson, J. J. Madden, F. Donahoe, D. A. Shafer, D. Gordon, P. Bokos, and A. Falek, *Clinical Immunol. Immunopathol.* **41,** 254–264 (1986).
41. H. F. Havas, M. Dellaria, G. Schiffman, E. B. Geller, and M. W. Adler, *Int. Arch. Allergy Appl. Immunol.* **83,** 377–383 (1987).
42. D. Fuchs, A. Hausen, G. Reibnegger, D. Schonitzer, B. Unterweger, H. G. Belcha, P. Hengster, H. Rossler, T. Schultz, and E. R. Werner, *Cancer Detect. Prev. Suppl.* **1,** 535–541 (1987).
43. E. S. Watson, J. C. Murphy, H. N. ElSohly, M. A. ElSohly, and C. E. Turner, *Toxicol. Appl. Pharmacol.* **71,** 1–13 (1983).
44. R. R. Watson, *J. Nutr.* **122(Suppl. 3),** 744–748 (1992).
45. O. Bagasra, and L. J. Forman, Biological role of cocaine in the development and expression of AIDS. *Int. Conf. AIDS.* **5,** 677 (abst) (1989).
46. M. C. Lopez, D. S. Huang, B. Watzyl, G. J. Chen, and R. R. Watson, *Life Sci.* **49,** 1253–1262 (1991).

[26] Immunological, Pharmacological, and Electrophysiological Detection of T-Cell-Modulating Properties of Substances of Abuse

Robert M. Donahoe, John J. Madden, Dorothy R. Oleson, and Charles B. Nemeroff

Introduction

Since the late 1800s, information has accumulated that opiates have immunomodulatory properties (1). This information has serious public health implications in that communicable diseases like viral hepatitis and acquired immunodeficiency syndrome (AIDS) are spread by drug addicts and immune deficits created by addiction could exacerbate this spread. In 1979, Wybran *et al.* (2) made a major breakthrough in understanding the nature of the immunomodulatory properties of opiates by showing that T lymphocytes are directly responsive to opiates *in vitro*. The main implication of this finding, that T cells have opiate receptors, has since been confirmed pharmacologically by various investigators (3). Despite such evidence, however, it is also clear that the *in vivo* effects of opiates on immune function involve more than their simple direct interaction with T cells. Opiates also interact, *in vivo,* with neuroendocrine (1, 4) and neural (1, 5) processes which influence T-cell activity. Moreover, opiates influence a variety of cells from the immune system besides T cells. Accordingly, opiates modulate immunity *in vivo* in complex ways that are difficult to elucidate because of the many interactive variables involved.

When studying the complexities involved with the *in vivo* effects of opiates and other substances of abuse like cocaine and alcohol, it is important to realize that the initial site of interaction of the immune system with such substances and the products they induce within the neuroimmune system is the surface membrane of the immune cell. To simplify studies of the etiology of these interactions, we have taken an *in vitro,* reductionistic approach aimed at determining the influence of opiates, other substances of abuse, and neuroimmune produces induced by these substances, on membrane-receptor and ion-channel phenomena. To further reduce the complexity of this task while maintaining the relevance of our studies to cell-mediated

Methods in Neurosciences, Volume 24

immune deficits encountered by substance abusers, we have targeted T cells for study. In the present report, we describe immunobiological, immunopharmacological, and immunoelectrophysiological techniques that are useful for *in vitro* reconstruction of the *in vivo* milieu associated with substance abuse. The techniques described are valuable also for analyses of direct effects of all types of behaviorally active substances on T-cell function.

T-Cell Preparations

T cells are far from homogeneous. It is their nature to express various distinctive surface molecules as they develop through differentiation processes in the thymus and, later, in the periphery, in response to antigen, which distinguish their functional attributes. A fundamental property of all T cells entering the circulation after differentiating in the thymus is their expression of CD2 (E-receptor) and T-cell receptor (TCR) molecules. The TCR is responsible for specific recognition of foreign antigen and is invariably complexed with the signal-transducing CD3 molecule. Progression of T-cell maturation in the thymus also involves the staged expression of CD4 and CD8 molecules from co-expression to singular expression before T cells enter the circulation (a few $CD4^+/CD8^+$ cells enter also). CD4 and CD8 molecules are required for the restricted intercellular recognition and binding of T cells to other cells through interaction with either class II or class I histocompatibility (HLA) molecules, respectively, so that the HLA molecules can effectively present antigen to the TCR. T cells expressing CD4 or CD8 molecules typically appear in the circulation in a 2/1 ratio and are generally associated with either helper–inducer or suppressor–cytotoxic function, respectively. T cells also express a variety of molecules involved in intercellular adhesion and in homing to various anatomical locations, as well as participating in various pathways of cell activation and deactivation. Such molecules are typified by the CD45 tyrosine phosphatase which is expressed in varying, functionally distinctive, molecular weight isoforms contingent on prior antigen exposure and cell activation.

Expression of all of the molecules mentioned above has been shown to be affected by opiates and/or substances of abuse. Because these molecules are expressed differentially in response to the developmental experiences of a particular T-cell type, it is essential that studies of the effects of substances of abuse on T cells be conducted with sensitivity to the variability inherent to this circumstance. This situation requires that such studies control for and/or reduce such variability—a goal that can be accomplished through the use of leukocyte preparations enriched for T-cell expression and through manipulation of the differential properties of such cells.

On an interindividual basis, T cells are likely to give variable responses to substances of abuse and other behaviorally active substances because of variability in the immunological experiences and immunogenetics of the donor host. Thus, when mechanistic explorations are being conducted, it is best to use a source of cells that can be sampled repeatedly to avoid problems inherent to interindividual variability. This requires repeated sampling from a given individual and, often, frozen storage of large aliquoted samples so that interassay variation can be reduced through use of a single lot of cryopreserved leukocytes. The ideal starting material for T-cell enrichment and cryopreservation is leukapheresed leukocytes.

Mononuclear Leukocyte and T-Cell Isolations

Mononuclear leukocytes (T cells, B cells, and monocytes) are isolated from whole blood by differential centrifugation of cells through Ficoll/sodium metrozoite (Ficoll/Paque) and/or Percoll gradients. Additional processing is required for isolation of T cells from such preparations. For bulk T-cell purification, the common techniques include the use of sheep erythrocyte (E) adsorption procedures involving gradient centrifugation of T cell/E conjugates and lysis of E to derive T cells from the conjugates or passage of the mononuclear cells over columns of nylon wool. Nylon wool columns are prepared following the method of Julius *et al.* (6), with slight modifications. Approximately 35 g of scrubbed nylon wool fiber (Polysciences, Inc., Warrington, PA) is washed in 4 liters of boiling deionized water, containing 0.2% (w/v) sodium bicarbonate and 0.2% (w/v) EDTA, for 10 min, rinsed with fresh buffered water, and allowed to soak overnight at 37°C. The washing procedure is repeated the next day, and nylon wool is allowed to dry for 2–3 days in a laminar flow hood. Columns are then packed and eluted according to the manufacturer's instructions. Advantages of the nylon wool method over the E-rosetting method are derived from better yields and avoidance of problems of T-cell activation through the E-receptor.

For cell isolations aimed at selecting subtypes of T cells based on their differential expression of surface antigenic markers, antibody-based affinity-labeling techniques are commonly used. These procedures typically involve either panning or magnetic separation of cells tagged with specific monoclonal antibodies to the T-cell markers of choice. Separation of T cells in this way is best done using a "negative selection" approach which involves the use of monoclonal antibodies that recognize a marker counter to the one for which T-cell isolation is desired. In this way nonreactive (negative) T cells are separated from those that react with the chosen monoclonal reagent (positively selected cells) so that biological activation of cells via receptor–antibody interactions is avoided. This approach is only feasible when a distinctive counterreceptor reagent is available. Otherwise, direct positive selection must be used in which even the confounding influence of cell activation can be limited by culturing the positively isolated cells for several hours before use in assays.

As mentioned previously, the state of cell activation is important in assessing the functional attributes of T cells. This situation can be exploited to better delineate the effects of substances of abuse and other behaviorally active substances on T-cell function by activating the cells *in vitro* to distinguish their responses in this state from the preactivated condition. Also, homogeneity of cell preparations used in a given assay can be improved by using activated T-cell cultures. In several of the procedures outlined below cell activation has been used to gain such advantages. Either enriched T cell or mixed mononuclear cell populations may be activated in the presence of phytohemagglutinin (PHA) and interleukin 2 (IL-2). Optimal concentrations of PHA and IL-2 vary according to lot and individual responsiveness. Final working concentrations of PHA range from 2 to 10 μg/ml and IL-2 concentrations range from 10 to 40 units/ml. Lymphocytes are cultured in complete medium [Roswell Park Memorial Institute (RPMI) 1640 medium supplemented with: 10% (w/v) fetal bovine serum (FBS), 2 m*M* L-glutamine, and 20 μg/ml gentamycin] at a concentration of 10^6 cells/ml and incubated at 37°C in a 5% CO_2 atmosphere. Every 72 hr, cells are counted and resuspended at 10^6 cells/ml, in fresh complete medium supplemented with IL-2.

T-Cell E-Rosette Formation

The formation of rosettes between T cells and sheep erythrocytes (E) has been shown to be very sensitive to substances of abuse and other behaviorally active compounds. The E-receptor is the CD2 molecule and its natural ligand is LFA3 which is expressed in high numbers on E as well as on other cells of the immune system. CD2 is expressed specifically on T cells and is known to be an integral mediator of both intercellular adhesion and signal transduction. T cells are distinguished by the number and ligand affinity of the CD2 they express at any given time since these features dictate the avidity of T cells for intercellular binding and their excitability in signal transduction. Accordingly, the rate of E-rosette formation is faster in cells that express high-affinity E-receptors and slower in cells that do not. Modulation of the number and affinity of E-receptors by substances of abuse and other behaviorally active substances, therefore, is one of the causes for modulation of T-cell function by these compounds. Because the E-rosette formation assay is defined by the interaction of two cell types, this assay allows unique observations about the nature of intercellular interactions that cannot be obtained through use of direct monoclonal antibody-staining techniques based on cytofluorometric technology. The following assay is used to determine rates of T-cell E-rosette formation.

Reagent Preparation

Mononuclear leukocytes or purified T cells prepared as described previously are used as a source of T cells in the E-rosette formation assay. Leukocytes are suspended in RPMI 1640 medium at 5×10^6/ml for use in this assay. Their exposure to substances of abuse can occur either *in vivo,* prior to cell isolation, or *in vitro* by incubation of the purified leukocytes with appropriate concentrations of the drugs of choice.

E are prepared fresh weekly for use in the assay. Commercially available E, suspended in Alsever's solution, are washed by placing 1 ml of a stock into a 50-ml conical tube along with sufficient Earle's balanced salt solution (EBSS) to fill the tube. The diluted cells are mixed by repeated gentle inversion of the tube. The tube is then centrifuged at 400*g* for 10 min. The supernatant is discarded and the pellet resuspended in EBSS, and the wash procedure is repeated at least two more times or until no hemolysis of E is apparent (the supernatant is clear). E prepared in this way are stored at 4°C and are stable for 1 week. However, if not used immediately after washing, the stored cells should be rewashed at least once on the day of assay. For the E-rosette assay, a pellet of washed E is suspended in 10 ml of EBSS and the E are counted by use of an electronic cell counter. Suspensions of E are then prepared in EBSS to contain 2.5×10^8 and 5×10^7 E/ml.

Fetal bovine serum used in the E-rosette formation assay must be preadsorbed against E. Using a packed cell pellet of E prepared by the washing procedure described above, 2 ml of E is mixed with 10 ml of fetal bovine serum by gentle inversion. The mixture is incubated for 30 min in a water bath set at 37°C and then held overnight at 4°C. The mixture of serum and E is then suspended, and the tube centrifuged at 400*g* for 10 min. The adsorbed-serum supernatant (FBSa) is removed, aliquoted in small portions, and stored at −20°C.

T-Cell E-Rosette Formation Assay

In each assay, two separate sets of reaction mixtures are prepared so that conditions are favorable for evaluation of both the rate of rosette formation and the total number of T cells in the circulation. For determinations of the rate of E-rosette formation, sets of mixed E and T cells are prepared so that kinetic analyses of E-rosette formation can be conducted. Each tube of cell mixture is comprised of 25 μl of leukocytes added to 25 μl of prewarmed (37°C) FBSa and added, in turn, to 50 μl of E, at 5.0×10^7/ml. This procedure yields an E/T ratio of 12.5/1. For total T cells, the same procedures and volumes of reactants are used except that the concentration of E added to the tubes is at 2.5×10^8/ml so that an E/T ratio of 50/1 is effected. The relatively low E/T ratio for the rate determinations is used to assure that low-affinity E-receptors on the T cell will be restricted in their capacity to bind to E early during the incubation so that distinctions in the rates of binding of E to T cells will be apparent. The higher E/T ratio used for evaluation of total T cells is to assure every opportunity for the T cell to react and bind to E. The cell mixtures are then incubated for 5 min at 37°C and immediately centrifuged at room temperature at 2000*g* for 20 sec. For rate determinations, incubations are at room temperature for brief durations (typically, 0, 2, 4, 8, 16, 32, and 64 min). For total T cells, incubations are at 4°C overnight. These different incubation conditions are employed also to enhance distinctions in the rates of binding of E to T as described above. After the respective incubations, the cell pellets from both the rate-determining and total T-cell procedures are gently disrupted by gentle back-and-forth rocking of the fluid contents of the tubes over the pellet. Then, 15 μl of methylene blue is added to each tube and mixed gently, and 13 μl of the cell suspension is placed on a microscope slide which is then covered with a coverslip. The lymphocytes are evaluated microscopically and those having three or more E attached are scored as T cells. The percentage of T cells in the preparation is then calculated as the number of rosettes formed compared to the number of lymphocytes counted (minimum of 100). Triplicate samples should be run for each time point evaluated and kinetic curves constructed from the arithmetic means of the responses.

Opiate Binding to T Cells and Component Fractions

One of the earliest assumptions about the activity of substances of abuse on T lymphocytes is that these cells have specific binding sites, or receptors, on their surface which provide the primary site of action for these drugs. The specificity of the known leukocyte, opiate receptors has already been reviewed (3) but new sites have been identified. There are also reports of internalization of many alkaloid drugs, e.g., morphine, which leave open the possibility of an internal site of action for these drugs as well. Because little is known about the subsequent steps beyond initial opiate binding, however, information is yet to be developed regarding the linkage of these external and internal binding sites to specific immunological alterations. Also, much remains to be learned about the immunological and pharmacological specificity and avidity of the binding sites themselves. The protocols below outline the basic methods for defining these binding sites using ligands previously used to specify opiate receptors of the central nervous system (CNS). Whether these "neural" ligands define identical binding sites on cells of the immune system is a subject of current investigation. This task is likely to be facilitated by the recent publications of the cloning of the CNS delta opiate receptor (7, 8), plus brief presentations at meetings of the cloning of the μ_1, μ_2 and κ opiate receptors (9). Such information suggests that molecular description of leukocyte opiate receptors should soon be forthcoming.

Specific opiate binding is defined as the difference between nonspecific binding and total binding. Nonspecific binding is measured as the amount of radioactive ligand which binds in the presence of a 1000-fold excess of nonradioactive ligand. Total binding is assessed as the binding of radioactive ligand alone. A typical binding curve contains six to eight concentration points spread over a 2–4 log concentration range. Plots, like the Scatchard plot (bound ligand concentration vs bound/free concentrations), can then be used to assess the affinity constant (K_D) and binding sites/cell (B_{max}). It is important to note that both the nonspecific binding values and variability at each point are considerably higher for lymphocyte material than typical values for neuronal membrane preparations. This variability and high background may be responsible for the nonlinear Scatchard blots frequently found for lymphoid membranes. Interestingly, lymphocyte microsomal preparations give more normal (i.e., linear) Scatchard plots than lymphocyte membrane fractions.

Preparation of Cell Fractions Used in Opiate-Binding Assays

At least two fractions derived from human T lymphocytes bind (−)-Morphine specifically, the cell membrane and the microsomal fraction. Membranes from G_0, peripheral lymphocytes have a low-affinity (K_D 300–400 nM) morphine-binding site and a high-affinity (K_D 50 nM) site for the opiate agonist naloxone (10). However, if lymphocytes are stimulated to proliferate by PHA and then maintained on IL-2, a high-affinity morphine-binding site appears on the membrane. The morphine binding at this site can be totally displaced by β-endorphin, while des-Tyr β-endorphin is only about half as effective in displacing morphine. This is the only reported lymphoid site at which there is an interaction between morphine and β-endorphin. Less is known about the binding of opiates to the microsomal fraction, but morphine binds with high specificity to microsomes, not only from lymphocytes but also kidney and neuronal tissue (11). The presence of internal opiate-binding sites may be accounted for by the ability of alkaloids like morphine to be transported into many types of human cells.

Membrane Preparations

Tubes containing T lymphocytes diluted to 2×10^8 cells/ml in Hanks' balanced salt solution (HBSS) are held in an ice bath (10). Five 20-sec sonic bursts from a No. 300 Virtis Cell Disrupter (Gardiner, NJ) are used to shatter >95% of the cells. Between bursts, the solution is stirred in the ice bath to prevent destruction of the binding site by heat. A membrane pellet is obtained by centrifugation at 70,000*g* for 10 min at 4°C and homogenized four times in the original solution volume of HBSS with the aid of an ice-cold glass homogenizer.

Microsomal Preparations

Lymphocytes (10^9 cells in 5 ml HBSS) are disrupted in a Parr cell disruption bomb (No. 4639) by raising the pressure to 1500 psi using nitrogen over a 5-min period and then maintaining the pressure for 10 min. Rapid depressurization fractures all of the cells. The N_2 cavitation procedure preserves subcellular structure to a greater degree than the sonication method described above. The microsomes are then isolated by differential centrifugation. Nuclei and membranes are removed from the solution by centrifugation at 600*g* for 10 min at 4°C. Supernatant from this procedure is then centrifuged at 1800*g* for 20 min to remove mitochondria and the resulting supernatant is centrifuged at 175,000*g* for 60 min to pellet the microsomal fraction which is harvested for study.

Procedure for Opiate-Binding Assay

Triplicate 0.1-ml samples of a cell fraction (equal to material from 2.5×10^6 cells) are mixed with 0.1 ml of varying concentrations of tritiated morphine (specific activity 40–60 Ci/mmol; concentrations typically would be 0.25, 0.50, 0.75, 1, 2, 5, and 10 n*M*) plus either HBSS alone, to determine total binding, or 1000-fold excess (10 μM) of unlabeled morphine, to determine nonspecific binding. The triplicates are incubated for 45 min at 4°C. The bound morphine is harvested on Whatman (Clifton, NJ) GF/C filters and washed twice with 4 ml ice-cold HBSS. The filters are counted in 0.5 ml of

0.1 *M* KOH and 10 ml Beckman Redi-Solv (Beckman Instruments, Inc., Fullerton, CA) in a scintillation counter.

Ligand Specificity

Morphine and β-endorphin can bind to several different sites on neuronal cells. To determine which receptor mediates the action of any particular opioid, various ligands have been synthesized which bind with very high degrees of specificity to individual neuronal receptors. Several reports have described the use of specific compounds to define the existence of different receptor types on lymphoid cells, but these reports do not provide affinity constants for the binding (12). However, studies using either β-endorphin (13) or morphine (14) as the radioactive ligand and various specific site ligands as displacers suggest that the opiate binding sites on human T lymphocytes have specificities significantly different from those of the CNS. Thus it is not yet clear that the specific ligands derived for the CNS can be expected to provide the same information for lymphocytes.

Media Conditions Which Promote Opiate Binding

Morphine binding to lymphocyte membranes is maximized by the presence of 0.15 *M* NaCl as opposed to CNS membrane where low salt concentrations favor morphine binding. The lymphocyte–morphine binding is inhibited by both sulfhydryl reagents and reagents which split S–S bridges, e.g., 2-mercaptoethanol and dithiothreitol, respectively. This latter consideration is important because many commonly used media like RPMI 1640 contain sulfhydryl compounds such as glutathione that inhibit measurement of morphine binding. Finally it is also important to note that the presence of platelets and macrophages in the initial cell preparation can mask specific binding by lymphocytes by significantly raising nonspecific binding of the membrane fraction (10).

Patch Clamping T Cells

Neher and Sakmann's patch-clamp technique revolutionized biophysics and brought small cells, such as lymphocytes, into the field of electrophysiology (15–17). Patch-clamp methods, ranging from how to construct a work station to controlling noise, have been compiled in Methods in Enzymology, Vol.

207, 1992. The present discussion will focus on applying the technique to lymphocytes.

Cells

Preparation of T cells for patching is accomplished by washing 3× in standard saline. Enzymatic cleaning of the cell surface is not necessary. Although lymphocytes can survive in saline for 24 hr or more, seal formation and viability during recording are increased by removing cells from culture every 2–3 hr. Both activated and quiescent T cells can be patch-clamped on a routine basis. Activating T cells with PHA and IL-2 increases the average diameter of cells from 6 to 11 μm, which is advantageous, and increases K conductance approximately twofold in human cells (18, 19).

Electrodes and Solutions

Standard electrodes of 3–5 megohms (MΩ) are fabricated from borosilicate glass with a micropipette puller, coated with Sylgard 184 (Dow Corning, Midland, MI) and fire-polished right before use. Alternative glass compositions and coatings are available and have been used successfully with lymphocytes (20, 21). Pipettes are typically pulled to a diameter of 2 μm with a taper length of 5 mm and fire-polished down to a diameter of less than 1 μm. Extracellular and intracellular solutions are varied according to experimental design and purpose. A common physiologic, extracellular solution is composed of (in m*M*): 140 NaCl, 5 KCl, 2 $CaCl_2$, 2 $MgCl_2$, and 10 Na-HEPES (pH 7.4, 290 mOsm); and an intracellular solution may consist of (in m*M*): 150 potassium aspartate, 4 NaCl, 2 $MgCl_2$, 0.55 $CaCl_2$, 1.1 EGTA (pCa 7), and 10 K-HEPES (pH 7.2, 295 mOsm). T-cell electrical properties remain most stable when fluoride is the major anion in the intracellular solution (22). However, since fluoride is distinctly nonphysiologic and activates G proteins in the presence of aluminum, potassium aspartate is a good second choice (22–24).

Equipment and Data Analyses

Cells are voltage-clamped by controlling the positive input of a current–voltage converter. Membrane voltage is clamped, or held at a specific level, and the currents required to maintain that voltage are recorded with an amplifier. Patch pipettes filled with internal solutions are positioned over AgCl wires and connected to a probe. Whole-cell currents are typically sampled every millisecond and filtered at bandwidths of 1–5 kHz. Data analysis is facilitated by using a digital oscilloscope, video tape recorder, and personal computer. Inverted microscopes are preferred due to longer working distances between condensers and objectives. Microscopes are placed on vibration-free tables, in Faraday cages, and illumination is converted to a direct current source to reduce noise. Convenient recording chambers are wet mount microscope slides and 35 mm plastic petri dishes. Coating petri dishes with 5% FBS prior to patching prevents T cells from flattening out against the plastic, and allows them to retain a spherical shape.

Formation of Gigaohm Seals

Lymphocytes generally seal quite readily against patch electrodes with gentle suction. Seal resistances of 10 GΩ and above are common. Seal formation is monitored by applying a repetitive voltage step; typical protocols contain a 10-mV step which is maintained for 10 msec and delivered every 100 msec. When sealing is difficult, voltage clamping the membrane and applying −40 to −60 mV and/or releasing the suction improve the chance of obtaining a gigaohm seal.

Recording Configurations

Whole Cell

Whole-cell configuration is achieved by applying brief bursts of negative pressure to the cell membrane within the electrode until it breaks. An abrupt increase in the capacitive transient of a test pulse, due to increased capacitance of the cell membrane, is used as an indication of access to the interior (23). Whole-cell configuration allows contents of the electrode and cell to exchange freely and is useful for introducing pharmacologic agents directly into cells. The most prevalent voltage-gated channel in T cells is highly selective for K ions (18–23) and has been cloned and expressed in *Xenopus* oocytes (24, 25). It is related to the *Drosophila* Shaker A channel and shares 60 to 70% of its amino acids with the Shaker core sequence (24). Alterations in potassium conductance (gK) occur during the first 10 min of whole-cell recording in T cells. These include a negative shift in the voltage associated with channel opening or threshold potential by 10–15 mV, acceleration in activation and inactivation kinetics, and an increase in cumulative inactivation (18, 22, 23). Therefore, whole-cell experiments are most frequently performed after waiting 15–20 min for potassium currents to stabilize. Ligand-gated calcium currents that occur following stimulation of TCR-CD3 also have been studied in whole-cell configuration, but not as extensively as for potassium channels (26, 27).

Perforated Patch

Perforated-patch configuration is a permeabilized membrane technique developed by Horn and Marty (28, 29). It makes use of a monovalent ionophore, nystatin, which allows electrical access to the cell interior while virtually blocking the diffusion of cellular constituents into the patch pipette. Nystatin pores are approximately 0.8 nm in diameter and allow passage of molecules less than 200 Da (28). Perforated-patch configuration is similar to whole-cell in that macroscopic currents, comprised of every ion channel in the membrane capable of being activated, are recorded. Nystatin-containing electrodes form gigaohm seals far less frequently than standard electrodes and do not always achieve an acceptable access resistance. Optimal working concentrations of nystatin range from 35 to 100 μg/ml, form pores within 10 min and produce an access resistance of 20–50 MΩ. Pore formation is monitored by observing the amplitude and decay of a capacitive current in response to a test pulse (23). Capacitance (C_m) measurements of T-cell membranes range from 2.7 to 5.2 pF in perforated-patch configuration and agree closely with the range for whole-cell recordings of 2.9–6.4 pF. Access (series) resistance (R_a) is approximately 4$\times$ higher during perforated-patch recordings, increasing the average time constant ($C_m R_a$) of the capacitive transient from 40 μsec (whole cell) to 160 μsec (perforated patch) (23). A caveat when performing perforated-patch experiments is that larger R_a values increase the potential drop across the patch in direct relation to the height of the current and shift I–V relationships in the depolarizing direction. Characteristics of T-cell voltage-gated potassium currents, comparing whole-cell and perforated-patch techniques, are presented in Ref. 23.

Cell-Attached Patch

Cell-attached patch configuration is the least invasive patch-clamp conformation. The electrode is sealed to the cell with suction, but, rather than rupturing or permeabilizing the membrane, the patch is left intact and the ion channels within it are studied. Using this technique, a number of ion channels have been identified in human T cells. These include nonselective cation channels, various chlorine channels, calcium-activated potassium channels, and non-voltage-gated potassium channels (20, 21, 30–33). Cyclic adenosine monophosphate (cAMP) elevating agents increase potassium channel activity in cell-attached patch configuration but fail to do so in whole-cell configuration (20, 33). Moreover, ethanol increases the number of simultaneously active potassium channels and subsequent current maxima in cell-attached patches, but does not affect macroscopic potassium currents in perforated-patch recordings (34). These results indicate that an intact cytosol is required by cAMP and ethanol to increase channel opening and suggest that either a diffusible cellular component (less than 200 Da) or an undisturbed ionic microenvironment is necessary for the normal functioning of potassium channels in T cells.

Inside-out and Outside-out Patches

Isolated patches of membrane are studied in these configurations. Inside-out refers to the cytosolic face of the membrane facing out, away from the pipette, and exposed to the bath. Outside-out is the opposite, the outer membrane faces the bath and the cytosolic side is exposed to the pipette solution. When forming isolated patches, it is best to begin by allowing T cells to attach strongly to plastic petri dishes in the absence of protein. Gigaohm seals are attained as outlined previously. After seals are formed, pulling the electrode swiftly up off the cell removes a piece of membrane, which quickly anneals into a vesicle. To form an inside-out patch, the vesicle is broken by either passing it close to the solution–air interface or out of the bath entirely and back in (16, 17). Unfortunately, seals are frequently lost when attempting to produce inside-out patches. Outside-out configuration is achieved with less effort by breaking the cell membrane, as in whole-cell configuration, prior to moving the electrode up and away from the cell.

References

1. R. M. Donahoe, *Adv. Neuroimmunol.* **3,** 31 (1993).
2. J. Wybran, T. Appelboom, J. P. Famaey, and A. Govaerts, *J. Immunol.* **123,** 1068 (1979).
3. J. J. Madden and R. M. Donahoe, *in* "Drugs of Abuse and Immune Function," (R. R. Watson, ed.), p. 213. CRC Press, Boca Raton, FL, 1990.
4. H. U. Bryant, E. W. Bernton, and J. W. Holaday, *NIDA Res. Monogr.* **96,** 131 (1990).
5. R. J. Weber, L. C. Band, B. DeCosta, A. Pert, and K. Rice, *NIDA Res. Monogr.* **105,** 96 (1991).

6. M. H. Julius, E. Simpson, and L. A. Herzenberg, *Eur. J. Immunol.* **3,** 645 (1973).
7. C. J. Evans, D. E. Keith, H. Morrison, K. Magendzo, and R. H. Edwards, *Science* **258,** 1952 (1992).
8. B. L. Kieffer, K. Befort, C. Gaveriaux-Ruff, and C. G. Hirth, *Proc. Natl. Acad. Sci. U.S.A.* **89,** 12,048 (1992).
9. Meeting of the College on the Problems of Drug Dependency, June 1993, Toronto, Canada.
10. J. J. Madden, R. M. Donahoe, J. Zwemmer-Collins, D. A. Shafer, and A. Falek, *Biochem. Pharmacol.* **36,** 4103 (1987).
11. B. L. Roth, M. B. Laskowski, and C. J. Coscia, *Brain Res.* **250,** 101 (1982).
12. R. T. Radulescu, B. R. DeCosta, A. E. Jacobson, K. C. Rice, J. E. Blalock, and D. J. J. Carr, *Prog. Neuroendocrinol. Immunol.* **4,** 166 (1991).
13. N. A. Shahabi, K. M. Linnear, and B. M. Sharp, *Endocrinology* **126,** 1442 (1990).
14. S. R. Roy, B.-L. Ge, S. Ramakrishnan, N. M. Lee, and H. H. Loh, *FEBS* **287,** 93 (1991).
15. E. Neher and B. Sakmann, *Nature (London)* **260,** 799 (1976).
16. O. P. Hamill, A. Marty, E. Neher, B. Sakmann, and F. J. Sigworth, *Pflugers Arch.* **391,** 85 (1981).
17. B. Sakmann and E. Neher, *Annu. Rev. Physiol.* **46,** 455 (1984).
18. C. Deutsch, D. Krause, and S. C. Lee, *J. Physiol.* **372,** 405 (1986).
19. C. Deutsch, M. Price, S. Lee, V. F. King, and M. L. Garcia, *J. Biol. Chem.* **266,** 3668 (1991).
20. S. C. Lee, D. I. Levy, and C. Deutsch, *J. Gen. Physiol.* **99,** 771 (1992).
21. M. P. Mahaut-Smith and L. C. Schlichter, *J. Physiol.* **415,** 69 (1989).
22. M. D. Cahalan, K. G. Chandy, T. E. DeCoursey, and S. Gupta, *J. Physiol.* **358,** 197 (1985).
23. D. R. Oleson, L. J. DeFelice, and R. M. Donahoe, *J. Membr. Biol.* **132,** 229 (1993).
24. J. Douglass, P. B. Osborne, Y. Cai, M. Wilkinson, M. J. Christie, and J. P. Adelman, *J. Immunol.* **144,** 4841 (1990).
25. S. Grissmer, B. Dethlefs, J. J. Wasmuth, A. L. Goldin, G. A. Gutman, M. D. Cahalan, and K. G. Chandy, *Proc. Natl. Acad. Sci. U.S.A.* **87,** 9411 (1990).
26. M. Kuno, J. Goronzy, C. M. Weyand, and P. Gardner, *Nature (London)* **323,** 269 (1986).
27. R. S. Lewis and M. D. Cahalan, *Cell Regul.* **1,** 99 (1989).
28. R. Horn and A. Marty, *J. Gen. Physiol.* **92,** 145 (1988).
29. S. J. Korn and R. Horn, *J. Gen. Physiol.* **94,** 789 (1989).
30. J. H. Chen, H. Schulman, and P. Gardner, *Science* **243,** 657 (1989).
31. P. A. Pahapill and L. C. Schlichter, *J. Membr. Biol.* **125,** 171 (1992).
32. L. C. Schlichter, *Can. J. Physiol.* **70,** 247 (1992).
33. P. A. Pahapill and L. C. Schlichter, *J. Physiol.* **445,** 407 (1992).
34. D. E. Oleson, L. J. DeFelice, and R. M. Donahoe, *Clin. Exp. Res.* **17,** 604 (1993).

Index